WORKING WITH CHILDREN
TO HEAL INTERPERSONAL TRAUMA

Working with Children to Heal Interpersonal Trauma

THE POWER OF PLAY

Edited by
ELIANA GIL

Foreword by Lenore C. Terr, MD

THE GUILFORD PRESS
New York　　London

© 2010 The Guilford Press
A Division of Guilford Publications, Inc.
72 Spring Street, New York, NY 10012
www.guilford.com

Printed in the United States of America

This book is printed on acid-free paper.

Last digit is print number: 9   8   7   6   5   4   3   2   1

Library of Congress Cataloging-in-Publication Data

Working with children to heal interpersonal trauma : the power of play /
edited by Eliana Gil.
    p. ; cm.
  Includes bibliographical references and index.
  ISBN 978-1-60623-892-9 (hard cover: alk. paper)
    1. Psychic trauma in children—Treatment.   2. Post-traumatic stress
disorder in children—Treatment.   3. Child abuse—Treatment.   4. Abused
children—Rehabilitation.   5. Interpersonal relations in children—
Psychological aspects.   6. Play therapy.   I. Gil, Eliana.
    [DNLM: 1. Child Abuse—therapy.   2. Play Therapy—methods.
3. Child.   4. Professional–Patient Relations.   5. Stress Disorders, Post-
Traumatic—therapy.   6. Survivors—psychology. WS 350.4 W926 2010]
  RJ506.P66W64 2010
  618.92′8521—dc22

                                                            2010018205

About the Editor

Eliana Gil, PhD, is Clinical and Educational Specialist for Childhelp, Inc., in Fairfax, Virginia. She is also a partner in a private group practice, the Gil Center for Healing and Play in Fairfax, Virginia, which provides mental health services to children and families with a variety of emotional, behavioral, and social problems, where she specializes in the treatment of traumatized children and their families. A well-known author, lecturer, and clinician, Dr. Gil has worked in the field of child abuse prevention and treatment for the last 37 years. Over the past decade, Dr. Gil directed sexual abuse treatment programs at the Kellar Center and Childhelp Inc., both in Fairfax, Virginia. She is also an adjunct faculty member at Virginia Tech's Family Therapy Department, a registered play therapy supervisor, a registered art therapist, and a licensed marriage, family, and child counselor. Dr. Gil has served on the Board of Directors of the American Professional Society on the Abuse of Children and the National Resource Center on Child Sexual Abuse, and is also a former president of the Association for Play Therapy.

Dr. Gil has written numerous books on child abuse and related topics and has several educational videotapes that feature her work (available from The Guilford Press) as well as a self-published videotape on family play therapy. Her most recent book is *Helping Abused and Traumatized Children: Integrating Directive and Nondirective Approaches*. Other books include *Cultural Issues in Play Therapy* (with Athena A. Drewes); *Treating Abused Adolescents; Systemic Treatment of Families Who Abuse; The*

Healing Power of Play; *Play in Family Therapy*; and *Sexualized Children: Assessment and Treatment of Sexualized Children and Children Who Molest* (with Toni Cavanagh Johnson). Several of her books have been translated into other languages, including Spanish. Originally from Guayaquil, Ecuador, Dr. Gil is both bilingual and bicultural. She consults and trains locally and across the country and currently conducts intensive 3-day trainings through the Starbright Training Institute for Child and Family Play Therapy in northern Virginia.

Contributors

David A. Crenshaw, PhD, ABPP, Founder and Director, Rhinebeck Child and Family Center, LLC, Rhinebeck, New York

Athena A. Drewes, PsyD, Director of Clinical Training, Astor Services for Children and Families, Poughkeepsie, New York; Adjunct Professor, Marist College, Poughkeepsie, New York

Eliana Gil, PhD, Clinical and Educational Specialist, Childhelp, Inc., Fairfax, Virginia; private practice, Gil Center for Healing and Play, Fairfax, Virginia; Adjunct Faculty, Family Therapy Department, Virginia Tech, Falls Church, Virginia

Myriam L. Goldin, LCSW, Bryant Adult Alternative High School and Alternative Learning Center, Fairfax County Public Schools, Fairfax, Virginia; private practice, Gil Center for Healing and Play, Fairfax, Virginia

Eric J. Green, PhD, Assistant Professor, Department of Counseling and Human Services, University of North Texas at Dallas, Dallas, Texas

Rosalind L. Heiko, PhD, Director, Pediatric and Family Psychology, PA, Cary, North Carolina

Nicole Erin Jalazo, LCSW, Therapist, Childhelp, Inc., Fairfax, Virginia; private practice, Gil Center for Healing and Play, Fairfax, Virginia

Christine R. Ludy-Dobson, PhD, Director of Programs and Research, ChildTrauma Academy, Houston, Texas

Vincent L. Pastore, PhD, private practice, Mooresville, North Carolina

Bruce D. Perry, MD, PhD, Senior Fellow, ChildTrauma Academy, Houston, Texas

Jennifer A. Shaw, PsyD, Therapist, Childhelp Inc., Fairfax, Virginia; private practice, Gil Center for Healing and Play, Fairfax, Virginia

Eva-Maria Simms, PhD, Associate Professor of Psychology and Director of Graduate Studies, Department of Psychology, Duquesne University, Pittsburgh, Pennsylvania

Barbara Sobol, LPC, ATR-BC, Director, Washington Art Therapy Studio, Washington, DC; Adjunct Faculty, George Washington University Graduate Program in Art Therapy, Washington, DC

Foreword

Looking at the effects of terrifying events across groups of children or on one child over time gives us the chance to understand how young people process traumas. How does a certain set of extreme situations affect a number of different children (Terr, 1990)? And how might an extreme situation affect only one child as the youngster moves—stage by stage—into adulthood (Terr, 2009)? Then, too, what might the mental health professional do about treating this early kind of trauma—immediately, during a youngster's childhood, or years later as an adult (Terr, 2008)?

In reading *Working with Children to Heal Interpersonal Trauma: The Power of Play*, you can't help but think of the hurts you suffered as a child, of the friends and families whom you knew when you were in school, of your earliest professional contacts with traumatized individuals who needed your help, and of concerns you hold today about your own future. Are your concerns the same as those of your peers? Did they change over time? Yes, there are usually striking similarities in people's lives. But the details of your life and the ways you handle life's small and large traumas are still unique to you, and they change as you change, as well.

Two examples from my psychiatric practice come to mind in the context of uniqueness. The first case (Terr, 1990) illustrates how a single traumatic event and its extended aftermath were processed by four siblings, who were all genetically similar but psychologically unique. The second case (Terr, 2009) shows how, over a period of more than 20 years, the mental challenges and meanings of an extended and complicated event changed in just one person's mind.

Let me present my first case, Holly, a mischievous, fun-loving child about to enter kindergarten. Holly is enjoying summertime in a California neighborhood kiddie pool, and she has discovered that a steel drain cover under the water moves. Beneath it, she feels some suction. "Is it a snake?" her burgeoning imagination inquires. She asks her 4-year-old brother, Duane, to join her in attacking the snake, but her fellow-in-mischief feels afraid and holds back. Her 7-year-old big sister, Cindy, is otherwise engaged but remains semiaware of Holly. And Winifred, the 2-year-old baby of the family, swimming about in her mother's arms, is too busy to notice. Then disaster hits! Holly sits down on the unprotected drain and is immediately captured by the pool's suction, which pulls out her intestines through her anal opening. She will die almost 3 years later after a heroic surgical attempt to give her a new liver and intestines. I work with these children for the next 2 years and for almost a year after Holly's death—until the little survivors and their newly divorced mother move across the Atlantic Ocean. I try to help the children as a group, but I find that each child has an individual need for treatment and an individual means of expression. I must see each one alone, if only for part of a shared psychiatric hour.

The four children in this family suffered posttraumatic disorders. Their behaviors and play were repeated; they experienced periods of detachment, sadness, anger, and guilt; they showed posttraumatic fears; and they had problems envisioning their futures. Most important for the purposes of this book, however, they reacted uniquely according to their personalities and stages of development. Holly, always a girl of action, remained so until she died. She endured a number of surgeries with bravery and determination. She went to school and got all A's while expertly learning how to read and do mathematics. We successfully worked on Holly's "snake" idea through play, but we had more trouble with the "witch" who Holly believed was in league with Mr. Snake. In fact, shortly before Holly died in Pittsburgh, Pennsylvania, she accused one of her home night nurses of slapping her. To prove it, she showed me three big bruises. I phoned Holly's pediatrician. Because her liver was severely diseased, he said that Holly was bruising spontaneously. Holly had found what in her mind represented a real witch. This nurse was dismissed with a good letter of recommendation and no child abuse charges.

Duane, Holly's brother and closest friend throughout her short life, was a great player and an imaginative little architect. He built toy swimming pools in my office and at home. Of course, building the pools alone could not remove the reality of the accident. We had to talk about the need for nailed-on drain covers and for maintenance people who take care of pools and drain them from time to time to check on the equipment, and about the need to watch the pools in which children swim. These realities, which Duane could not have known as a pre-schooler, resolved his swimming pool issues and he was able to stop his architectural game. Later, he constructed tons of harmless and funny practical jokes to keep Holly busy and amused. I briefly stopped seeing Duane. When Holly died, however, Duane began experiencing all sorts of pranks from Holly's "ghost," such as slamming doors and weather changes. Duane's newfound ghost gave him a double-sided opportunity: the chance to disengage from his lost sister while simultaneously keeping her close to him. Holly's ghost was unique to Duane, who as an individual had to deal with it over time.

Cindy, the oldest sister, had always been a meticulous person. A good student and a well-behaved child, Cindy saw "strings" coming out of Holly after her sister's facial expression in the pool changed from joy to surprise. At home, although nobody noticed, Cindy began collecting strings. Any yarn, thread, or "find" out in the street found its way into a growing ball. The ball turned into a massive dirty object, but it was simultaneously Cindy's masterpiece. This latency-age child had become string obsessed. As she waited to see me in my waiting room, she played cat's cradle. But this was not an obsessive–compulsive disorder per se; it was trauma. We needed to turn Cindy's posttraumatic play into a mechanism of cure rather than an expression of endless repetition.

Shortly after Holly died, I was asked to see Winifred, now 5, who had supposedly been spared the trauma because she never saw Holly's accident. But young Winifred was not spared. She had a vivid picture-memory of the accident that was based on what she had heard about it. Winifred then began a strange game with trains. It was frequently played, unstoppable, and grim. All trains traveled from west to east and terminated in Pittsburgh. A large city had become Winifred's primary worry. It stood for death. The train was the mechanism by which one would travel to meet one's demise.

So now, looking back, what do snakes, witches, pool architecture, balls of string, and Pittsburgh have in common? Can this panoply of repetitive symptoms be treated with one medication or 10? Might a treatment manual or 8 or 20 therapy sessions organized on a certain timetable and with a certain series of exercises have worked for this particular family? These questions inspire books like the one you now hold in your hand. But, before we come to any preliminary conclusions, we look at the same questions from one more angle—the angle of time— in the second case.

This case involved a beautiful, young mother who recently brought her 8-year-old daughter to my office for, she hoped, a quick cure for the girl's fear of using her elementary school's toilets. They "smell bad," the child said. Yes, she was right. But the child was so overly concerned about bathroom odors that she developed painful urinary infections as a result of bladder retention for all the hours she was at school. It seemed to me that some cognitive-behavioral techniques would work, with not more than a few treatment sessions (and "homework" in between). "Good!" the mother proclaimed in response to my assessment. "It took you only a few sessions to cure me when I was 3 and kidnapped by my father!"

I never recognized her! Of course, her surname was now her married name. Also, the treatment had been only six sessions years before. But this woman, now a mother herself, had been kidnapped as a young child by her father, the noncustodial parent, and taken to a distant state where she was hidden, was told that her mother did not want her, was asked to look out for the police because they were "bad," and then became a witness to the "bad" police taking her father away. Afterward, she slept in a group foster home—for her, a house full of strangers. The next day her mother came for her.

I remembered that the main themes of this woman's play as a preschooler had been "bad police" and "ghostiss [sic] in milk." We had played repeated games with "good police" finding children for their mothers who really wanted them. And we had talked about fathers who were mixed up about their kids and sometimes made mistakes. But mostly it was the corrective play with police cars that appeared to make the difference. As to "ghostiss in milk"—we never did figure that one out.

So what happened 20 years later? Well, this young woman was concerned personally about only one problem when we spoke about her trauma. Her mother, who lived with her, wished to give the house to her daughter and retire to the mountains. But the young woman could not give her mother up. "I don't know if I can stand her moving away," she told me. Here was an issue that had festered long after a "successful" treatment during early childhood. The implanted idea "Mom doesn't want you" had haunted this young woman. It had changed over time, yet persisted.

What this young mother needed from me was a short hearkening back to what her father had told her during the months they were running from the police. If she could understand "Mom doesn't want you" as a trauma-causing lie, she could bear her mother's departure for retirement. It worked. Her mother left and the young woman's 8-year-old daughter successfully learned to use the school's bathroom facilities. As for her father, this young woman told me that when she turned 18, he phoned her, wanting to restart their relationship. She said, "Never call me again!" and hung up. On her own, this teenager had decided who was really evil—her father.

These two examples vividly depict what Eliana Gil and her colleagues discuss in a more scholarly, annotated, and enriched fashion throughout this book. No one program for posttraumatic problems in children is perfect. What works for a child immediately may not work years later. What successfully erases a certain youngster's fears may not suffice for another young child's fears, even if the other child shares a similar genetic background and family environment and the same trauma. Some children like to talk. But many other children prefer art, play, poetry, drama, and music. In other words, we still need individual assessments and specifically individualized modes of treatment for traumatized youngsters. We need a complete armamentarium of techniques along with treatment manuals, a choice of medications, and books like this very wonderful one. We need to give traumatized kids "time" and perhaps even annual psychological checkups. Most important, we must keep our minds open—and we must open and peruse good books like this one.

LENORE C. TERR, MD
Clinical Professor of Psychiatry
University of California San Francisco
School of Medicine

REFERENCES

Terr, L.C. (1990). *Too scared to cry*. New York: Basic Books.

Terr, L.C. (2008). *Magical moments of change*. New York: Norton.

Terr, L.C. (2009). The use of context in the treatment of traumatized children. *Psychoanalytic Study of the Child, 64*, 275–298.

Contents

PART ONE

The Extent of the Problem and Its Impact

CHAPTER 1

Introduction

ELIANA GIL

> After 4 months of therapy, 6-year-old Miranda came into my office with a Ping-Pong paddle in her hand, announcing, "Here, this is for you!" "Oh, what is it?" I asked, and she said, "It's a paddle." When I then inquired what the paddle was for, she said, "For you to hit me," in a matter-of-fact way. "Why would I want to hit you?" I responded with shock, and she quite earnestly replied, "You like me, don't you?"

This vignette illustrates one of the most insidious lessons of child abuse: People who love you hurt you. The unfortunate reality is that children who are abused and maltreated can develop expectations of the world as unsafe and grow to believe that interpersonal relationships carry inherent dangers that will surface predictably. As Lieberman and van Horn (2008) so poignantly explain, "The child's normative tendency to seek protection from the parent is violated by the stark realization that the parent is the source of danger. The child is torn between approach and avoidance, between seeking out comfort and fighting off danger"(p. 23).

Little 6-year-old Miranda had already learned at her young age to expect some kind of injury at the very point that she felt nurtured. For her, love or affection went hand in hand with physical injury. Once she was assured of someone's positive regard for her, her entire body began to cue her that something bad would happen. Miranda, however, was a very resilient and smart young girl, a girl who worked hard to establish some kind of predictability in her world: As she began to sense anticipatory anxiety about the inevitable danger she faced at the hands of someone who liked her, she took charge of when and how the injury would happen. Thus she brought me the weapon with which I would hit her and requested that I get it over with so we could proceed with our relationship and she could calm her body. What a sad and amazing behavior for a child who had been beaten by her mother since she was 3 years of age (and likely before) and had learned that once her mother beat her, she would hold her in her arms and rock her, sometimes for hours.

This was not the extent of how Miranda had learned to take care of herself. She also developed a unique ability to scan her mother's face for signs of tension, pinpointing how close her mother was to becoming explosive. Miranda was infinitely talented in finding a way of provoking an incident that would elicit her mother's release of tension (an explosion) and create for her a shortcut to mother's repentant arms and the warmth of the comfort she seemed unable to generate at other times. Unfortunately, Miranda had quickly learned to both expect and elicit negative responses in order to reap the rewards of her mother's fleeting guilt.

I was eager to meet Maria Lourdes, a 4-year-old child who had been abused sexually by a confused, distressed, and young drug-addicted mother who prostituted herself for drug money. It is hard to understand how mothers can reach such depths of pain as to turn to their young children to get their own needs met. From what could be deciphered, the mother was confused about her sexuality, far gone into the world of drugs, and had recently taken her daughter from her father in order to extract more financial help from him to support her habit. She'd only had this child for about 1 full month, but during that time, the child witnessed sexual activity by her mother and her customers, was left alone to fend for herself for days without food, and was witness to her mother's severe beating by an unknown male, likely a drug supplier, angry at not being paid. From what this child was able to communicate verbally to police, her mommy was "gone now," and she repeatedly asked for her father.

When I first met with this child, she appeared healthy and full of curiosity. It appeared that she was very comfortable with her father, who came into the play therapy office with her so that she could see the room that he had described to her prior to coming to therapy.

Once the door was closed and her father had left, Maria Lourdes took off her underwear and sat across from me, spreading her legs so that I could see her vagina. Few moments in my professional life have left me as stunned as I was with little Maria Lourdes. I had an immediate realization that I had to act. I took her underwear from the floor, handed it to her, and stated firmly and gently, "This is a place where you keep your underwear on and I keep my underwear on!" I repeated this statement only one other time, and the behavior ceased; however, it was a behavior I would never forget. Here again, this child had learned an interaction with her mother that she could neither forget nor understand. As a result, it's likely that she was conditioned to view private situations with adult women as situations that often included some sharing of sexual interactions. Once her father left the room and she was alone with me, she was clearly triggered to recreate an interaction that at this point she both expected and feared. As I later decoded the child's behavior, she was clearly asking "Is this what you want?" and "Will you do these sexual things to me as well?" The experience of being alone with me and hearing me say that we would "play" together in this room obviously moved us into perilous ground. I believe that Maria Lourdes, anxious at being left alone with a woman, was now taking action to decrease her anxiety and make the situation more predictable and more within her control.

To understand how children can construct these very complex ways of interacting with their abusive caretakers, and later others, it is important to underscore some of the important lessons that Miranda and Maria Lourdes demonstrated too well: Children are most attentive and receptive to their parents' interactions with them. In fact, as their parents exhibit tenderness, anger, or indifference, children are captive students to their very first lessons about the world. The very broad and prolific field of bonding and attachment has been quite definitive on this topic. In fact, Bowlby was the first to define and develop the concept of "internal working models," emphasizing the concept that an "individual developing within himself one or more working models representing principal features of the world about him and of himself as an agent in it . . . such working models determine his expectations and forecasts and provide him with tools for constructing plans of action" (Bowlby, 1989, p. 140). When discussing parental behaviors such as neglect, rejection, threats of not loving a child, and a range of threats to abandon the child, Bowlby further states that these experiences "can lead a child, an adolescent or an adult to live in constant anxiety lest he lose his attachment figure and, as a result, to have a low threshold for manifesting attachment behavior . . . anxious attachment" (Bowlby, 1989, p. 163).

Children can have multiple responses to inconsistent caretaking: Some develop anger toward parents that turns to unexpressed resentment; others withhold expectations in order to avoid disappointment; still others may constantly try to alter their own behaviors in the hopes of finally eliciting the love and affection they crave. Left unresolved, these attachment difficulties, which begin in the context of a parent–child relationship, can become the substantive root of many relational difficulties throughout the child's development (see Shaw, Chapter 2, this volume). In what appear to be random or erratic ways, children with attachment issues may reject those they most want, may elicit negative responses from those they desire to feel cared for, and may be unable to sustain an investment in another in any kind of successful manner. In fact, research suggests that interpersonal trauma "is especially destructive to children's attachment relationships" and that "maltreated children have higher rates of insecure and disorganized attachment and are less able to rely on their caregivers for emotional and behavioral regulation, have relationship problems associated with dysregulations in children's stress hormone systems, and the fact that they cannot turn to their parent for help (because the source of protection is simultaneously the agent of terror) creates what Main and Hesse (1990) call an 'unsolvable dilemma'" (Lieberman & van Horn, 2008, p. 48).

Recent work in the area of neurobiology expands our understanding of attachment to include the physiological changes that take place internally as attachment behaviors are activated and exhibited through emotions, verbal declarations, and behaviors. Badenoch (2008), describing early attachment processes and citing the work of Cozolino (2006), Goleman (2006), and Siegel (1999), states that "our brains are genetically hard-wired for attachment, seeking the interpersonal sustenance needed to structure our brains for personal well-being and healthy relationships" (p. 52). She goes on to state that "the sympathetic nervous system dominates over the parasympathetic during this early period of life, fueling the infant's efforts to reach and connect" (p. 52). Schore (2003) and Sigel (1999) note "that the way our parents approach us shapes the structure of our developing brain" (as cited in Badenoch, 2008, p. 53).

Daniel Siegel's (1999) book *The Developing Mind* catapulted the focus on the relational aspect of the brain to new heights, and others have followed suit. Bruce D. Perry has made a great contribution to our understanding of the value of recognizing brain science and has postulated a structured and sequential approach to therapy called the neurosequential model of therapy (Perry & Szalavitz, 2007). He strongly emphasizes early attachment relationships and the importance of activating attachment impulses in children who sustain early injuries through interpersonal trauma with attachment figures.

CHILDREN AND TRAUMA: PLAY OR ACT IT OUT

In Chapter 4 I discuss posttraumatic play by children in greater detail. Suffice it to say that children who undergo traumatic injuries at the hands of parents and trusted caretakers often have powerful challenges ahead. The fact is that young children, as recipients of abuse, are ill equipped to process psychological stress on their own. In fact, the younger they are, the more global the impairment can be, given their inability to protect themselves from physical and emotional injuries. So somewhere, somehow, some issues must be repaired in order for the child to meet his or her full potential. Lenore Terr (1991) stated that traumatized children "play it out or act it out," and this observation rings true from my years of clinical work with children. The child who can perceive and identify his or her distress, worries, and problems and who can then seek help, communicate clearly, and find a positive resolution on his or her own, is a rare youngster indeed. More common is the youngster who is emotionally and behaviorally dysregulated or the one who is utilizing play to depict stories replete with pain, catastrophic outcomes, or palpable anxiety and who represents danger and death and pessimism. Thus, our clinical responses have to be ample enough to recognize that children may not approach problems in only one way and that they may elicit the very negative attention that they seek to repel. The child victim of interpersonal trauma is highly compromised in his or her ability to seek and receive help (see Dobson & Perry, Chapter 3, this volume). At the very core of the problem is that child victims of interpersonal complex trauma often long for and fear the very same thing: an intimate and safe relationship with a trusted and caring individual. Clinicians are thus advised to be patient, hopeful, and above all, prepared to engage fully with children who may push them away, or worse, children who find or create obstacles at every turn.

TRAUMAS NEED RESOLUTION

This is an exciting and promising time to be a clinician working with traumatized children. The amount of information that is immediately available is unprecedented. Emerging data are available to us in record fashion, and practitioners appear persistent, dedicated, and consistent in their efforts to tackle important issues regarding the mental health needs of traumatized children.

Several evidence-based approaches now guide and shape our responses. The Child Study Group of the National Center for Child Traumatic Stress (NCCTS) has reached a consensus about specific areas for mental health treatment, further increasing our chances of assisting our child clients to resolve their trauma-based problems, restore their developmental trajectory, and develop positive outlooks for the future.

It has been incredibly helpful to the emerging field of trauma studies to have several groups in positions of national leadership. Great strides have been made with the organizational efforts, direction, and focused attention of the National Child Traumatic Stress Network (NCTSN), the International Society for the Study of Traumatic Stress Studies (ISTSS), and the formidable group of professionals of Division 56 of the American Psychological Association. Substantive efforts have been made to increase the refinement of diagnostic categories related to trauma and children (van der Kolk, 2005; van der Kolk & Courtois, 2005) as well as increase the quality of mental health services provided to abused and traumatized children across the nation. Many research studies have yielded valuable data, and we are now in the best possible position to continue to augment the efforts already undertaken.

At the same time, as the research studies, treatment models, and mental health options and possibilities continue to emerge, clinicians will likely always be well served by expanding and building upon any single theory and approach. Common sense dictates that children benefit the most from multimodal approaches that can provide the flexibility to help them with their unique developmental, gender-related, and cultural needs, as well as those with cognitive and linguistic differences. I believe it is imperative that we continue to embrace the information produced by countless professionals on the front line of service provision and to inform ourselves of the many evidence-based programs that show great potential for helping our child clients—for example, trauma-focused cognitive-behavioral therapy (Cohen, Mannarino, & Deblinger, 2006); child–parent psychotherapy (van Horn & Lieberman, 2008), cognitive-behavioral interventions for traumatized students (Kataoka et al., 2003), parent–child interaction therapy (Eyberg, 1988), and child–parent relationship therapy (Landreth & Bratton, 2006), to name a few. In addition, several treatment models have surfaced in the last decade that contribute greatly to our state-of-the-art knowledge about service delivery to this population; see, for example, the Chadwick Center's pathways assessment-based trauma model (*www.chadwickcenter.org*), Lanktree's integrative treatment of complex trauma and self-trauma (*clanktree@memorialcare.org*), Perry's neurosequential model of therapeutics (*www.childtraumaacademy.org*), and Cincinnati Children's Medical Center's integrated model for treatment of early abuse (*www.cincinnatichildrens.org*; call 513-558-9007 to receive the manual).

The goal of this book is to suggest that some children might be receptive to a play therapy context in which they can design and implement their own treatment direction and strategy. As the title suggests, this is a book about interpersonal complex trauma and one way that children can implement a reparative strategy. Needless to say, not all young children have the capacity or drive to engage in this play. It is something that clinicians may sometimes underestimate, overlook, or distract children away from, and definitely something that deserves to be explored, encouraged, and perhaps at times tolerated by those who are not trained in child or play therapy and who may feel more comfortable taking a more active, directive, or predictable route.

My impression has always been that the conclusions that children arrive at on their own are probably equal to, or surpass, the conclusions that are provided to them by their therapists. Sometimes our insistence to provide children with ready conclusions is met with compliance and agreement, yet such a response does not mean that these children have made internal shifts in their understanding or that they can translate that understanding into positive change. I believe that the healing process is very personal and has a multitude of idiosyncratic factors unique to each person. Thus reparation, by definition, is multifaceted and best sought via multiple paths leading to the same agreed-upon outcome.

SUMMARY

Children who suffer traumatic abuse or neglect at the hands of trusted attachment figures must negotiate multiple needs in the course of their treatment. Because they cannot protect themselves from the substantial harm of interpersonal trauma, children are left to defend themselves in varied and creative ways. Traumatized children access amazingly defensive strategies that serve them well in the short run but may cause long-term difficulties and challenges. Other chapters talk more in depth about the impact of interpersonal trauma on the developing child (see Dobson & Perry, Chapter 3, this volume).

Healing from interpersonal trauma is a complex and idiosyncratic process that needs to stay open and flexible in order to accommodate intrinsically unique abilities related to developmental, cognitive, linguistic, gender, and cultural factors that can influence children's abilities to self-repair successfully. Although there is a consensus about the areas of treatment that must be explored when working with traumatized children, there continues to be animated discussion about the relative merits of integrating evidence-based approaches (Ford & Cloitre, 2009) with other clinically sound therapies that rely on craft knowledge, best-practice guidelines, promising tests, and a vast, informative literature. Several authors suggest that multimodal approaches might maximize our chances of reaching young children, who are, after all, limited in their ability to describe their ailments and seek assistance on their own.

This book honors children's reparative processes by emphatically valuing their own healing strategies. Clinical interventions that allow children opportunities to find their own way toward healing may prove to be extremely helpful and child-friendly.

REFERENCES

Badenoch, B. (2008). *Being a brain-wise therapist: A practical guide to interpersonal neurobiology.* New York: Norton.

Bowlby, J. (1989). *The making and breaking of affectionate bonds.* New York: Routledge.

Cohen, J. A., Mannarino, A. P., & Deblinger, E. (2006). *Treating trauma and traumatic grief in children and adolescents.* New York: Guilford Press.

Cozolino, L. (2006). *The neuroscience of human relationships: Attachment and the developing brain.* New York: Norton.

Eyeberg, S. (1988). PCIT: Integration of traditional and behavioral concerns. *Child and Family Behavior Therapy, 10,* 33–46.

Ford, J. D., & Cloitre, M. (2009). Best practices in psychotherapy for children and adolescents. In C. A. Courtois & J. D. Ford (Eds.), *Treating complex traumatic stress disorders: An evidence-based approach* (pp. 59–81). New York: Guilford Press.

Goleman, D. (2006). *Social intelligence: The new science of human relationships.* New York: Bantam.

Kataoka, S., Stein, B. D., Jaycox, L., Wong, M., Escudero, P. Tu, W., et al. (2003). A school-based mental health program for traumatized Latino immigrant children. *Journal of the American Academy of Child and Adolescent Psychiatry, 42,* 311–318.

Landreth, G. L., & Bratton, S. C. (2006). *Child parent relationship therapy (CPRT): A ten- session filial therapy model*. New York: Routledge.

Lieberman, A. F., & van Horn, P. (2008). *Psychotherapy with infants and young children: Repairing the effects of stress and trauma on early attachment*. New York: Guilford Press.

Main, M., & Hesse, E. (1990). Parents' unresolved traumatic experiences are related to infant disorganized attachment status: Is frightened and/or frightening parental behavior the linking mechanism? In M. T. Greenberg, D. Cicchetti, & M. Cummings (Eds.), *Attachment in the preschool years: Theory, research and intervention* (pp. 121–160). Chicago: University of Chicago Press.

Perry, B. D., & Szalavitz, M. (2007). *The boy who was raised as a dog: And other stories from a child psychiatrist's notebook*. New York: Basic Books.

Schore, A. N. (2003). *Affect regulation and the repair of the self*. New York: Norton.

Siegel, D. J. (1999). *The developing mind: How relationship and the brain interact to shape who we are*. New York: Guilford Press.

Terr, L. C. (1991). Childhood traumas: An outline and overview. *American Journal of Psychiatry, 148*, 10–19.

van der Kolk, B. A. (2005). Developmental trauma disorder. *Psychiatric Annals, 35*, 439–448.

van der Kolk, B. A., & Courtois, C. A. (2005). Editorial: Complex developmental trauma. *Journal of Traumatic Stress, 18*(5), 385–388.

van Horn, P., & Lieberman, A. F. (2008). Using dyadic therapies to treat traumatized children. In D. Brom, R. Pat-Horenczyk, & J. D. Ford (Eds.), *Treating traumatized children: Risk, resilience, and recovery* (pp. 210–224). London: Routledge.

CHAPTER 2

A Review of Current Research on the Incidence and Prevalence of Interpersonal Childhood Trauma

JENNIFER A. SHAW

Before reviewing the incidence and prevalence of childhood interpersonal trauma, it is important to briefly discuss the evolution of the word *trauma,* particularly the context in which it was introduced to the mental health field and how it is currently used in the professional literature. For three decades the term *psychological trauma* has been expanded in the literature and is currently applied in enough contexts that it has lost some of its original meaning (Briere & Scott, 2006). Clinical exploration into the short- and long-term effects of trauma was prompted, in part, by observed and reported difficulties of veterans of the Vietnam War, and continued with renewed curiosity throughout the 1970s (Courtois & Gold, 2009). An increase in public awareness of violence against women and children in tandem with the knowledge gained from veteran experiences resulted in the inclusion of posttraumatic stress disorder (PTSD) and the dissociative disorders (DDs) in the third edition of the *Diagnostic and Statistical Manual of Mental Disorders* (DSM-III; American Psychiatric Association, 1980). The inclusion of PTSD in the DSM-III (along with five DDs (fugue, dissociative amnesia, depersonalization disorder, multiple personality disorder, and dissociative disorder, not otherwise specified; American Psychiatric Association, 1980) was welcomed not only by those treating combat trauma but also researchers investigating other types of trauma, such as rape, domestic battering, and child abuse and neglect (Courtois, 2008). Initiated primarily by an investigation into Vietnam combat trauma, the study of posttraumatic stress reactions first focused on abnormal events in adulthood (Ross, 2007). Criteria for PTSD were derived directly from the study of adult males exposed to war trauma, and subsequent researchers found that the effects of child abuse trauma, although posttraumatic in nature, were significantly different from PTSD as defined in the DSM-III (American Psychiatric Association, 1980; Courtois, 2008).

Professional debates regarding the nature and scope of diagnostic criteria as well as the clinical utility of the label have continued to influence both practitioner and scholar since the introduction of PTSD to the diagnostic nomenclature. Influenced by research findings and clinical curiosity within the last decade, definitions of traumatic events and experiences (also known as *traumatic stressors*; Courtois & Gold, 2009) were expanded to include events within the range of normal experience that are capable of causing death, injury, or threaten the physical integrity of the child or loved one (American Academy of Child and Adolescent Psychiatry [AACAP], 1998). Following the inclusion of PTSD in the DSM-III, clinical exploration of psychological trauma flourished (Courtois & Gold, 2009). The essential feature of PTSD remains the development of characteristic symptoms following an extreme stressor. The *Diagnostic and Statistical Manual of Mental Disorders*, 4th edition, text revision (DSM-IV-TR; American Psychiatric Association, 2000, p. 463) defines a traumatic stressor as

> involving direct personal experience of an event that involves actual or threatened death or serious injury, or other threat to one's physical integrity; or witnessing an event that involves death, injury, or a threat to the physical integrity of another person; or learning about unexpected or violent death, serious harm, or threat of death or injury experienced by a family member or other close associate (Criterion A1). The person's response to the event must involve intense fear, helplessness, or horror (or in children, the response must involve disorganized or agitated behavior) (Criterion A2).

Intense fear, helplessness, or horror are reactions that are well understood to be potential responses to trauma, but stress reactions are proven to be far more dynamic and complex than Criterion A2 suggests (Briere & Scott, 2006). Since there are also events and experiences that may be traumatic yet not include "threatened death or serious injury, or other threat to one's physical integrity," the definition of trauma by the DSM-IV-TR is criticized by many as too limiting (Briere, 2004). With its focus on traumatic events, the conventional definition of trauma is considered by experts in the field to be incomplete or misleading. In his discussion on the problem of comorbidity in psychiatry in the context of *the trauma model,* Ross (2007) argues that the deeper trauma for the child victim is not the traumatic event but rather the absence of love, affection, attention, care, and protection. The trauma for many children, particularly those who have suffered interpersonal violence and multiple victimizations, is the experience of "not being special to mom and dad . . . it is the errors of omission by the parents, not the errors of commission, which are the fundamental problem" (Ross, p. 61). In Levine and Kline's (2007) review of the effects of trauma on the nervous system, trauma is defined as the antithesis of empowerment and as *any* experience that "stuns us like a bolt out of the blue; it overwhelms us, leaving us altered and disconnected from our bodies. Any coping mechanisms we may have are undermined, and we feel utterly helpless and hopeless. It is as if our legs are knocked out from under us" (p. 4). Current research strongly supports the premise that children are more vulnerable to traumatic experiences than adults. Studies suggest that the lifetime incidence in a total adult population of PTSD ranges from 3 to 14%. Similar studies in adolescents vary between 2 and 5%. The numbers drastically increase when applied to children. Between 15 to 90% of children exposed to traumatic events develop PTSD, depending on the nature of the event (Perry, 1999).

The measurement of trauma is said to be a technical problem, not a conceptual one (Ross, 2007), and whether the nature or specific type of event has to satisfy diagnostic definitions of trauma to be considered "traumatic" continues to be a source of discussion (Briere & Scott, 2006). The following proposal for the definition of *traumatic* is repeated in current literature regarding the effects of traumatic stressors on children: "An event is traumatic if it is extremely upsetting and at least temporarily overwhelms the individual's internal resources" (Briere & Scott, 2006, p. 4). The current language reflects a change from the formerly held belief (in part, promoted by the language of the DSM) that traumatic symptoms are equivalent to the type and severity or enormity of an external event to a broader and much more complex definition of trauma. The magnitude of the stressor continues to be understood as an important factor, but it is now argued that this factor cannot define trauma, nor can the size or scope of events be used to inform a clinician as to whether or not the effect on the child was, in fact, traumatic. The current focus on describing and categorizing trauma is less on the event or experience than on the complex psychobiological responses (Briere & Scott, 2006). As summarized by Levine and Kline (2007), "Trauma is not in the event itself; rather, trauma resides in the nervous system" (p. 5).

THE SCOPE OF CHILDHOOD TRAUMA

Approximately 25% of children in the United States are believed to experience at least one potentially traumatic event in their lifetime, including natural disasters, life-threatening accidents, maltreatment, assault, and family and community violence (Costello, Erkanli, Fairbank, & Angold, 2002; Pynoos & Fairbank, 2003). However, the true prevalence of childhood trauma, including abuse and neglect, is not fully represented in the crime data. In a critical review of the status of violence, crime, and abuse in the lives of young people in America, Finkelhor (2008) clearly illustrates how difficult it is to determine the prevalence of violence and abuse of young children. It is well understood that offenses against children are far less reported than other kinds of victimization, and children are among the least likely victims to make a report to the police. However, the extent of the underrepresentation of children in crime statistics remains fairly undetermined—which, according to Finkelhor (2008), creates an added victimization burden on children.

Frequently used by the federal government and conducted by the Bureau of Census for the U.S. Department of Justice, the National Crime Victimization Survey (NCVS) is a highly regarded source of statistical information on crime and victimization in the United States (Finkelhor, 2008). This particular survey was not designed with young people in mind as respondents, and it does not capture crime victimizations in children under the age of 12 years. Even though it is frequently used to estimate crimes against youth, the NCVS does not mandate that respondents be interviewed in private; therefore, the survey likely undercounts incidents of domestic violence. NCVS interviewers are also permitted to hold proxy interviews with caregivers instead of talking to the youth involved, regardless of what caregivers may or may not know about the extent of victimization. In spite of the methodological weaknesses of the NCVS as it pertains to crimes against youth, the statistics still clearly illustrate an increased vulnerability of children. For violence overall, including aggravated assault and rape, the rate was 2.6 times higher for youth than adults in the 1990s. Based on extrapolations from the Federal Bureau of Investigation (FBI) data, 1.3 million violent crimes against children were reported to police in 2004. In the same year, there were approximately 872,000 cases of substantiated child abuse and neglect, and not all would be considered crimes; 17% were physical abuse and 10% were sexual abuse (Finkelhor, 2008). Children and adolescents are frequently reluctant to disclose abuse. Parents and caregivers are the primary source of information about abuse of younger children. Since there is often much these caregivers may not know about or may be reluctant to disclose (Finkelhor; Levine & Kline, 2007), violence against children is at least underestimated. Considering that other forms of abuse are even more difficult to quantify in terms of incidence and prevalence, such as psychological abuse and neglect (Herman, 1992), the total burden of victimization on children is absent from official crime estimates (Finkelhor, 2008).

A telephone survey of youth between the ages of 10 and 16 years (slightly younger than the ages of victimized youth in the NCVS estimates) resulted in 40.5% of respondents reporting an experience of violent victimization, attempted kidnapping, or attempted sexual assault (Boney-McCoy & Finkelhor, 1995). Designed to assess for the presence of all types of traumatic events as defined by the DSM-IV criteria for PTSD, a 2007 community sample of 1,420 children, ages 9, 11, and 13 years, followed longitudinally, showed an even higher prevalence than reflected in the study by Boney-McCoy and Finkelhor (1995). In this study by Copeland, Keeler, Angold, and Costello (2007), 67.8% were found to have been exposed to a traumatic experience (as defined by the DSM-IV) by age 16 (Courtois & Gold, 2009).

Bruce Perry (1999) estimates that more than 5 million children in the United States experience an extreme traumatic event each year, including natural disasters, motor vehicle accidents, life-threatening illness and associated painful medical procedures, sexual assault, physical abuse, witnessing domestic or community violence, or kidnapping and sudden death of a parent. Perry found that approximately 40% of the children who experience an extreme traumatic event are at risk for developing a chronic neuropsychiatric problem, the majority of which are classified as anxiety disorders, with most meeting criteria for PTSD.

FAMILIAL ABUSE AND INTERPERSONAL CHILDHOOD TRAUMA

Physical, sexual, and emotional abuse are prevalent forms of violent crime against children in America. As characterized by Finkelhor (2008), children are an extremely crime-victimized segment of the population. According to 1995 FBI crime data, 27% of all violent crime involved violence within families, with 48% perpetrated by acquaintances of the family and the violent act occurring inside the home. Considering the low rate of reporting and undercounting involved in the crime estimates, the actual incidence of domestic violence is likely much higher than indicated by FBI data (less than 5% of domestic violence is thought to be reported to police; Levine & Kline, 2007). Given that the most common source of a traumatic event for a child tends to involve an older family member or another familiar adult (Levine & Kline), for many children the home is the most violent place in America (Finkelhor, 2008). Approximately 30% of children living with two parents are exposed to domestic violence (McDonald, Jouriles, Ramisetty-Mikler, Caetano, & Green, 2006), and the lifetime prevalence of exposure to aggression between parents is likely even higher, considering the need to include children and adolescents whose parents have separated or divorced (Margolin & Vickerman, 2007). Severe physical abuse alone is estimated to victimize between 5 and 10% of children each year, and over 50% are believed to experience corporal punishment (Straus, Hamby, Finkelhor, Moore, & Runyan, 1998).

According to Briere and Scott (2006), childhood sexual and physical abuse (ranging from fondling to rape and from severe spankings to life-threatening beatings, respectively) is found to be quite prevalent in the United States. Retrospective studies of child abuse reports suggest that approximately 25–35% of women and 10–20% of men report experiences consistent with physical abuse (Briere & Elliot, 2003). Studies suggest that, if asked, 35–70% of female mental health patients report a history of childhood sexual abuse (Briere, 1992). Children's exposure to violence is even more difficult to quantify; if not the direct victims, children are frequently witnesses to violent crime (Finkelhor, 2008; Levine & Kline, 2007).

Familial abuse (i.e., spousal and child abuse) occurring in the home is frequently noted as one of the most severe adverse events during childhood (Margolin & Gordis, 2000). Whether the primary victim experiences the events directly or is witness to them, the experience has the potential to cause major posttraumatic emotional/psychological and physical repercussions (Courtois & Gold, 2009). For many young victims of domestic violence, one or both parents are not able to offer protection or safety. The compromised emotional state of the parent(s) is an added characteristic of family violence as a traumatic stressor (Margolin, 1998; van der Kolk, 2005). In many cases of interpersonal trauma, the betrayal, secrecy, and additional shame involved when the experience is at the hands of someone the child has trusted to protect them (e.g., family member, neighbor, teacher, religious leader), is in itself overwhelming (Levine & Kline, 2007).

COMPLEX PSYCHOLOGICAL TRAUMA

Given that traumatic stressors take many forms and the impact can be devastating and complex, the literature has refined terminology and revised criteria based on the field's expanding knowledge base of the impact of trauma on human development. Exposure to domestic violence and/or child abuse falls into the category of *complex traumas* (van der Kolk, 2005), a conceptualization characterized by chronic or repeating traumatic events (Margolin & Vickerman, 2007), usually occurring over a period of time and within specific relationships and contexts (Courtois, 2008). As defined by van der Kolk (2005), complex trauma refers to the experience of "multiple, chronic, and prolonged, developmentally adverse traumatic events, most often of an interpersonal nature (e.g., sexual or physical abuse, war, community violence) and early life onset" (p. 401). Ford and Courtois (2009) recently defined complex psychological trauma as "resulting from severe stressors that (1) are repetitive or prolonged, (2) involve harm or abandonment by caregivers or other ostensibly responsible adults, and (3) occur at developmentally vulnerable times in the victim's life, such as early childhood or adolescence (when critical periods of brain development are rapidly occurring or being consolidated" (p. 13). Estimated to occur in as many as 1 in 7 to 1 in 10 children, complex trauma is more prevalent than is typically recognized (Ford & Courtois, 2009).

Lenore Terr (1991) first distinguished trauma between two types: "Type I" single-incident trauma and "Type II" complex or repetitive trauma, which has since been more broadly characterized into (1) "acts of God" and (2) acts of humans (Courtois & Gold, 2009). Type II includes ongoing abuse, domestic violence, community violence, war, or genocide (Ford & Courtois, 2009), and frequently occurs cumulatively. Events that are human-induced involve premeditation, planning, and deliberateness in their implementation, which would include "all forms of sexual and physical assault, psychological and verbal abuse, bullying, acts of terrorism and torture, combat and genocide, human trafficking, and so forth" (Courtois & Gold, 2009, p. 5). *Betrayal trauma* is a similar conceptualization of trauma used to describe a form of complex psychological trauma. A traumatic event of an interpersonal nature usually involves a fundamental betrayal of trust in primary relationships and is considered an especially severe form of interpersonal violence "involving major perfidy of a kinship or a role relationship" (see also, Courtois & Gold, 2009, p. 5; Freyd, 1996). Betrayal trauma includes relational/ attachment trauma, domestic violence, and all forms of child abuse (including incest and neglect) perpetrated by relatives or acquaintances (Courtois & Gold, 2009).

When traumatic events are accidents or natural disasters, parental support for the child is proven to be a crucial buffer in minimizing symptoms of posttraumatic stress (AACAP, 1998). Human-induced traumatic events can be a result of accident, negligence, or human error but are too frequently deliberate acts against children without a parental buffer. Even though the effect can be damaging to the victim whether or not the act or event was intentional (Courtois & Gold, 2009), when the event is deliberate and involves betrayal and interpersonal violence, the result is frequently a greater severity of response (Herman, 1992). The more severe response and greater psychological damage are thought to stem from the "deliberate and willful and/or due to human error, negligence, or disregard" (Courtois & Gold, 2009, p. 6).

Victims of interpersonal traumas are determined to be at statistically greater risk of additional interpersonal traumas and revictimization (Briere & Scott, 2006). Children who have suffered one kind of victimization are found to be at substantially higher risk for multiple victimizations, referred to as *polyvictimization* (Finkelhor, Ormrod, & Turner, 2007). Polyvictimization is associated with an increased likelihood of adverse traumatic symptoms (Ko et al., 2008), including chronic mental health problems and poor outcomes. According to Finkelhor's (2008) analyses of crime estimates and childhood victimization, out of the children who had experienced any victimization in the previous year, two-thirds had experienced two or more victimizations (average of three victimizations, with total victimizations ranging up to 15; Finkelhor). Finkelhor argues that polyvictims should be of particular concern to professionals, as they harbor the greatest amount of distress.

EFFECTS OF INTERPERSONAL TRAUMA IN CHILDHOOD

Traumatic stress can result in significant disruptions in child or adolescent development and exert profound long-term consequences. As stated by Judith Herman (1992), traumatic events are extraordinary "not because they occur rarely, but rather because they overwhelm the ordinary human adaptations to life" (p. 32). Extreme traumatic stress in childhood is associated with increased use of health and mental health services and increased involvement with other child-serving systems, including the child welfare and juvenile justice systems. Due to their disproportionate experience of violence, academic failure, and insufficient access to mental health care, ethnic-minority and low-income youth are found to be particularly vulnerable to the adverse effects of trauma (Ko et al., 2008). A variety of factors contributes to a child's vulnerability to trauma, particularly age and trauma history. In general, the younger the child, the more likely that the child will be overwhelmed by common occurrences that may not affect an older child (Levine & Kline, 2007). Chronic or repeated exposure to traumatic experiences can alter psychobiological development and is associated with increased risk of low academic performance, engagement in high-risk behaviors, and difficulties in relationships (Ko et al., 2008). Examples of such stressors are extended child abuse, torture, captivity as a prisoner of war or concentration camp internee, and chronic spousal abuse (Levine & Kline, 2007).

The clinical presentation and evolution of trauma-related symptoms are typically complex (Perry, 1999), and children's exposure to interpersonal violence is now recognized as a potential precursor to posttraumatic stress reactions (Margolin & Vickerman, 2007). The following six domains of potential impairment are consistently associated with complex trauma: (1) affect regulation; (2) information processing, including attention, concentration, learning difficulties, and consciousness; (3) self-concept, including guilt and shame; (4) behavioral control, including aggression and substance abuse; (5) interpersonal relationships, including trust and intimacy; and (6) biological processes, including somatization and delayed sensorimotor development (van der Kolk, 2005; Margolin & Vickerman, 2007). Van der Kolk (2002) includes alterations in the systems of meaning and loss of sustaining beliefs as additional potential impairments. Psychological trauma has been termed the affliction of the powerless; "at the moment of trauma, the victim is rendered helpless by overwhelming force" (Herman, 1992, p. 33). According to van der Kolk et al. (1996), the more complex posttraumatic outcomes arise from severe, prolonged, and repeated trauma, most often of an interpersonal nature. The effects impact the psychological structures of the self as well as the systems of attachment and meaning that link individual and community (Herman, 1992).

Ross (2007) describes trauma as a complex interaction of events and the organism's response to those events. Responses of fear and helplessness are considered particularly overwhelming when the threatened or actual injury is caused by a parent and directed toward the child or a family member (Margolin and Vickerman, 2007). For children who have experienced the overwhelming dysregulation secondary to complex trauma, Margolin and Vickerman (2007) state that even minor stressors can lead to serious distress. The aftermath includes potential damage to the survivor's faith and sense of community and is "particularly severe when the traumatic events themselves involve the betrayal of important relationships" (Herman, 1992, p. 55). Steven Stosny (1995) described attachment as "the psychobiological glue that holds the family together" (p. 13). In the case of child abuse by a primary caregiver, from the perspective of attachment theory the child is in a position of powerlessness and is likely to respond to the threatened or actual injury with disorganized attachment because the parent or caregiver is both the source of safety and the source of danger (Lieberman & van Horn, 2005). According to Herman (1992), it is within this climate of unpredictability, danger, and disrupted relationships that the child faces a formidable developmental task: to form attachments to caregivers who are either dangerous or, from the child's perspective, negligent.

From the perspective of trauma therapy, trauma to the attachment systems during childhood, particularly the betrayal of trust, can be more hurtful than the abusive event itself (Ross, 2007). According to Herman (1992), children in this type of chronically abusive environment develop the ability to scan their environment for warning signs; they become attuned to their abusers' inner states, recognizing subtle changes in facial expression, voice, and body language as signals of anger, sexual arousal, intoxication, or dissociation. Eventually this non verbal automatic communication occurs outside of the child's conscious awareness, and the child learns to respond even when not able to name or identify the warning signals (Herman, 1992). For the purposes of accurately assessing potential impairment and family treatment planning, Eliana Gil (1996) distinguished cumulative from current (acute) abuse in her review of the impact of abuse on adolescents. Compared to abuse starting in late childhood or during adolescence, Gil finds cases of chronic abuse to be less responsive to crisis intervention and generally to require long-term treatment; those who have been abused throughout their lives are likely to have much greater difficulty both emotionally and behaviorally. Additionally, Gil finds that nonoffending parents of these youth are more likely to be unable or unwilling to make the necessary efforts to effect a positive change. For an older child, adolescent, or adult victim of childhood interpersonal violence, an immature system of psychological defenses is/was constructed to compensate for the absence of adult protection and care (Herman, 1992). Due to the longstanding abuse, "abilities to trust, feel safe, or be receptive to a new environment may be greatly endangered" (Gil, 1996, p. 52). These children attempt to "preserve a sense of trust in people who are untrustworthy, safety in a situation that is unsafe, control in a situation that is terrifyingly unpredictable, power in a situation of helplessness" (Herman, 1992, p. 96).

SUMMARY

Up to 5 million children in the United States are exposed to a traumatic event each year (Levine & Kline, 2007; Perry, 1999), and up to 40% of those children are at risk for developing a chronic neuropsychiatric problem (Perry, 1999). For many children, extremely stressful events become customary experiences (Margolin & Vickerman, 2007). Exposure to interpersonal trauma is increasingly accepted as a potential precursor to posttraumatic stress reactions in children and adolescents. A review of the literature indicates that there is an increasingly sophisticated understanding of childhood trauma that continues to challenge current diagnostic nomenclature. Research indicates a shift from the view of traumatic stress as limited to extraordinary events or experiences to a broader context that includes the contribution of interpersonal violence and complex psychological trauma. Physical, sexual, and emotional abuse are found to be prevalent forms of childhood victimization in the United States. Interpersonal childhood trauma, with its complex psychobiological repercussions, appears to be much more prevalent in the United States than is reflected in official crime estimates (Finkelhor, 2008).

As stated by Levine and Kline (2007), the complicated mixture of multiple traumas and multiple symptomatic responses to trauma is well known to trauma-focused clinicians. Clinicians who work with childhood interpersonal trauma can find it difficult to discriminate trauma-related symptoms from less trauma-specific symptoms (Levine & Kline, 2007) and can be unclear about how to describe a client with significant posttraumatic symptoms (Briere & Scott, 2006). As stated by Herman (1992), the environment of childhood abuse forces the development of extraordinary capacities, both creative and destructive: "It fosters the development of abnormal states of consciousness in which the ordinary relations of body and mind, reality and imagination, knowledge and memory, no longer hold" (p. 96). According to Gil (1996), one of the greatest difficulties for a clinician to contend with is these children's distrust of adults; they often enter therapy "with years and years of pain, feelings of helplessness, well-entrenched defenses, and enormous distrust of adults (and of human interactions in general)" (p. 203). It is within the holding environment of therapy that the recovery process can begin with the establishment of safety and security.

In addition, the focus of treatment has become clearer over time. As Herman (1992) asserts, "The core experiences of psychological trauma are disempowerment and disconnection from others. Recovery, therefore, is based upon the empowerment of the survivor and the creation of new connections. Recovery can take place only within the context of relationships; it cannot occur in isolation" (p. 133). Children need support to release this highly charged state, given how susceptible they are to trauma's effects (Levine & Kline, 2007), and we must continue to find ways to ensure that our efforts are developmentally appropriate and fully engaging for children of varied chronological and emotional ages.

REFERENCES

American Academy of Child and Adolescent Psychiatry. (1998). Practice parameters for the assessment and treatment of children and adolescents with posttraumatic stress disorder. *Journal of the American Academy of Child and Adolescent Psychiatry, 37*, 4–26.

American Psychiatric Association. (1980). *Diagnostic and statistical manual of mental disorders* (3rd ed.). Washington, DC: Author.

American Psychiatric Association. (2000). *Diagnostic and statistical manual of mental disorders* (4th ed., text rev.). Washington, DC: Author.

Boney-McCoy, S., & Finkelhor, D. (1995). Psychosocial sequelae of violent victimization in a national youth sample. *Journal of Consulting and Clinical Psychology, 6*, 726–736.

Briere, J. (1992). *Child abuse trauma: Theory and treatment of the lasting effects.* Newbury Park, CA: Sage.

Briere, J. (2004). *Psychological assessment of adult posttraumatic states: Phenomenology, diagnosis, and measurement* (2nd ed.). Washington, DC: American Psychological Association.

Briere, J., & Elliot, D. M. (2003). Prevalence and symptomatic sequelae of self-reported childhood physical and sexual abuse in a general population sample of men and women. *Child Abuse and Neglect, 27*, 1205–1222.

Briere, J., & Scott, C. (2006). *Principles of trauma therapy: A guide to symptoms, evaluation, and treatment.* Thousand Oaks, CA: Sage.

Copeland, W. E., Keeler, G., Angold, A., & Costello, E. J. (2007). Traumatic events and posttraumatic stress in childhood. *Archives of General Psychiatry, 64,* 577–584.

Costello, E. J., Erkanli, A., Fairbank, J. A., & Angold, A. (2002). The prevalence of potentially traumatic events in childhood and adolescence. *Journal of Traumatic Stress, 15*(2), 99–112.

Courtois, C. A. (2008). Complex trauma, complex reactions: Assessment and treatment. *Psychological Trauma: Theory, Research, Practice, and Policy, S*(1), 86–100.

Courtois, C. A., & Gold, S. N. (2009). The need for inclusion of psychological trauma in the professional curriculum: A call to action. *Psychological Trauma: Theory, Research, Practice, and Policy, 1*(1), 3–23.

Finkelhor, D. (2008). *Childhood victimization: Violence, crime, and abuse in the lives of young people.* New York: Oxford University Press.

Finkelhor, D., Omrod, R., & Turner, H. (2007). Poly-victimization: A neglected component in child victimization. *Child Abuse and Neglect, 31,* 7–26.

Ford, J. D., & Cloitre, M. (2009). Best practices in psychotherapy for children and adolescents. In C. A. Courtois & J. D. Ford (Eds.), *Treating complex traumatic stress disorders: An evidence-based guide* (pp. 59–81). New York: Norton.

Ford, J. D., & Courtois, C. A. (2009). Defining and understanding complex trauma and complex traumatic stress disorders. In C. A. Courtois & J. D. Ford (Eds.), *Treating complex traumatic stress disorders: An evidence-based guide* (pp. 13–30). New York: Norton.

Freyd, J. (1996). *Betrayal trauma: The logic of forgetting childhood abuse.* Cambridge, MA: Harvard University Press.

Gil, E. (1996). *Treating abused adolescents.* New York: Guilford Press.

Herman, J. L. (1992). *Trauma and recovery: The aftermath of violence—from domestic abuse to political terror.* New York: Basic Books.

Ko, S. J., Ford, J. D., Kassam-Adams, N., Berkowitz, S. J., Wilson, C., Wong, M., et al. (2008). Creating trauma-informed systems: Child welfare, education, first responders, health care, juvenile justice. *Professional Psychology: Research and Practice, 39*(4), 396–404.

Levine, P. A., & Kline, M. (2007). *Trauma through a child's eyes: Awakening the ordinary miracle of healing.* Berkeley, CA: North Atlantic Books.

Lieberman, A. F., & van Horn, P. (2005). *"Don't hit my mommy!": A manual for child–parent psychotherapy with young witnesses of family violence.* Washington, DC: Zero to Three.

Margolin, G. (1998). Effects of domestic violence on children. In P. K. Trickett & C. J. Schellenbach (Eds.), *Violence against children in the family and the community* (pp. 57–102). Washington, DC: American Psychological Association.

Margolin, G., & Gordis, E. B. (2000). The effects of family and community violence on children. *Annual Review of Psychology, 51,* 445–479.

Margolin, G., & Vickerman, K. A. (2007). Posttraumatic stress in children and adolescents exposed to family violence: I. Overview and issues. *Professional Psychology: Research and Practice, 38*(6), 613–619.

McDonald, R., Jouriles, E. N., Ramisetty-Mikler, S., Caetano, R., & Green, C. E. (2006). Estimating the number of American children living in partner-violent families. *Journal of Family Psychology, 20*, 137–142.

Perry, B. D. (1999). Stress, trauma, and post-traumatic stress disorders in children. *Child Trauma Academy: Interdisciplinary Education Series, 2*(5).

Pynoos R., & Fairbank, J. (2003). The state of child trauma in America, 2 years out. *Brown University Child and Adolescent Behavior Letter, 19*, 1–7.

Ross, C. A. (2007). *The trauma model: A solution to the problem of comorbidity in psychiatry*. Richardson, TX: Manitou Communications.

Stosny, S. (1995). *Treating attachment abuse: A compassionate approach*. New York: Springer.

Straus, M. A., Hamby, S. L., Finkelhor, D., Moore, D. W., & Runyan, D. (1998). Identification of child maltreatment with the Parent–Child Conflict Tactics Scales: Development and psychometric data for a national sample of American parents. *Child Abuse and Neglect, 22*, 249–270.

Terr, L. (1991). Childhood traumas. *American Journal of Psychiatry, 148*, 10–20.

van der Kolk, B. A. (2002). The assessment and treatment of complex PTSD. In R. Yehuda (Ed.), *Treating trauma survivors with PTSD* (pp. 127–156). Washington, DC: American Psychiatric Association.

van der Kolk, B. A. (2005). Developmental trauma disorder. *Psychiatric Annals, 35*, 401–408.

van der Kolk, B. A., Pelcovitz, D., Roth, S., Mandel, F. S., McFarlene, A., & Herman, J. L. (1996). Dissociation, somatization, and affect dysregulation: The complexity of adaptation of trauma. *American Journal of Psychiatry, 153*(Suppl.), 83–93.

CHAPTER 3

The Role of Healthy Relational Interactions in Buffering the Impact of Childhood Trauma

CHRISTINE R. LUDY-DOBSON
BRUCE D. PERRY

Humans are social creatures. We live, work, and grow up in social groups. For the vast majority of the last 200,000 years, humans have lived in multigenerational, multifamily hunter-gatherer bands characterized by a rich and continuous relational milieu; the concept of personal space and privacy is relatively new. Child mortality during our history was high; children were highly valued by the band and in these groups of 40–60 members, there were roughly four developmentally more mature potential caregivers for each child under the age of 6. This enriched relational ratio helped the group protect, nurture, educate, and enrich the lives of each developing child.

These living groups were the source of safety and sustenance for individuals in a dangerous world. Survival depended upon the ability to communicate, bond, and share with and receive from other members of the band. Then, as today, the presence of familiar people projecting the social–emotional cues of acceptance, understanding, compassion, and empathy calmed the stress response of the individual. We feel safest in the presence of familiar and nurturing members of our family and community. These powerful regulating effects of healthy relational interactions on the individual—mediated by various key neural networks in the brain—are at the core of relationally based protective mechanisms that help us survive and thrive following trauma and loss. Individuals who have few positive relational interactions—a child without a healthy family/clan—during or after trauma have a much more difficult time decreasing the trauma-induced activation of the stress response systems. The result is an increased probability of developing trauma-related problems. Further, children in a relationally impoverished setting will likely be unable to recover or heal from these effects without a change in the relational milieu. Positive relational interactions regulate the brain's stress response systems and help create positive and healing neuroendocrine and neurophysiological states that promote healing and healthy development both for the normal and the maltreated child.

There is another aspect to the interconnectedness of the stress response and relational neurobiology. Human history, to this very day, is characterized by clan on clan, human on human competition for limited resources. Indeed the major predator of humans has always been other humans. In our competitive, violent past, encounters with unfamiliar nonclan members were as likely to result in harm as harmony. As the infant becomes the toddler and the toddler becomes the child, the brain is making a catalogue of "safe and familiar" attributes of the humans in his or her clan; the language, the dress, the nonverbal elements of communication, the skin color of the family and clan become the attributes of "safe and familiar," which, in future interactions with others, will tell his or her stress response networks to be calm. In contrast, when this child interacts with strangers, the stress response systems activate; the more unfamiliar the attributes of these new people, the greater the activation. In some cases, a clan's beliefs may have exacerbated this response; if the child grows up with ethnic, racial, or religious beliefs and values that degrade or dehumanize others, the stress activation that results in an encounter with different peoples can be extreme. In this case, relational interactions activate and exacerbate trauma-related stress over activation. A recent study by Chiao and colleagues (2008), for example, has shown that fear-related social cues from individuals from one's own group/ethnicity have greater "power." We are more tuned into people in our own "group." Fear of a member in our group will induce greater amygdalar activation than similar cues from nongroup members.

The social milieu, then, becomes a major mediator of individual stress response baseline and reactivity; nonverbal signals of safety or threat from members of one's "clan" modulate one's stress response. The bottom line is that healthy relational interactions with safe and familiar individuals can buffer and heal trauma-related problems, whereas the ongoing process of "tribalism"—creating an "us" and "them"—is a powerful but destructive aspect of the human condition that only exacerbates trauma in individuals, families, and communities attempting to heal.

THE IMPACT OF CHILDHOOD EXPERIENCES

The experiences of early life have the profound ability to shape the infant, child, adolescent, and ultimately the adult. Each child has his or her own unique genetic potential, yet this potential is expressed differentially depending upon the nature, timing, and patterns of developmental experience (see Perry, 2001, 2002). An understanding of how early experiences shape neurodevelopment is imperative if we seek to impact the lives of children with whom we live and work. This is especially true in the case of children growing up in homes plagued by violence, maltreatment, and neglect.

For many, childhood is a very violent time; for others, childhood is permeated with unpredictability, chaos, threat, and other forms of adverse developmental experience. There is a wealth of research describing the negative impact of childhood trauma on the physical, behavioral, cognitive, social, and emotional functioning of children (Perry & Pollard, 1998; Bremner & Vermetten, 2001; Read, Perry, Moskowitz, & Connolly, 2001; Malinosky-Rummell & Hansen, 1993; Fitzpatrick & Boldizar, 1993; Graham-Berman & Levendosky, 1998; Margolin & Gordis, 2000; Sanders-Phillips, 1997; Berenson, Wieman, & McCombs, 2001; Anda et al., 2006). Children exposed to trauma have increased neuropsychiatric problems (e.g., posttraumatic stress disorder [PTSD], depression, dissociation, conduct disorders), school and academic failure, involvement with the juvenile justice system, drug and alcohol use, antisocial behaviors, and engagement in high-risk sexual behavior and teenage pregnancy. The impact of early trauma is so profound because it occurs during those critical periods when the brain is most rapidly developing and organizing. Because the experiences of early life determine the organization and function of the mature brain, going through adverse events in childhood can have a tremendously negative impact on early brain development, including social and emotional development.

THE HUMAN BRAIN AND THE IMPACT OF TRAUMA

The brain of a newborn is composed of billions of neurons and glial cells that, from conception, have been changing—dividing, moving, specializing, connecting, interacting, and organizing. This organization takes place from the bottom, simplest area (brainstem) to the highest, most complex (cortex). The various functions of the brain parallel this structure: The brainstem regulates the simplest reflexive functions (e.g., body temperature and heart rate), and the cortical areas mediate complex functions such as abstract thought and language (Perry, 2001). The brain is a use-dependent organ that changes in response to patterned, repetitive activity. Thus the more any neural network of the brain is activated, the more that part will change. Among other things, this process is the basis for memory, learning, and development.

All experience, therefore, changes the brain—even if in the subtlest, microscopic ways. Yet experiences in childhood have disproportionate power in shaping the brain. Early in life the brain organizes at an incredible rate, with more than 80% of the major structural changes taking place during the first 4 years. Experiences that take place during this window of organization have a greater potential to influence the brain—in either positive or negative ways. Because the majority of brain growth and development takes place during these first years, early developmental trauma and neglect have a "disproportionate influence on brain organization and later brain functioning" (Perry & Hambrick, 2008; see also, Perry, 2008). Unfortunately, traumatic experiences that take place during this critical window impact the brain in multiple areas and can actually change the structure and function of key neural networks, including those involved with regulating stress and arousal (Perry, 2008). These stress response systems in the brain are designed to sense and respond to threats, either from internal (body) or external sources. Thus, the end effect is that children who are exposed to chronic threat develop overactive and overly reactive stress response neural systems. In short, they live in a persistent state of fear. Although these neuronal changes are useful and protective when the child is living in an abusive environment, they lead to problems in other settings. For example, a hyperaroused child is often preferentially alert to nonverbal cues, which is adaptive with an unpredictable, violent parent but maladaptive in a classroom where the child will miss much of the verbal information presented by a teacher.

As the brain develops in a use-dependent manner, it requires stimulation at specific times in order for the systems to function at their best (see Perry, 2001; Perry & Szalavitz, 2007). If these sensitive periods of development are missed, "some systems may never be able to reach their full potential" (Perry & Szalavitz, 2007, p. 85). Inconsistent, abusive, or neglectful caregiving in early childhood alters the normal development of neural systems involved in both relationships and the stress response. It is through patterned, repetitive neural stimulation provided by consistent, nurturing, predictable, responsive caregivers that the infant's brain receives what is needed to develop the capacity for healthy attachment and self-regulation capabilities. The caregiver becomes the external stress regulator for the infant. However, if the caregiver is depressed, stressed, "high," inconsistent, or absent, these two crucial neural networks (relational and stress response) develop abnormally. The result is a child more vulnerable to future stressors and less capable of benefiting from the healthy nurturing supports that might help buffer stressors or trauma later in life.

These early developmental experiences with caregivers create a very literal template or set of associations for the child's brain about what humans are. The brain of a child growing up in a home with attentive, attuned caregivers will create a template of humans as safe, predictable, and a source of sustenance, comfort, and pleasure. The brain of a child living in a home plagued by domestic violence and whose primary caregiver is preoccupied and chaotically neglectful will create a template in which humans are unpredictable and a source of fear, chaos, pain, and loss. Children carry these templates created by their initial caregiving experiences into all future relational interactions, either increasing or decreasing their capacity to benefit from future nurturing, caring, and invested adults. Relationships in early childhood, then, can alter the vulnerability–resilience balance for an individual child. Negative or neglectful primary caregiving relationships have the capacity to increase the likelihood that the child will have a more vulnerable, dysregulated stress response network and a less receptive relational capacity to buffer and heal following trauma as the child grows.

SOCIAL AND EMOTIONAL DEVELOPMENT

Understanding healthy social and emotional development in children underscores why disruptions to, or disorganization in, early attachment has such far-reaching implications. *Attachment* is defined as an enduring relationship with a specific person that is characterized by soothing, comfort, pleasure, and safety. It also includes feelings of intense distress when faced with the loss, or threat of loss, of this person. By far the most important attachment relationship is that of mother and infant. Even before birth, the emotionally healthy mother begins the process of attaching to her baby as she grows attuned to its patterns of movement and the way it responds to stimuli such as sound (Greenspan & Wieder, 2006). Bowlby (1969) describes maternal–infant attachment as a reciprocal relationship. Greenspan and Wieder (2006) note that "the rhythmic, near-synchronous patterns of movement and vocalization between infant and caregiver enable the infant to begin attending to and appreciating the world" (pp. 14–15). In fact, many have aptly described this mother–infant relationship as a dance, the moves of which will be used with many partners throughout the child's life.

The importance of healthy attachment has been extensively studied. Research in this area has identified four categories of attachment: secure, insecure-resistant, insecure-avoidant, and insecure-disorganized/disoriented. Securely attached children feel a consistent, responsive, and supportive relation to their mothers even during times of significant stress. Children with insecure attachment feel inconsistent, punishing, unresponsive emotions from their caregivers and feel threatened during times of stress. Ainsworth, Blehar, Waters, and Wall (1978) posited that the type of attachment a child develops is dependent on the kind of caregiving received during the first year of life. A solid and healthy attachment with a primary caregiver predicts healthy relationships with others as the child grows.

Development in many other areas is rooted in the development of a healthy attachment to a primary caregiver. These areas include development of emotional, social, cognitive, and self-regulatory capabilities. These first relationships, including those formed with other significant people during early childhood, "are the prism through which young children learn about the world, including the world of people and of the self" (Thompson, 2002, p. 10). These early experiences literally provide the organizing framework for the infant/child. Regulation of the infant's emotional states develops through the repeated appropriate responses of an attentive, attuned caregiver to the baby's changing emotional states (e.g., fear, anger, distress). Through this consistent, predictable, and repetitive nurturing the child develops the capacity to self-regulate these emotional states as well as to communicate his or her emotions (Emde, 1998). These nurturing behaviors also provide feelings of safety and security. According to Lyons-Ruth and Spielman (2004), a mother's capacity to regulate her infant's distress and fear is vital to the child's ultimate sense of security.

The timing of relational interactions is critically important for the development of attachment and social–emotional functioning. An absence of nurturing during the first 3 years of life can lead to disorganization of the neural systems that mediate social–emotional functioning (Perry, 2002). Without the vitally important relational input from caring, attuned caregivers, children may develop as if the entire world were a cold, dangerous place. Not surprising, many studies have found that maltreated infants exhibit disturbed or insecure attachment (Carlson, Cichetti, Barnett, & Braunwald, 1989; Crittenden, 1985; Lamb, Gaensbauer, Malkin, & Schultz, 1985; Schneider-Rosen, Braunwald, Carlson, & Cichetti, 1985). Children who have experienced abuse and neglect in infancy and early childhood are at greater risk for developing maladaptive behaviors and mental health problems as they get older.

CASE 1: CAREGIVER ISSUES IMPACTING BONDING AND ATTACHMENT

Mark, age 2, was brought to our clinic by his adoptive mother due to concerns that he may have an attachment disorder. He had been adopted at 10 months of age from a small Eastern European orphanage, where he had been placed at birth. His adoptive mother, Sarah, had no knowledge of Mark's biological parents but reported that the orphanage seemed "better than most," as Mark had relatively stable caregivers to whom he appeared attached and areas in which he could explore and play. She reported that her difficulties with Mark began almost immediately upon returning home. According to Sarah, he would not look her in the eyes, didn't enjoy being held, and didn't engage in exploratory play. In an effort to strengthen the attachment bond, she had taken Mark to multiple therapists specializing in attachment. Further, she had been trained in holding therapy and had read countless books on the subject.

In an effort to get to know Sarah and Mark better, clinicians observed their interaction over the course of the first two interview sessions. During the initial interview Sarah sat and talked with the lead clinician while Mark explored the room. Mark quickly discovered that he could climb from the chair to the desk, and within minutes he was happily walking on top of the desk and onto the adjoining table. The observing clinicians watched in dismay as Sarah continued the interview with no acknowledgment of her son's precarious situation. Only when the suggestion was made that Mark might fall and injure himself did she remove him from the table.

During the second interview, Sarah offered to demonstrate the activities she was currently implementing to increase her son's attachment to her. She picked Mark up and held him tightly in her arms, her hand under his chin, in an effort to force him to look directly into her face. The child squirmed and fought to get loose; eyes closed, he turned his head violently in an effort to avoid her gaze. The more he fought and screamed the more resolute she became. Finally, she looked at the clinician and said, "See, this is exactly what I've been dealing with." However, to the clinician, Mark's reaction was not a surprise. When infants or young children are distressed due to pain, pervasive threat, or a chaotic environment, they will have difficulty participating in even a supportive caregiving relationship (Perry & Pollard, 1998)—which this obviously was not.

A second clinician participated in the third session with the family. While the primary clinician talked with Sarah about healthy development, the second clinician sat on the floor with Mark, who was playing with a large plastic dinosaur. The second clinician engaged in parallel play with another dinosaur. Within a short time, Mark had moved close to the clinician, interjecting his dinosaur into her play. He interacted easily with the clinician, making appropriate eye contact and happily describing the dinosaur's activity. In subsequent sessions it became clear that the issue was not centered in the child but in the parenting behavior. Sarah had experienced abuse at the hands of her own mother as a child. Relationships, it seemed, had been difficult for her throughout her adult life, but her hope was that by adopting a child she would fill this relational void. Unfortunately, it is not uncommon that caregivers who themselves experienced trauma or maltreatment as children carry these experiences into their own maternal–child relationships. The frightened or frightening behaviors of such a caregiver often creates a contradiction that is impossible for the child to resolve: The caregiver is both the source of, and solution to, the child's distress (Main & Hess, 1990). Without an acknowledgment of the impact that their own childhood experiences have on their parenting, these caregivers are unlikely to change their behavior. This was the case with Sarah. Attempts to help her better understand how her own trauma history impacted her ability to respond to her son's needs and to teach her appropriate nurturing activities ultimately were unsuccessful, leading ultimately to her decision to relinquish her parental rights. Mark was later adopted by another family who was more open to understanding the impact of his early experiences and to providing the necessary reparative experiences that would allow him to grow into a healthy happy child.

CASE 2: THE DEVASTATING IMPACT OF MALTREATMENT ON SOCIAL–EMOTIONAL DEVELOPMENT

Sydney never knew her biological parents. She had been removed from their care at birth due to the severe physical abuse of her three older siblings by her mother and father. Sydney was fortunate. She was placed in a loving home with foster/adoptive parents who cared for her as if she were their own child. Sydney thrived in the care of these nurturing, attentive, and attuned caregivers. In her mind, they were her mommy and daddy, and that's what she called them. Tim and Jan thought of Sydney as their child even though they had been reminded, time and time again by her caseworker, that there was no guarantee that they would be able to adopt her. Despite torturing their older children, the parental rights of Sydney's parents had not been terminated. The Child Protective Services (CPS) caseworker was concerned about the ethnic differences between the foster parents and Sydney, although that difference was only noticeable to those who didn't know them. They were a very happy family.

Then when Sydney was 3 years old the judge made a surprising decision. Her biological parents had completed all of the requirements placed upon them by CPS, including parenting classes, anger management classes, and domestic violence and drug and alcohol counseling. It now seemed that after several years they had finally gotten their act together and were once again ready to parent their four children. Sydney did know her brothers and sister; they had monthly visits during their time in foster care, although the infrequency of the time together did little to forge a sibling bond. Her parents, on the other hand, had rarely made the parental visits. However, this made little difference as the judge handed down his decision. They were her biological parents and that's what mattered. Tim and Jan hired an attorney, and they fought Sydney's removal from their home with all they had—but biology won out. On a crisp February morning, Sydney was taken from them. Jan later described how Sydney's screams haunted her day and night.

But that was just the beginning of the trauma for Sydney. She had been taken from her mommy and daddy and given to two people whom she didn't know. They said that they were her "real" mommy and daddy, but she knew that wasn't true, so she called them by their names. That was only one of the things that infuriated them about her. Within a short period of time, the torture began: beatings, burning with cigarettes, being locked in her room, and denied food. Sydney's world had completely changed and her 3-year-old mind couldn't begin to understand why.

Thankfully, Tim and Jan never gave up. They were not able to see Sydney but, based upon the reports when her siblings initially came into care, they could only imagine what she was going through. They continued to fight. They told Sydney's story to the media and sought the help of children's rights groups. But ultimately it was a neighbor who put an end to Sydney's suffering. She had seen Sydney only on rare occasions over the year and a half that the children had been back in the home. The older children went to school and played in the neighborhood park, but not Sydney. One day she witnessed the father kicking Sydney as she tried to walk out onto the front porch. The neighbor immediately called the police. When they arrived with CPS there was little doubt of the abuse suffered by this child. She was rushed to the hospital. Both parents were arrested, and her brothers and sister were once again placed in foster care.

When Jan and Tim entered the hospital room, they barely recognized their little girl. Her once beautiful hair was now matted to her head and was completely gone in some places. He eyes, once so sparkling and full of life, stared right through them. She didn't speak. Ultimately the results of days of tests and X-rays told the horrible truth. Sydney had suffered countless beatings that ended in broken bones that were never treated. She would have to endure multiple surgeries to chip away the calcium deposits that had formed on the healed bones in her legs. She had regressed in every developmental domain, and she exhibited severe PTSD.

It wasn't until she returned home that the healing could begin. Her room was just as she left it—the consistent, nurturing, and safe home was waiting for her. She would need hours of physical and occupational therapy and the efforts of therapists experienced in working with traumatized children. Most important, she needed the love and care of her family to provide the patterned, repetitive, and reparative experiences that would help build the developmental capacities that anger and cruelty had stolen from her. Ultimately Sydney did heal from all this early trauma because of her strong spirit and the parents who never gave up on her.

CASE 3: NEGLECT IN INFANCY
AND THE DEVELOPMENTAL CONSEQUENCES

Haley was adopted from an orphanage outside of the United States when she was 9 months old. While the information her adoptive parents had about her past was minimal, they did know that she had spent the first 2 months of her life with her biological mother, who was a known alcoholic. At the time she was placed, Haley had a serious illness and several bruises on her legs, and she spent at least a month in the hospital. Haley's adoptive parents had an opportunity to tour the facility, which they described as a "typical" orphanage—a cold place with large rooms filled with rows of cribs or beds and only a few caregivers.

Upon returning home with their new baby, the parents were surprised by her behavior. She cried very little during the day; she would often just sit and stare into space. At night, however, she would wake several times screaming uncontrollably. No matter what they tried, they were rarely able to comfort or soothe her when she was upset. She didn't like to be touched or held. and her eating was always rushed, as if she hadn't eaten in days and didn't know when she would eat again. Haley would often hurt herself by banging her head or pulling her hair until it came out, and she would also try to hit or bite anyone who tried to hold her.

Haley's adoptive parents, Kristy and Sam, worked to make home a safe place. Kristy quit her job to stay home with her daughter. They hired a psychologist to come into their home and teach them appropriate attachment techniques such as cuddling, gentle holding, and rocking. They worked very hard to build routines and predictability into Haley's day. Over time, Haley's self-injurious behaviors began to diminish, although they did not completely go away. However, following an outing to visit family out of state, Haley's behaviors regressed significantly. Once again she was rageful, hitting everyone within reach, touch averse, and exhibiting severe sleep disturbances. Only through limiting her exposure to those outside of the family and not venturing outside the home did her behaviors get better.

Haley seemed to be making progress. A massage therapist had worked with the family and now both parents used massage as a way to help soothe and calm their daughter. They built rocking and music and movement into their daily routine. They followed every recommendation to the letter—they were doing everything right. But without warning, Haley's behaviors began to escalate into severe mood swings. Her parents describe her as exceptionally gentle and loving one minute and defiant, rageful, rejecting, and hurtful the next. Despite all of the empathy, patience, and nurturing, Haley did not seem to be getting better. What Sam and Kristy didn't know was that the absence of critical organizing experiences during Haley's neglectful first 8 months was a major contributing factor to the devastating developmental problems they witnessed on a daily basis.

THE POWER OF RELATIONSHIPS TO HEAL

Understanding the power of traumatic events to shape the brain helps us to better determine what a child needs to heal. Although negative early life relational experiences have the ability to shape the child's developing brain, relationships can also be protective and reparative (see Figure 3.1). The cases of Mark and Syndey are examples of the power of relationships both to injure and to heal. There exists a wide body of research suggesting that social connectedness is a protective factor against many forms of child maltreatment— including physical abuse, neglect, nonorganic failure to thrive—as well as a means of promoting prosocial behavior (Belsky, Jaffee, Sligo, Woodward, & Silva, 2005; Caliso & Milner, 1992; Egeland, Jacobvitz, & Sroufe, 1988; Rak & Patterson, 1996; Travis & Combs-Orme, 2007; Chan, 1994; Coohey, 1996; Guadin, Polansky, Kilpatrick, & Shilton, 1993; Hashima & Amato, 1994; Pascoe & Earp, 1984; Altemeier, O'Connor, Sherrod, & Vietze, 1985; Benoit, Zeanah, & Barton, 1989; Crnic, Greenberg, Robinson, & Ragozin, 1984; Gorman, Leifer, & Grossman, 1993). Sydney's early experiences had taught her that home was a place where she was safe and loved. Her foster/adoptive parents and their extended family supplied her with the emotional connections, healthy interactions, and nurturing that provided a strong basis for surviving the horrors of life with her biological parents. We can only infer that Mark had something similar built in by his first caregivers in the orphanage that helped buffer the experiences with his first adoptive mother.

Haley, unfortunately, missed out on the nurturing, touch, and love that she needed in order to grow into a healthy, secure little girl. Her brain, literally, was a reflection of the severity of her neglect, likely combined with some type of physical maltreatment. Her stress response system overly active, Haley spent most of her time either hyperaroused or dissociating when her little system could take no more. Also, not surpris-

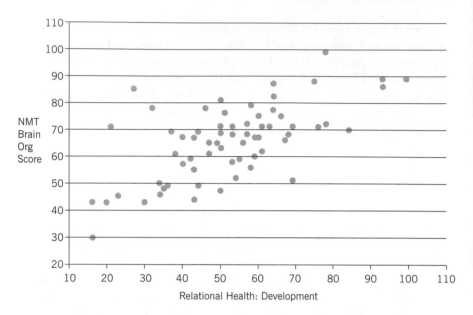

FIGURE 3.1. Relational health during development is protective. This graph is from research with a group of maltreated children. A retrospective measure of the presence, quality, and number of relational supports during each child's development was obtained as part of a clinical assessment (Relational Health: Development) using an approach called the Neurosequential Model of Thera-peutics (NMT; Perry, 2009). This is plotted against a measure of the develop-ment and functional capabilities of 28 brain-mediated functions (NMT Brain Organization [org] Score). A clear relationship between the relational health scores and overall quality of brain organization and functioning is seen.

ingly, the strategies that helped her survive in the environment of the orphanage made it more difficult for her to "take advantage of good-quality, loving and responsive" caregiving in her new home (Howe & Fearnley, 2003, p. 372). Experience in her earliest caregiving relation-ships had taught her that adults were frightening, hurtful, unpredict-able, and confusing. Children with early neglect histories and subse-quent attachment-related problems rarely feel safe when placed in new, healthy caregiving situations. Instead, they work to avoid close relation-ships, often becoming aggressive and controlling as a way to protect themselves from further hurt. Howe and Fearnley (2003) aptly describe the situation this way.

Close relationships are the one thing these children avoid. Their developmental agenda is to control and not to engage people. This denies them exposure to the very experiences they need. So long as they remain unable to relinquish control and relate fully and accurately with their carers and therapists, the children make little emotional or developmental progress (p. 380).

Sydney's case, in particular, provides an example of how healthy caregiving and strong attachments can help protect children from the lasting impact of traumatic events. That is not to say that all of the scars disappear or that the memories of trauma no longer exist, only that the reestablishment of predictable routines, reconnections with attentive, attuned, committed caregivers, and solid therapeutic treatment provide the opportunity for children to heal.

PRACTICE AND POLICY IMPLICATIONS

Our current mental health, child welfare, and judicial systems, as well as child-placing agencies deal with traumatized and maltreated children as if they were completely unaware of these essential findings in development, attachment, and trauma. We have few metrics to measure the number, quality, and patterns of healthy (or unhealthy) relational interactions; we move traumatized children from therapist to therapist, school to school, foster home to foster home, community to community. Indeed our systems often exacerbate or even replicate the relational impermanence and trauma of the child's life (see Figure 3.2). We expect "therapy"—healing—to take place in the child via episodic, shallow relational interactions with highly educated but poorly nurturing strangers. We undervalue the powerful therapeutic impact of caring teacher, coach, neighbor, grandparent, and a host of other potential "cotherapists."

Future effective therapeutic interventions—both preventive and healing—must be developmentally informed and trauma sensitive. There is much to learn, yet we know enough now to begin to evaluate and modify our current therapeutic practices, programs, and policies to take full advantage of the biological gift of the healing power of relationships.

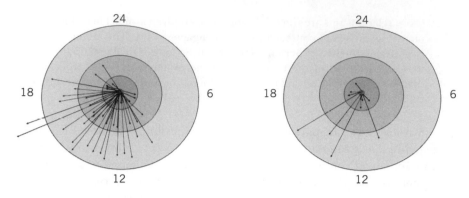

FIGURE 3.2. Positive relational interactions: Typical and foster child. These two figures are representative 24-hour relational contact maps examining the number of positive relational interactions in two children. Arrows represent positive interactions (as rated by observer and child); arrows ending in the inner circle represent interactions with family; additional circles represent friends, then classmates/acquaintances. Arrows outside the circle represent interactions with strangers. The figure on the right is based on a 10-year-old boy in foster care who was moved in the middle of the school year to a new foster home away from extended family and community. This figure is the best 24-hour map for a 2-week period for this child. Several days were completely devoid of any positive relational interaction. The relational poverty played a major role in this child's inability to progress; symptoms related to trauma and neglect persisted and increased while he was in relationally impoverished settings. Once in a stable placement with positive relationships created in school and the community, he stabilized and improved.

REFERENCES

Ainsworth, M., Blehar, M., Waters, E., & Wall, S. (1978). *Patterns of attachment: A psychological study of the Strange Situation.* Hillsdale, NJ: Erlbaum.

Altemeier, W., O'Connor, S. M., Sherrod, K. B., & Vietze, P. M. (1985). Prospective study of antecedents for nonorganic failure to thrive. *Journal of Pediatrics, 106,* 360–365.

Anda, R. F., Felitti, R. F., Walker, J., Whitfield, C., Bremner, D. J., Perry, B. D., et al. (2006). The enduring effects of childhood abuse and related experiences: A convergence of evidence from neurobiology and epidemiology. *European Archives of Psychiatric and Clinical Neuroscience, 256*(3), 174–186.

Belsky, J., Jaffee, S. R., Sligo, J., Woodward, L., & Silva, P. A. (2005). Intergenerational transmission of warm-sensitive-stimulating parenting: A prospective study of mothers and fathers of 3 year olds. *Child Development, 76,* 384–396.

Benoit, D., Zeanah, C. H., & Barton, M. (1989). Maternal attachment disturbances and failure to thrive. *Infant Mental Health Journal, 10,* 185–202.

Berenson, A., Weiman, C., & McCombs, S. (2001). Exposure to violence and
associated health-risk behaviors among adolescent girls. *Archives of Pediatric Adolescent Medicine, 155,* 1238–1242.

Bowlby, J. (1969). *Attachment and loss: Vol. 1. Attachment.* New York: Basic Books.

Bremner, J. D., & Vermetten, E. (2001). Stress and development: Behavioral and
biological consequences. *Development and Psychopathology, 13,* 473–489.

Caliso, J. A., & Milner, J. S. (1992). Childhood history of abuse and child abuse
screening. *Child Abuse and Neglect, 16,* 647–659.

Carlson, V., Cichetti, D., Barnett, D., & Braunwald, K. (1989). Disorganized/
disoriented attachment relationships in maltreated infants. *Developmental
Psychology, 25,* 525–531.

Chan, Y. (1994). Parenting stress and social support of mothers who physically
abuse their children in Hong Kong. *Child Abuse and Neglect, 18,* 261–269.

Chiao, J. Y., Iidaka, T., Gordon, H. L., Nogawa, J., Bar, M., Aminoff, E., et al.
(2008). Cultural specificity in amygdala response to fear faces. *Journal of
Cognitive Neuroscience, 20*(12), 2167–2174.

Coohey, C. (1996). Child maltreatment: Testing the social isolation hypothesis.
Child Abuse and Neglect, 20, 241–251.

Crittenden, P. M. (1985). Maltreated infants: Vulnerability and resilience. *Journal of Child Psychology and Psychiatry, 26,* 85–96.

Crnic, K., Greenberg, N., Robinson, N., & Ragozin, A. (1984). Maternal stress
and social supports: Effects on the mother–infant relationship from birth
to eighteen months. *American Journal of Orhospychiatry, 52,* 550–557.

Egeland, B., Jacobvitz, D., & Sroufe, L. A. (1988). Breaking the cycle of abuse.
Child Development, 59, 1080–1088.

Emde, R. N. (1998). Early emotional development: New modes of thinking for
research and intervention. *Pediatrics, 102*(5) Supplement, 1236–1243.

Fitzpatrick, K. M., & Boldizar, J. P. (1993). The prevalence and consequences of
exposure to violence among African American youth. *Journal of the American Academy of Child and Adolescent Psychiatry, 32*(2), 424–430.

Gaudin, J., Polansky, N., Kilpatrick, N., & Shilton, P. (1993). Loneliness, depression, stress, and social support in neglectful homes. *American Journal of
Orthopsychiatry, 63,* 597–605.

Gorman, J., Leifer, M., & Grossman, G. (1993). Nonorganic failure to thrive:
Maternal history and current maternal functioning. *Journal of Clinical
Child Psychology, 22*(3), 327–337.

Graham-Berman, S. A., & Levendosky, A. A. (1998). Traumatic stress symptoms in children of battered women. *Journal of Interpersonal Violence, 13*(1),
111–128.

Greenspan, S. I., & Wieder, S. (2006). *Infant and early childhood mental health: A
comprehensive developmental approach to assessment and intervention.* Washington, DC: American Psychiatric Association.

Hashima, P., & Amato, P. (1994). Poverty, social support, and parental behavior. *Child Development, 65,* 394–403.

Howe, D., & Fearnley, S. (2003). Disorders of attachment in adopted and fostered children: Recognition and treatment. *Clinical Child Psychology and Psychiatry, 8*(3), 369–387.

Lamb, M.E., Gaensbauer, T. J., Malkin, C. M., & Schultz, L. A. (1985) The effects of child maltreatment on security of infant–adult attachment. *Infant Behavior and Development, 8,* 35–45.

Lyon-Ruth, K., & Spielman, E. (2004). Disorganized infant attachment strategies and helpless-fearful profiles of parenting: Integrating attachment research with clinical intervention. *Infant Mental Health Journal, 25*(4), 318–335.

Main, M., & Hesse, E. (1990). Parents' unresolved traumatic experiences are related to infant disorganized attachment status: Is frightened and/or frightening parental behavior the linking mechanism? In M. Greenberg, D. Cicchetti, & E. Cummings (Eds.), *Attachment in the preschool years: Theory, research, and intervention* (pp. 161–182). Chicago: University of Chicago Press.

Malinosky-Rummell, R., & Hansen, D. J. (1993). Long-term consequences of childhood physical abuse. *Psychological Bulletin, 114*(1), 68–79.

Margolin, G., & Gordis, E. B. (2000). The effect of family and community violence on children. *Annual Review of Psychology, 51,* 445–479.

Pascoe, J., & Earp, J. (1984). The effect of mothers' social support and life changes on the stimulation of their children in their home. *American Journal of Public Health, 74,* 358–360.

Perry, B. D. (2001). The neuroarcheology of childhood maltreatment: The neurodevelopmental costs of adverse childhood events. In K. Franey, R. Geffner, & R. Falconer (Eds.), *The cost of maltreatment: Who pays? We all do* (pp. 15–37). Binghamton, NY: Haworth Press.

Perry, B. D. (2002). Childhood experience and the expression of genetic potential: What childhood neglect tells us about nature and nurture. *Brain and Mind, 3,* 79–100.

Perry, B. D. (2008). Child maltreatment: The role of abuse and neglect in developmental psychopathology. In T. P. Beauchaine & S. P. Hinshaw (Eds.), *Textbook of child and adolescent psychopathology* (pp. 93–128. New York: Wiley.

Perry, B. D. (2009) Examining child maltreatment through a neurodevelopmental lens: Clinical application of the neurosequential model of therapeutics. *Journal of Loss and Trauma, 14,* 240–255.

Perry, B. D., & Hambrick, E. P. (2008). The neurosequential model of therapeutics. *Reclaiming Children and Youth, 17,* 38–43.

Perry, B. D., & Pollard, R. (1998). Homeostasis, stress, trauma, and adaptation: A neurodevelopmental view of childhood trauma. *Child and Adolescent Psychiatric Clinics of North America, 7,* 33–51.

Perry, B. D., & Szalavitz, M. (2007). *The boy who was raised as a dog; and other stories from a child psychiatrist's notebook: What traumatized children can teach us about life, loss and healing.* New York: Basic Books.

Rak, C. F., & Patterson, L. E. (1996). Promoting resilience in at-risk children. *Journal of Counseling and Development, 74,* 368–373.

Read, J., Perry, B. D., Moskowith, A., & Connolloy, J. (2001). The contribution of early traumatic events to schizophrenia in some patients: A trauamagenic neurodevelopmental model. *Psychiatry, 64,* 319–345.

Sanders-Phillips, K. (1997). Assaultive violence in the community: Psycholgical responses of adolescent victims and their parents. *Journal of Adolescent Health, 21*(6), 356–365.

Schneider-Rosen, K., Braunwald, K. G., Carlson, V., & Cicchetti, D. (1985). Current perspectives in attachment theory: Illustration from the study of maltreated infants. *Monographs of the Society for Research in Child Development, 50*(1–2, Serial No. 209), pp. 194–210.

Thompson, R. A. (2002). The roots of school readiness in social and emotional development. In Kaufman Early Education Exchange, *Set for success: Building a strong foundation for school readiness based on the social–emotional development of young children.* (pp. 8–29). Kansas City: Ewing Marion Kaufman Foundation.

Travis, W. J., & Combs-Orme, T. (2007). Resilient parenting: Overcoming poor parental bonding *Social Work Research, 31*(3), 135–149.

CHAPTER 4

Children's Self-Initiated Gradual Exposure

The Wonders of Posttraumatic Play and Behavioral Reenactments

ELIANA GIL

Lenore Terr chronicled and studied the dramatic events in Chowchilla, California, in 1979. Three would-be abductors seeking a large ransom created an elaborate plan in which they successfully kidnapped a school bus with 26 elementary school children on board. The children were moved to a van, which was then buried in a hole. This was a remarkable feat both for its boldness and for its unusual plan. The kidnappers dug a hole large enough to drive in a white van, filled with children on their way home after a regular school day. What followed was the amazing escape and rescue of the children, all physically unharmed. This story was masterfully narrated in the book *Too Scared to Cry* (Terr, 1990) and included the recounting of Terr's interviews with the child victims 4 and 8 years after the events occurred.

I lived in California when this kidnapping occurred, and the news reports were, frankly, unbelievable. I remember being riveted to Terr's book, and as I read, wanting to know exactly what these children experienced and what accounted for their bravery and ability to rally personal resources during this event. I also wanted to know what happened to these children after this event: How much fear and anxiety did they carry with them? Were some scared enough to want to stay home? How did their parents react to these events? And were there some identifiable factors that made this intensely stressful incident more difficult for some than for others? What became clear as I read this book with fascination was that the children had idiosyncratic ways of facing this traumatic event: Some had the audacity to imagine an escape and then were able to mobilize resources on their own behalf to make concerted efforts to gain freedom. Others were able to mobilize helping resources and assisted others who began to make efforts to escape. Still others most closely fit the definition of traumatized children: Their capacity to cope was overwhelmed by strong affect that debilitated them and created great obstacles in their ability to help themselves.[1] These children exhibited variations of the fight–flight–freeze responses and an assortment of interesting behaviors—symptoms, in some instances, of underlying, unspoken worries.

Terr has a longstanding interest in childhood traumas and how they develop a life in the mind of the child victim throughout his or her development (Terr, 1991). She knew intuitively that a substantive study of childhood trauma would be necessary to amass the necessary data to attract or renew attention to the plight of the traumatized child (especially in her field of psychiatry). Due to geographic location, Terr was able to conduct a longitudinal study of the horrifying event when these young children were kidnapped and to collect important data about the short- and long-term impact of childhood abuse, mediating factors, and what could be described as children's individualized resiliency in the face of an overwhelming stressor. In addition, her study took a deeper look into posttrauma play. She documented how many of these children took small cars and buried them in the dirt over and over—they felt compelled to reenact the events literally, and their play at these times appeared stilted and joyless.

Another tragedy well documented in the media was the crash of the Uruguayan rugby players in the Andes mountains in October, 1972. Both in the book and in the film *Alive*, there was a clear distinction in survivors' responses to overwhelming stress. For some, the fight response

---

[1]Perry was recently asked, "Where does one draw the line between psychological stress and psychological trauma?" He responded: "Two people can have the same experience, but for one person the level of stress is so high that it is traumatic and for the other person it is not. From a neurobiological perspective, events become traumatic when stress response systems are activated in such an extreme way that they go from being adaptive to being maladaptive" (Perry, 2008, p. 2).

crystallized immediately, allowing some of the survivors to plan and implement actions designed to stay alive. For others, the challenges posed by the crash—the freezing cold, the environmental starkness, and the apparent likelihood of survival—overwhelmed their perception of coping options, and some became ill, gave up, or struggled greatly. Here again, the fight–flight–freeze responses were in full display. Of course these victims were adults, young men who likely had more coping strategies and prior life experience than young children.

There is no real accounting for the continuum of responses in individuals who face the overwhelming terrors that are inherent in traumatic events, whether they are human-made assaults, natural catastrophes, or interpersonal traumas. What is clear is that both the objective and subjective experience of the victim must be explored and understood (Pynoos, Steinberg, & Goenjian, 1996). Many reasons have been cited for why some people do better than others in overcoming tragedies and hardships. Some have written about the resilient nature of children (Rubin, 1996; Katz, 1997) and families (Walsh, 2006) in the face of harsh realities. But the reality is that we can never assume or predict with certainty how any individual will respond to trauma, and we can never underestimate the range and persistence of the survival instinct as well as the innate drive to make meaning and to self-repair.

NATURAL HEALING MECHANISMS

One needs only be observant in life to discover the myriad ways that people choose to address and resolve their personal injuries. Following disasters of any type—those occurring naturally as well as those human-made—people suffer differently and recover in different ways. After the tragedy of 9/11 in New York, Philadelphia, and Washington, DC, many children created art that painfully chronicled what they had witnessed. These art renditions are moving and compelling and seem to capture single moments, feelings, and thoughts that many people experienced. Theater groups coalesced and street plays were performed throughout the city, inviting people to participate in both the acknowledgment of the pain and the beginning of healing.

I firmly believe that children can often find natural ways to address their wounds if given the proper environment (*container*) and the presence of a calm, patient, and hopeful other, sometimes a therapist. Many of the children whom I saw after the tragedy of 9/11 (family victims

of the Pentagon deaths) constructed villages that were attacked by air-
planes and houses that were consumed by fire. Eventually these scenes
incorporated the presence of ambulances, police cars, and especially
firemen who began to rescue people, take them to the hospital, and
return buried toy people to their families. Jackson, Susser, and Hoven
(2001), teachers involved in the evacuation of some of the schools in
New York City, talked about their students' building blocks and tearing
them down, building and tearing them down, as if they were reconstructing the World Trade Center. Another child, after living through
Hurricane Hugo in 1989, sat at her dining room table eating dinner and
pretended that her broccoli stalks were big trees and the gravy was rush-
ing water toppling them over (Sleek, 1998). Goodman (1999) states:

> Children leave their mark on the world in any number of ways. They
> come to know they exist by seeing the results of their actions. They make
> a mud pie after a rain storm, scribble a free-form circle with a chunk of
> crayon, and build a sand castle at the water's edge. The evidence is clear,
> something that originated from within becomes public. There is curios-
> ity, learning, exploration, skill, and delight. They realize that feelings and
> thoughts can be communicated to the outside world. Art made by children
> provides a window into their world: It offers a view of who they are, regard-
> less of the suffering or pain they may endure. Because children struggle
> in their quest to cope with a challenge, or strive to compete with forces
> that mitigate the natural order of things, children in turmoil create with a
> discernible purpose and need. (p. 12)

In my work over the last three decades, I respect more and more
that this *purpose and need* is a mastery drive that children seem to possess after exposure to harsh and senseless acts of cruelty at the hands of
those who claim to love them. At the same time, I recognize that there
are other variables that can play a part in children's positive recovery.

Terr (1992) talked about the importance of the family's responses
to children—responses that could increase or decrease children's anxiety and/or adaptation. Parental reactions to trauma are also embedded
in their cultural beliefs about how to negotiate personal or external
crises, how to grieve, and what resources are most viable during a crisis. In fact, as Lewis and Ippen (2004) point out, culture can be both
a source of protection and a risk factor, and it *always* seems to provide
meaning to the lived experience of trauma. Engaging parents in open
discussions about how their traumas are experienced in the context of
their culture is always an important dialogue. Not only does it inform us

about individual attitudes and approaches to coping with trauma but it also provides us with useful information about what social and religious rituals might be considered valuable reparative resources for the family and traumatized child.

And there are other things people do when injured emotionally. Sometimes in times of great distress, people lift their voices in song or move their bodies in dance or use simple or sophisticated instruments to make music. Meditation, mindfulness, massage, yoga, and relaxation exercises seem to be very useful as well. Writing is valued by many. Engel (1995) states that "we use stories to guide and shape the way we experience our daily lives, to communicate with other people, and to develop relationships with them" (p. 25). Many a heart-wrenching poem has been composed when people are suffering as well as when they are in the heights of glowing emotions. Still other people find it helpful to engage in physical activities such as walking or running, climbing, working out, gardening, or swimming. It is not accidental that animal-assisted therapy (van Fleet, 2008; Chandler, 2005) has become a much more recognized therapeutic strategy with traumatized children. Finally, and by no means suggesting a limited list, reaching out to a higher power; praying; going to churches, temples, or mosques; or consulting spiritual leaders is also quite common when people are suffering.

What is the motivation behind these activities and why do some people find them easily, whereas others have to be encouraged toward them? The motivation seems to stem from an acute drive toward health and growth, articulated most often and loudly (in the field of psychology) by Piaget, Maslow, Carl Rogers, Mr. Rogers, Carl Jung, and Milton Erickson. These individuals all emphasized the human motivation toward growth and health, and they also asserted that human beings possess within them the healing properties that they require.

What appears certain is that many people are interested, indeed compelled, to express themselves; to understand, discharge, and release negative emotions; and to reach toward the light. One of my child clients, severely abused and frightened, made a depiction that clearly illustrated her desire to rise above her pain (Figure 4.1).

Just as plants reorient toward light, children seem to seek out and respond to kindness, to positive regard, to being treated with dignity and respect. As we know, they are biologically hardwired to attach to others. And their ability to keep trusting, to keep reaching out, to keep striving to feel better and more connected is, in and of itself, a tribute to the inherent drive toward health and to the presence of resiliency.

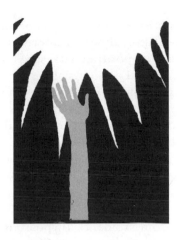

FIGURE 4.1. Reaching for the light.

CHILDREN, PLAY, AND POSTTRAUMATIC PLAY

When children play, their most natural of all activities, they discover its many curative benefits, including play as a way to communicate, a way to solve problems, a way to test out roles, a way to compensate for real-life difficulties, and a way to advance their developmental tasks (Schaefer, 1995). Partly this is true because play affords them an opportunity to externalize the thoughts, picture images, feeling states, and accompanying sensations that are often impossible to put into words for adults, let alone children, whose relationship to language takes developmental leaps as they grow and/or later choose verbal communication, to one degree or another, as their primary form of communication. Children's exposure to their challenging experiences and their consequent understanding or adaptation to events can feel overwhelming, far-reaching, complex, fragmented, or difficult to either perceive accurately or describe successfully. When children don't play, it usually signals that something is wrong. I have worked with children who show tremendously constricted play, don't interact with objects in a playful way, and don't appear to have creative instincts toward play. In all these instances, the children had been severely neglected, and the absence of positive attachment to another human being was clearly detrimental to their physical and emotional growth.

The DSM-IV (American Psychiatric Association, 2000) provides the most relevant information about the aftereffects of trauma in both children and adults with its posttraumatic stress disorder (PTSD) category, which cites the mental and physiological reexperiencing of the trauma, with signs of arousal and avoidance. Although PTSD was *not* a diagnostic category intended primarily for children, and few children meet the full criteria for PTSD, it is a common diagnosis when working with abused children, and several symptoms of PTSD are usually present in young traumatized children. In an effort to address that gap in relevance for young children, an inclusion was made about the fact that young traumatized children may exhibit repetitive reenactments of their trauma through play and that children can move back and forth along the continuum from avoidance (hypoarousal) to hyperarousal. In addition, Scheeringa, Zeanah, Drell, and Larrieu (1995) suggest that when assessing very young children, an altered criteria of PTSD should be applied that does not require self-reports of fear or helplessness and that includes posttraumatic play, play reenactments, and constriction of play.

INVITING POSTTRAUMATIC PLAY

Because it is certain that children can and do spontaneously utilize posttraumatic play and because they have other natural reparative potential, my initial work with them is always nondirective, inviting, and implicitly encouraging them to look around the room, at their own pace, and make use of whatever reparative approaches that they have at their disposal, including posttraumatic play. Osofsky (2004) agrees that nondirective play therapy "is an effective tool in enlisting the avoidant child to participate in therapy" (p. 149). She goes on to say that "following the child's lead ensures that therapy will not push the child into painful or retraumatizing material too quickly" (p. 149). In fact, Herman's (1997) words have always served as a guiding principle for me. She noted that there are two substantive errors when working with adult survivors: "Though the single most common therapeutic error is avoidance of the traumatic material, probably the second most common error is premature or precipitate engagement in exploratory work, without sufficient attention to the tasks of establishing safety and securing a therapeutic alliance" (p. 173). This principle applies to children as well: Direct inquiry too quickly may elicit children's resistance, whereas allowing them the time to develop comfort and trust is a necessary foundation for moving toward discussion or work regarding more personal material and its accompanying emotions.

I have always highlighted the possibility and the potential of post-traumatic play in my work (Gil, 1991, 2006). It's easy to miss it, and it's easy to get in its way, but once awareness of posttraumatic play exists, and you develop a trust that it can both occur and be useful, you will find yourself expecting it, delighting in its presence, trusting its twists and turns, and eventually feel increasingly competent in knowing how to discover it, work with it, and marvel at its self healing properties. This confidence in children's ability to draw on posttraumatic play by no means suggests that all children are capable of, or interested in, jumping into this type of play. Some children don't take to it, resist it, or plain delay it until much later in therapy when they feel more comfortable with the setting and the clinician or after they have processed the material in other ways. Many children with whom I have worked have never employed posttraumatic play, so while this book is replete with examples of children who can take advantage of this natural reparative strategy, some children will require a multitude of starts and stops with a variety of different therapeutic approaches before they can make full use of its therapeutic benefits. Indeed, some children remain distant and uninvolved throughout the entire therapy process and may need to be referred for additional, collateral services, such as occupational therapy, focused attachment work, psychopharmacology, trauma-focused cognitive-behavioral therapy, family therapy, etc.

THE MULTIMODAL APPROACH TO PLAY THERAPY

When I first thought about creating this volume, my goal was to provide a range of examples of children in treatment who were able to lead the way to their own recovery process—children who had a keen sense of what they needed to do to address their interpersonal injuries. Children who have such a predisposition to avail themselves of posttraumatic play may appear in clinical situations more often than we know, but they can be missed or redirected through immediate application of set agendas, procedures, protocols, and specific requests to do predetermined activities or engage in scripted interview schedules or therapy dialogues. Thus a common clinical response to children beginning therapy is to invite them, encourage them, cojole them, require them, or direct them to engage in therapist-led activities, rather than allow them a period of time to be completely free of expectations, a time to allow their bodies and minds to orient to the environment, to the clinical relationship, and to the task of self-repair. Child-centered play therapists have long recognized the value of the nondirective approach, and they are quite sensitive to following the child's lead at every step. However, because of a strong compulsion to avoid painful thoughts and feelings, children with trauma histories may find it facile to find shelter in a play therapy office and avoid thorny emotional work. Thus a purely nondirective approach may be limiting when attempting to help children process trauma. In addition, several experienced practitioners have suggested that an open discussion is essential to mastering the anxiety that often accompanies traumatic memories (Pynoos & Eth, 1986). Benedek (1985), in fact, states that "retelling is equivalent to reworking [and is] one attempt at mastery of an experience" (p. 11). From my point of view, and the general view of play therapists is that when the child plays, his or her language and communication are on display. When I observe, document, or help the child process posttraumatictic play, I am witnessing the creation of a narrative, sometimes out of full conscious awareness, sometimes without verbal expression, but a narrative nevertheless. So while I agree that children's verbal communication is essential and desirable, as a play and art therapist I regard the child's play or art as a form of communication, equal in value to words. Nader (2004) also states that the child can process traumatic memories by using drawings or paintings in play therapy, and the use of art with trauma survivors is well documented (see, e.g., Malchiodi, 2003).

In addition, I believe that processing traumatic material (with positive outcomes) can also be accomplished by employing diverse tactics. Rather than thinking of nondirective play therapy as an exclusionary form of treatment with traumatized children, many therapists suggest an integrated, prescriptive, or *multimodal* approach that inevitably presents our clients with the best possible therapeutic assistance. The overall goal, of course, is to help the child retell or rework or process traumatic experiences so that the child regains a sense of control (Shelby & Tredinnick, 1995; Herman,1992). While mental health practitioners and researchers seem to have reached consensus about the treatment goals when working with complex trauma cases (Cook et al., 2005), and there are definitive, specific, evidence-based treatment approaches for working with abused children (Cohen, Mannarino, & Deblinger, 2006), craft knowledge continues to be documented (Osofky, 2004; Gil, 2006; Goodyear-Brown, 2010) and more clinicians are conducting research on specific treatment models (e.g., Ford & Russo, Target, 2006; Kagan, real life heroes, 2008).

HOW WE RECOGNIZE THE ELEMENTS
OF POSTTRAUMATIC PLAY

Terr (1991) cited features of posttraumatictic play that distinguished them from children's generic play. One of the most salient of these features is the literal nature of the play. Children who have been in a car crash, for example, might require miniatures of cars, street lights, stop signs, passengers, and drivers. If children have been through an earthquake, they might require toy structures that can be taken down and rebuilt. Children seem to have the urge to recreate what has traumatized them by using literal rather than symbolic representations. This point seems important because clinicians must remain attuned to providing children with objects that might suit *their* specific needs.

Terr also talked about the robotic, repetitious nature of children's posttraumatic play, a type of play that is devoid of affect, spontaneity, and the usual evolving quality of children's play. Posttraumatic play is repetitive and sequential and, to the observer, can look uncanny in its attention to detail and precise duplication. Yet there is something very impressive about children's sullen control of this play, something that seems useful, although not immediately evident to the observer. Children seem very intent in exercising fastidious movements and reiterating precise sequences over and over. They appear completely self-absorbed in the play—the typical interactive style of children's play is markedly absent. Sometimes children appear to be in trance, and clinicians must intervene to elicit their cooperation in ending the session. Some children even show clear periods of "spacing out" as if they enter dissociative states—a very exceptional type of play indeed.

Most children don't appear to consciously choose to play out their traumas; rather, it is as if the trauma material finds its way out of their unconscious into concrete form. Some children may have other possible outlets, such as verbal discussion with family or friends. Others "act out" their traumatic experiences by engaging others in repetitive, reenactive behaviors, some of which possess literal elements of their traumas, particularly interpersonal ones. Terr (1990) describes case after case study demonstrating trauma through behavior or play. The behavioral or literal play reenactments can signal that something about their traumatic experiences remains conflictual, worrisome, or unresolved.

In essence, this behavior or play exists because it is necessary for the child. Through this repetitive play, children often appear to inoculate themselves against the stress of remembering what occurred, allowing themselves instead to face what may have felt unbearable and to create pathways to healing. What I find most remarkable is that this ability to use posttraumatic play is *initiated by* the traumatized child; it is the *child's* creation, and the child can reap the benefits.

GRADUAL EXPOSURE

I have stated elsewhere (Gil, 2006) that posttraumatic play can be understood as children's natural means of achieving gradual exposure to their traumatic experiences. Clinicians don't often need to introduce this cognitive-behavioral technique because the child can initiate this work on his or her own. Gradual exposure is a very well-recognized therapeutic strategy in the cognitive-behavioral approach to treatment. Indeed, desensitization strategies and gradual exposure are the treatments of choice when addressing a variety of behaviors, including phobia. This technique is proposed and implemented by trained clinicians, who lead the client through structured activities designed to produce incremental exposure to feared stimuli. The basic concept is that the introduction of that which is feared (in gradually increasing dosages) allows the individual to tolerate and/or manage his or her affect over time; clients who succeed on one level are introduced to increasingly higher levels of anxiety-producing material. Eventually, clients feel better able to overcome adverse responses to a feared object.

I once worked with a mother who was debilitated by her fear of elevators, especially because her employment was on the 12th floor of a highrise. Although she was adept at walking up and down the stairs, she often had to run errands for her employer and sometimes became irritable when asked to leave the building. This woman and I spent time watching people go up and down on elevators. We then moved to going into the elevator and opening and shutting the door. Eventually, she went up one floor and got out, later two. Finally, she was able to decide when she felt confident enough to take the elevator and when she wanted to walk. This gradual exposure to elevator riding was very beneficial to her and, as simple as it sounds, it was meticulous work that spanned a 6-month time frame of weekly sessions. In addition, her anxiety at the beginning was so intense as to provoke sweats, dizziness, and headaches, so the work was approached very carefully and in coordination with her physician.

HOW WE ADVANCE POSTTRAUMATIC PLAY
AND OVERSEE ITS BENEFITS

With traumatized children, it is important to prepare the room for them based on a thorough understanding of their traumatic experience. For example, I was once referred a case in which a 3-year-old boy had been sitting at a breakfast diner when a waiter dropped boiling water in his lap. He endured second-degree burns and was unable to sit in a bathtub, drink hot drinks, or play comfortably with other children in any water-related sports, such as swimming on hot summer days. For 6 months after the accident, he seemed unusually afraid of getting hurt, and he had regressed developmentally. In order to encourage his posttraumat-ictic play, I bought a little round table with chairs around it, a café store-front sign, a small set of cups and saucers, and most importantly, a toy waiter carrying a tray. I then found a small steel water container, similar to the one that had carried hot water to his table on the day of his burn. These objects were placed in the play therapy office, in a small dollhouse (now with a café sign) that sat on a table. I took him around the office to show him all the toys in the room, and one of the things I showed him (in a matter-of-fact way) was the café with the family having breakfast and the waiter bringing them food. This child immediately sat in front of the little café and began playing with the people figures, moving them around so that the child was sitting on the mother's lap. Slowly but surely, over a 3-month period, he was able to show me repeatedly what had happened to him both at the café and later at the hospital. Eventually, this child engaged in water play and carefully maneuvered small amounts of cold, warm, and slightly hot water in a medicine dropper until he could mix waters to the temperature of his liking. His ability to engage with the literal symbols of his trauma facilitated a process of mastery. In fact, mastery is the overriding goal of posttraumatic play, and it is a feeling of mastery and control that is likely the most central benefit of this play.

However, sometimes the goal of mastery cannot be easily achieved and when that occurs, children may need more clinical intervention. Marvasti (1994) wrote about positive and negative types of posttraumatic play, conceptualizing that when positive play occurred, the child was able to modify negative components of the play (often with clinical help). Conversely, when negative play occurred, the child's attempts to relieve anxiety were unsuccessful and, in fact, the symptoms worsened—the play brought little resolution or closure to the child. In previous work (Gil, 1999) I have referred to these differences in posttraumatic play as *dynamic* and *toxic*: dynamic posttraumatic play meets its basic intent of achieving a sense of mastery for the client; toxic posttraumatic play is play that becomes stuck, without movement, without relief, devoid of new options, explorations, or release.

Over the years I've focused substantial efforts on understanding this phenomenon better. I have carefully documented children's posttraumatic play and looked for slight variations that suggest movement. I've learned that it is not possible to predict how long it will take for children to experience benefits in the play, and clinical interventions to move the play along are usually met with irritability and signs of resistance. In fact, some children with whom I've worked have literally reversed their play to its very beginning in direct response to something I've said. Children have literally trained me to stay quiet during the serious play, as they incubate for as long as they need to do so. As a much younger clinician I would grow weary of waiting. As a much more seasoned clinician, I've learned to trust that good things come to all who wait.

My current understanding of toxic posttraumatic play is that the play becomes "stuck" because it does not have the proper distance from the child. In posttraumatic play, the externalization and miniaturization of the process makes it a feasible undertaking to a child who may be unable to fully tolerate his or her feelings, thoughts, or physical responses when traumatic memories began to emerge intrusively. The process of play allows children to identify with small objects of their choosing and then project specific emotions, infusing the play with their own issues in a cushioned and protected way. Vulnerable children can show that vulnerability by using objects that they then enliven with special traits or characteristics. A very frightened child, for example, might choose a turtle who can retract its head or a very small deer that runs away from most everything. The child can then create scenarios and stories in which these frightened creatures experience dangers and eventually retrieve some sense of bravery. In doing so, the child begins to learn coping strategies and finds alternatives to feeling so scared that he or she can only hide, and the stories grow with possibility. The beauty of the play is that the child is able to introduce and initiate work that is relevant to him or her in a way that protects, buffers, and emboldens. One very important benefit of the play is that it is once-removed from the traumatic experience so that the frightened child can remain safe and comfortable as he or she begins to expose him- or herself to those deepest worries and concerns—so deep, he or she cannot yet show them to anyone except in disguised fashion. It is wonderful to see how well children can remain distant from the stories they create in their play even when those stories closely resemble real-life experiences and situations.

When posttraumatictic play becomes toxic, something in this safety cushion is insufficient and flawed. Instead of the child feeling sheltered by the play, the usual invisible barrier that creates a sense of distance does not take hold.

I was working with a little girl who was clearly experiencing toxic posttraumatic play. She was compelled to make the precise scene over and over again, and yet there was no resolution whatsoever—her symptoms were increasing at home and at school, and during the play she became dissociative for brief, intermittent periods, particularly occurring at specific intervals. Her foster parents reported that the child was sinking into behaviors present when she was first placed. I grew concerned and began to understand that the play was actually retraumatizing for this child and that she was reliving, rather than remembering, the abuse. I felt it was important to try different interventions, but most of them had very little impact. It was as if she was intensely connected to the play, and it showed in her physical posture, in her fixed stare, and in her stilted breathing. I decided that I needed to interpose some separation from the play, so I videotaped the next session of her static play and then asked her to review the tape with me the following week. She was initially miffed that I was asking her to do something other than simply allow her to play as she wanted. But when she saw herself setting up the play on the television screen, she was immediately fascinated and sat with me to watch. I showed her how to use the reverse and forward buttons, and she took delight in moving the tape back and forth. Eventually, I asked her to stop the tape to engage her in general conversation about what she noticed in the picture, what she thought might be going on, how she felt looking at the picture on the screen, etc. Suddenly, this child became interactive with me and descriptive of the play. Her behavior changed completely, and I learned from her about the importance of being removed enough from the play to optimize its full potential.

I haven't always had a video camera available for recording children's posttraumatic play. Other means of creating this sense of distance include placing mirrors near the play scenario on which the child is working. I've also drawn a storyboard for children that depicts what I see in their play (sequence and action) and that is presented to them in comic book form—yet another way that the play material is available but a little more removed.

PROCESSING POSTTRAUMATIC PLAY

There are times when children utilize posttraumatic play in a silent fashion, over a long period of time, with multiple and evolving variations in their work, and with concomitant changes in their attitudes, behaviors, affective expression, and in their interactions with clinicians and others. Their parents or caretakers report that the children's problems have diminished, and a sense of well-being is apparent in them. In other words, and simply put, kids get better! It is quite apparent in these instances that children have truly profited from the therapy, as well as from other countless factors, including the passage of time, the absence of abuse, and the presence of loving caretakers. How large a part the therapy plays is never clear, but what is clear is children's delight in coming to therapy, their positive regard for their treatment providers, and the way their moods appear lighter as they leave the sessions. One important gauge is parental observation; just as parents can be quick to inform you that no positive changes are taking place, they are equally vociferous about improvement. In addition, our routine use of assessment instruments also provides us with clear indicators that positive changes are occurring. In these cases, following children's leads might be warranted such that clinical activity is limited to serving as a silent witness, a resonating figure, a person with the capacity for emotional connection, and a steady, consistent, empathic presence.

Other children may use posttraumatic play intermittently and very briefly and may incorporate this play into a much ampler therapy experience that includes other modalities and activities. Clinical posture, activity, and direction are therefore varied, and because no single approach will fit all children, flexibility and comfort with shifting from nondirective to directive approaches are good skills to hone, particularly when working with children who have experienced trauma (Shelby & Felix, 2005).

Over the years I've learned to be more or less active as children engage in posttraumatic play, and while my preference is to allow children to evolve their play without much interruption on my part, other clinicians prefer a more active approach. Dripchak (2007), for example, using an Ericksonian model, assists clients by introducing new endings or solutions for some of the stories that children tell. Dripchak suggests the use of "refractions (which is the process of the therapist speaking through dolls or puppets, while the child infers the meaning), reflective statements, interspersed suggestions (emphasizing through play certain words or phrases to create a different direction or emphasis), and direct suggestions" (p. 127). By providing these interventions, Drip-chak (2007) states, "the child both guides and is guided by the play therapy process" (p. 127). She concludes that in her approach, when used appropriately, the play will not retraumatize the child. Dripchak and Marvatsi (2004) describe their work as follows: "The child is guided by the therapist to emphasize her strengths rather than weaknesses, pos-sibilities rather than losses, hope rather than despair, solutions rather than problems, and healing power rather than pathology" (as cited in Dripchak, 2007, p. 130).

Goodyear-Brown (2010) also processes play in a more active way by utilizing what she calls experiential mastery play. She employs carefully chosen questions, encourages active engagement with or disposal of a perpetrator symbol, and uses active physical manipulation of an art or sand creation or directly invites the child to dispose of the troublesome content in a way that is meaningful to him or her (p. 222). Both these highly experienced clinicians propose a more directive role for the ther-apist and find positive results in their work. It is clear that even though approaches may differ, restoring a sense of control in the child is the common goal. Herman (1992, 1997) cites Adam Kardiner as defining the role of the therapist as that of an assistant whose goal it is to "help the patient complete the job that he is trying to do spontaneously and to reinstate the element of renewed control" (p. 134).

SUMMARY AND CONCLUSIONS

Posttraumatic play is a remarkable tool most accessible to young chil-dren who bring to the forefront their life experiences in a way that is both visible, tangible, and evocative. There appears to be an interesting paradox as children bring forth their stories and play action: They are both exposed and shielded simultaneously. When children play natu-rally, their play is replete with liveliness, role playing, joy, and sponta-neity, and they invite and cojole peers and caretakers into participa-tion and interaction. When children suffer a myriad of interpersonal traumas, they are often left alone with whatever thoughts, feelings, and bodily sensations they experience and they may feel confused, fright-ened, and isolated. Thus, their play can appear grim, flat, isolating, and robotic.

Young traumatized children are in need of help to cope with highly stressful experiences that are compounded by conflicting feelings of love and dependency on their parents or caretakers, often the very same people who have injured and hurt them inexplicably. Because of cognitive, linguistic, and emotional limitations, youngsters may struggle to find a way to work through the subsequent pain and anxiety that may linger.

Posttraumatic play is a viable option for many children because it provides them with a natural and comfortable way to communicate, express, and arrive at an understanding of what they have endured. By introducing them to miniaturized depictions of the very things that provoke fear and discomfort, they are able to gradually develop coping strategies and allow themselves to discharge emotion. The end result is a situation in which children feel a sense of mastery from telling or showing what is on their minds, from expressing how they feel, by developing a coherent story that they understand, and by feeling a restored sense of well-being. Indeed, posttraumatic play may be driven by children's natural reparative mechanisms. The therapist's ultimate goal is to help the child move forward while acknowledging the hurts of the past.

Posttraumatic play occurs in natural settings as well as clinical ones. Therapists are advised to both facilitate engagement with posttraumatic play (by providing items that represent the child's traumatic experience) as well as assist the child in processing the play that emerges in the therapy setting. Processing or working through traumatic material can be done in a variety of ways; some clinicians prefer to exercise patience and allow the child the time to find his or her own solutions and options, whereas other clinicians engage more actively with the play to promote the child's growth and avoid retraumatization.

Because posttraumatic play often takes its own time, it is impossible to predict how long it will take for the child to achieve the goal of mastery; however, careful clinical attention may provide guidance about the evolution of the play. Measuring minuscule alterations in the play in a highly structured way may provide clues as to the positive (dynamic) or toxic (static or negative) state of the play. Dynamic play will take its course and usually produce quite positive results, whereas static play is potentially dangerous and needs to be interrupted. Even how this play is interrupted varies among professionals and can range from distracting the child away from the play, to videotaping sessions, to using dramatic techniques to present new options to the child.

Posttraumatic play is one of the most effective natural healing strategies available to children and, as such, it should be the focus of clinical interventions. In fact, therapists who work with child trauma will find it beneficial to identify, encourage, invite, and honor posttraumatic play and its potential to help children heal. As a child-initiated activity, posttraumatic play is a sterling example of the power of play.

REFERENCES

American Psychiatric Association. (2000). *Diagnostic and statistical manual of mental disorders.* (4th ed., text rev.). Washington, DC: Author.

Benedek, E. (1985). Children and psychic trauma: A brief review of contemporary thinking. In S. Eth & R. S. Pynoos (Eds.), *Post-traumatic stress disorder in children* (pp. 1–16). Washington, DC: American Psychiatric Association.

Chandler, C. K. (2005). *Animal assisted therapy.* New York: Routledge.

Cohen, J. A., Mannarino, A. P., & Deblinger, E. (2006). *Treating trauma and traumatic grief in children and adolescents.* New York: Guilford Press.

Cook, A., Spinazzola, J., Ford, J. D., Lanktree, C., Blaustein, M., Cloitre, M., et al. (2005). Complex trauma in children and adolescents. *Psychiatric Annals, 35,* 390–398.

Dripchak, V. L. (2007). Posttraumatic play: Towards acceptance and resolution. *Clinical Social Work Journal, 35,* 125–134.

Dripchak, V. L., & Marvasti, J. A. (2004). Treatment approaches for sexually abused children and adolescents. In J. A. Marvasti (Ed.), *Psychiatric treatment of victims and survivors* (pp. 155–176). ILL: Charles C. Thomas.

Engel, S. (1995). *The stories children tell: Making sense of the narratives of childhood.* New York: Freeman.

Ford, J. D., & Cloitre, M. (2009). Best practices in psychotherapy for children and adolescents. In C. A. Courtois & J. D. Ford (Eds.), *Treating complex traumatic stress disorders: An evidence-based guide* (pp. 59–81). New York: Guilford Press.

Ford, J. D., & Russo, E. (2006). A trauma-focused, present-centered, emotional self-regulation approach to integrated treatment for post-traumatic stress and addiction. *American Journal of Psychotherapy, 60,* 335–355.

Gil, E. (2006). *Helping abused and traumatized children: Integrating directive and nondirective approaches.* New York: Guilford Press.

Gil, E. (1999). Understanding and responding to post-trauma play. *Association for Play Therapy Newsletter, 17*(1), 7–10.

Gil, E. (1991). *Healing power of play: Working with abused children.* New York: Guilford Press.

Goodman, R. F. (1999). Introduction. In H. S. Koplewicz & R. F. Goodman (Eds.), *Childhood revealed: Art expressing pain, discovery, and hope* (pp. 12–15). New York: Abrams.

Goodyear-Brown, P. (2010). *Play therapy with traumatized children: A prescriptive approach.* New York: Wiley.

Herman, J. (1992). *Trauma and recovery.* New York: Basic Books.

Herman, J. (1997). *Trauma and recovery* (2nd ed.). New York: Basic Books.

Jackson, H., Susser, E., & Hoven, C. (2001). Terrorism and mental health in school: The effects of 9/11/2001 on New York City's school children. New York: NYC Board of Education Study, Columbia University.

Kagan, R. (2008). Transforming troubled children into tomorrow's heroes. In D. Brom, R. Pat-Horrenczyk, & J. D. Ford (Eds.), *Treating traumatized children: Risk, resilience, and Recovery* (pp. 255–268). London: Routledge.

Katz, M. (1997). *On playing a poor hand well: Insights from the lives of those who have overcome childhood risks and adversities.* New York: Norton.

Lewis, M. L., & Ippen, C. G. (2004). Rainbows and tears, souls full of hope: Cultural issues related to young children and trauma. In J. D. Osofsky (Ed.), *Young children and trauma: Intervention and treatment* (pp. 11–46). New York: Guilford Press.

Malchiodi, C. (Ed.). (2003). *Handbook of art therapy.* New York: Guilford Press.

Marvasti, J. A. (1994). Please hurt me again: Posttraumatic play therapy with an abused child. In T. Kottman & C. Schaefer (Eds.), *Play therapy in action: A casebook for practitioners* (pp. 485–525). Lanham, MD: Jason Aronson.

Nader, K. (2004). Treating traumatized children and adolescents. In N. B. Webb (Ed.), *Mass trauma and violence: Helping children and families cope* (pp. 50–74). New York: Guilford Press.

Osofsky, J. D. (Ed.). (2004). *Young children and trauma: Intervention and treatment.* New York: Guilford Press.

Perry, B. (2008). Healthy families, healthy communities: An interview with Bruce D. Perry, M.D., Ph.D., by James E. McCarroll, Ph.D. *Joining Forces: Joining Families, 10*(3), pp. 1–8.

Pynoos, R. S., & Eth, S. (1986). Witness to violence: The child interview. *Journal of the American Academy of Child and Adolescent Psychiatry, 25,* 306–319.

Pynoos, R. S., Steinberg, A. M., & Goenjian, A. (1996). Traumatic stress in childhood and adolescence: Recent developments and current controversies. In B. A. van der Kolk, A. C. McFarlane, & L. Weisaeth (Eds.), *Traumatic stress: The effects of overwhelming experience on mind, body, and society* (pp. 331–358). New York: Guilford Press.

Rubin, L. B. (1996). *The transcendent child: Tales of triumph over the past.* New York: Basic Books.

Schaefer, C. E. (Ed.). (1995). *The therapeutic powers of play.* New York: Jason Aronson.

Scheeringa, M. S., Zeanah, C. H., Drell, M. J., & Larriew, J. A. (1995). Two approaches to the diagnosis of PTSD in infancy and early childhood. *Journal of the American Academy of Child and Adolescent Psychiatry, 34*(2), 191–200.

Shelby, J. S., & Felix, E. D. (2005). Post-traumatic play therapy: The Need for an integrated model of directive and nondirective approaches. In L. A. Reddy, T. M. Files-Hall, & C. E. Schaefer (Eds.), *Empirically-based play interventions for children* (pp. 79–103). Washington, DC: American Psychological Association.

Shelby, J. S., & Tredinnick, M. G. (1995). Crisis intervention with survivors of natural disasters: Lessons from Hurricane Andrew. *Journal of Counseling and Development, 73*(5), 491–497.

Sleek, S. (1998). After the storm, children play out fears. *APA Online, 29,* 6.

Terr, L. C. (1991). Childhood traumas: An outline and overview. *American Journal of Psychiatry, 148,* 10–19.

Terr, L. (1990). *Too scared to cry.* New York: Basic Books.

van Fleet, R. (2008). *Play therapy with kids and canines: Benefits for children's developmental and psychosocial health.* Practitioner's Resource Series.

Walsh, F. (2006). *Strengthening family resilience* (2nd ed.). New York: Guilford Press.

Clinical Responses

PART TWO

Clinical Acupuncture

CHAPTER 5

Silent Grieving in a World without Words

A Child Witnesses His Brother's Murder

ELIANA GIL

CASE REFERRAL INFORMATION

Four-year-old Wilson's grandmother called me to explain a tragic family situation that had resulted in Wilson developing selective mutism. Initially, she was difficult to understand because she had not yet mastered the English language. Lilly had come from Korea, a recent widow, after her son (as well as her adult daughter and her family) and her daughter-in-law had established themselves near the Washington, DC, area. Lilly had been tasked with locating me and making an initial appointment for Wilson's parents. She told me that a colleague of mine had referred her to me for "play work" with her grandson. I empathized with Lilly having to communicate this important initial information to me, and she apologized many times for not having command of English. I apologized for not knowing Korean and told her I was in no rush, to take her time, and that I was perfectly capable of understanding her and asking questions when I didn't.

Lilly seemed to develop more ease as she found that I could understand what she was telling me. She reported that Wilson, her 4-year-old grandson, had unfortunately witnessed the killing of his brother Sam by their other brother, Cliff. Cliff was 17 years old and was currently in a juvenile detention facility; Sam was 14 on the day of his violent death, now 2 months prior. No one really knew what had precipitated this random act of violence, although Lilly made mention that drugs were suspected. She went on to tell me that her daughter and son-in-law were distraught and that they needed help. She said, "They want him to forget but Wilson, he can't forget easy." As she offered some details of the death, I was able to discern that Sam had been beaten to death with a baseball bat on top of the washer and dryer in the basement. Wilson had seen everything. She added, "I iron, I no hear screaming with radio on. Me fault I not hear." I offered some encouraging words to Lilly, but it was clear she was shouldering a lot of the responsibility for what had occurred, a feeling shared by many survivors of murdered loved ones. She said that Wilson "lie on floor, no move, lie like ball" when he was found by police. I offered Lilly an appointment for the next day, and she called back to confirm that Wilson's parents (her son Steven and his wife, Ann) would attend the appointment. I encouraged her to come as well, but she noted that she would stay with Wilson while his parents came to the appointment. I gave her the address, and she said her son had already found it on the Internet. I agreed to meet the parents who had lost two children in one brief moment, and I braced myself for an emotional meeting hoping I would find some words of comfort for them.

The grief of Wilson's parents was palpable and distressing—they sat separate from each other with their hands folded in front of them. They tearfully described how they had removed every single reminder of their son Sam. They did not want to upset Wilson any more than he had already been upset, and they thought that moving forward with their lives was the right thing to do for this young child. I learned from Steven and Ann that they had not talked to Wilson directly about Sam's death or where his brother Cliff was, and they reported that Wilson had not asked about or mentioned either of his brothers since their death. Wilson had been sent to live with his grandmother Lilly and Aunt Kim (Steven's sister) for the first month after his brother's death and they had instructed Lilly and Kim to avoid discussing Sam's death within Wilson's earshot. In this way the parents sought to regain some control and hoped to protect their youngest child from the profound pain they now endured.

I listened to these grief-stricken parents as they described being unable to sleep, how they felt distant from each other, and how they were filled with ambivalence toward their son in juvenile detention.

They told me that they were seeing a psychiatrist friend of Steven's who had not given any guidance about Wilson, except telling the parents that they had to keep their grief hidden from their child so that Wilson did not worry about his parents. This psychiatrist had also recommended me to Steven and Ann and said that I specialized in working with very young children and that I would know how to advise them. Steven and Ann had known intuitively to maintain Wilson's routines at preschool and day care and had him spend additional time with his Grandmother Lilly. They were concerned that Wilson had stopped talking to people, and they expressed grave concern that it could affect his entering kindergarten in the fall.

Steven and Ann referred to the murder as "the accident" and seemed reluctant to give much detail. I did ask a few important questions both because I thought their answers would help me to help Wilson and also because I wanted to model that it was important to speak about death and its impact openly. Of course, that was much easier for me to do since I was not in the throes of profound grief. I asked Ann and Steven if they could tell me who was in the house when the fight erupted between their sons. Ann told me that Lilly always babysat during the day since both parents worked outside the home. Ann added that her job was part-time and that she often came home early in the afternoon. She also told me that she took Wilson to preschool three mornings a week and on those days, worked only until noon. This violent event had occurred on one of the days that Ann was out of the house longer and Lilly was the primary caretaker; however, Ann had come home and was preparing dinner when "the accident" happened. Lilly was upstairs ironing (as she had told me on the phone), Ann was making dinner, and Steven had not yet arrived from work. Lilly had the radio on (Ann said that it was a custom of hers to listen to a Korean news radio), and Ann had opened the doors to the deck while she cooked. She added, "Sometimes it's noisy when I open the doors, but I like the air to come in—maybe that's why I didn't hear anything from downstairs." Steven piped in that Ann had heard "something" but didn't know what it was. Ann nodded her head in agreement that she had heard "something" but couldn't make it out. The expression in her eyes changed when her husband interrupted her to clarify/correct what she had told me. "I should have stopped what I was doing and gone downstairs . . . maybe then—." It seemed that Lilly and Ann were sharing the guilt of being unable to stop the death of their grandson and son. I quickly told Ann, "I'm sure that if you had known what was going on, or that one of your children needed protection, you would have stopped what you were doing and you would have rushed downstairs." Steven touched her hand and said, "Of course, you would have. I told you, no need for you to feel responsible." Ann looked at him squarely and said, "You say that now, but you also remind me all the time that I heard something. It's like you're telling me I should have known." Steven removed his hand and looked away. I told both parents that after accidents and losses occur, it is very common for surviving family members to try to find explanations or even to place blame. I added that "hindsight is 20/20," and they needed to forgive themselves for not knowing there was trouble brewing downstairs. Ann had held her tears back quite efficiently, but at that moment, she put her hands to her face and sobbed. I gestured to Steven to move closer to his wife, and he was able to hold her and stroke her hair. I went to get Ann some water and reassured her that I would try to help Wilson. I also encouraged them to continue to see the psychiatrist because this was one of the most difficult experiences anyone could endure. I also told them that I would ask them to come in from time to time once I began to work with Wilson, and that I thought Lilly might also need some assistance. They told me that Lilly would be leaving soon to return to her native Korea because her sister had become ill. My heart ached for Wilson because this was yet another impending loss. I quickly told them that they should take special precautions so that Wilson knew when Grandmother would return: Perhaps a calendar that showed him clearly when she would leave and return. The parents followed this and every other directive I gave them.

My final question to them was what, if anything, they had told their son about his brothers. They explained what Lilly had already told me: They wanted to protect Wilson from having more pain, they wanted him to forget what he had seen, and thus they had not mentioned anything to him. They quickly added, "He has not asked, he doesn't want to know." I offered an alternate explanation: "Children take their cues from the important adults in their lives. Maybe he does not want you to feel more pain, and maybe since you have not mentioned anything to him, he thinks it's not okay to talk about his brothers." Steven and Ann listened, but it was clear that telling Wilson about his brothers felt overwhelming. "This is something we can work on together," I said. "Let me meet him first, start our work, and then let's talk again about how to do this, keeping your concerns in mind." I gave them a book to read about how parents can help children with grieving. They never did follow through with readings. I also asked for a release of information so that I could speak with their psychiatrist. "Maybe he and I can talk a little about how to help you find something useful to say to Wilson about his brothers." I mentioned that there was a distinct field of study regarding the impact of grief and loss on both family members and children, and that it would be important for them to get the help they needed because they were having very normal reactions (Cohen, Mannarino, & Deblinger, 2006; Fiorini & Mullen, 2006; Webb, 2010).

The look of relief was obvious. Steven and Ann needed to know that others before them had dealt with, and recovered from, the death of a child. They also needed guidance on what to do about Wilson, and they dreaded the idea of talking directly to him about what had occurred. They were still having trouble speaking with each other about the death of one son and the incarceration of the other.

I explained nondirective play therapy, particularly the fact that I would not pressure Wilson to speak to me; rather, I would get to know him through his play. I told them that children sometimes "play out" traumatic experiences, and I trusted that this would occur on some level. I then gave the parents a brochure to read about play therapy, *Why Play Therapy?* (published by the Association for Play Therapy, 2001), and told them that I would be in touch with them after I got to know their child a little better.

FORMULATION OF THE PROBLEM

Play therapists are a perfect fit for children with selective mutism because play therapists welcome children's more ample forms of nonverbal communication and don't rely so much on verbal exchanges. Selective mutism has been discussed more in the last two decades, and the importance of differential diagnosis is noted. Several theories have been posited about its origins, including it being a response to family neurosis (e.g., over protective mothers or remote fathers), a manifestation of unresolved psychodynamic conflict, a reaction to trauma (including abuse, death of a loved one, frequent relocations), a social phobia, or related to anxiety and obsessive–compulsive disorder (Spasaro & Schaefer, 1999). In my clinical experience, many of these factors can be present or contributory, as well as other factors: I have also worked with children showing selective mutism who had extreme anger and an excessive desire and need for control or attention. In Wilson's case, it was clear that his mutism was in direct response to an acute trauma that had likely left him feeling horrified, overwhelmed, and terrified. To add insult to injury, his parents had not known how to comfort or reassure him and, misguidedly, both sent him away for one full month thinking it best that the child not witness their distress (with no contact during that time) and opted to avoid their shared reality. I felt it imperative for this child to have some kind of release from the traumatic thoughts, feelings, and sensations that he likely constricted and suppressed. Specifically, I hoped to invite and facilitate posttraumatic play so that Wilson could "play out" the traumatic scene he had witnessed in the basement of his home. The best way I knew to do this was to provide him with the specific items that he could use to reenact the traumatic event that he had witnessed. After learning that Sam, 14, had been beaten to death with a baseball bat by Cliff, 17, on top of the washer and dryer in the basement, I purchased a miniature washer and dryer and provided something resembling a baseball bat and three male children of different sizes. I also made sure that Asian parent and grandparent figures were available for him to use (he chose to use white male figures instead).

INVITATION TO PLAY THERAPY: MEETING THE BOY WITHOUT WORDS

Wilson seemed compliant and lifeless. He took my hand and walked with me to the play therapy office with barely a goodbye or glance at his mother. She had told me that he seemed sad lately, a change from his playful attitude prior to his brother's death, but I wasn't prepared to see a child this young surrender so easily to walking with a stranger.

When we got into the room I repeated some of the things I had said when I greeted him and his mother in the waiting room: "Like I told you outside, my name is Dr. Gil, and I know, Wilson, that right now you are not using your words. I want you to know that this is a place where you decide what to do and what to say. I won't be asking you to use words, and chances are, I won't use too many words either. Let me show you around the room so you can see what you would like to play with today." I showed him around the room, and he followed easily as I introduced the art materials, the hospital, the dollhouse, the sand tray, the miniatures, the puppets, and a few random toys in a cabinet.

When Wilson walked with me to the dollhouse, his face leveled off with the second floor of the house. "This is a house, Wilson, and people and families can live in this house. Upstairs are bedrooms and a bathroom. Downstairs is a kitchen, a place to eat or watch television, and a place where parents can wash clothes, in a washer and a dryer. In some houses these things are in a basement." No response. "Here are some people who might live in the houses. There are white people, black people, and here are some Korean people like you."[1]

After I showed him everything in the room, I sat down and told him that he could decide what to do and what to play with. He looked around and moved very slowly, finally settling for some colorful, large Legos, which he took out and pushed together. His play was quite solitary and devoid of any outward signs of enjoyment—he didn't attempt to construct anything with the Legos, he simply moved them around listlessly. Wilson went to the door with about 15 minutes left in the session, signaling that he was ready to go. His mother greeted him warmly, but Wilson remained rather constricted in affect, and they left the building without much animation from Wilson.

I called the mother during the week, and she said that Wilson appeared the same. I was curious how he would respond to coming to see me again and asked her to mention to him that next Tuesday, she would once again bring him to see Dr. Gil.

Wilson seemed to separate from his mother too easily on this second session as well as the next three. During these sessions, I noticed an interesting pattern: Wilson pulled up a little chair and situated himself on it with his back turned to the dollhouse, but coincidentally, he was always that way. At first I thought I had imagined this, but as I paid attention to his placement, I found this practice quite meaningful.

By the eighth session I was convinced that I was working with a child who had definitively compartmentalized the traumatic event he had witnessed and was now in full avoidance of any remembrance of this event. It was, of course, hard to know if he was having intrusive thoughts and flashbacks, but his parents reported that he was having "strong dreams" from which he awakened in a sweat.

It was clear to me that Wilson was having the avoidance and numbing symptoms of PTSD, and the hyperarousal features appeared through nightmares. I considered how I might gently "tickle the defenses" of this child and offer him an opportunity to begin to process this traumatic incident that likely had him feeling bound up and isolated in his silent world. I decided that I would make his defensive strategies explicit by doing a very simple act: I covered the dollhouse with a blanket. I was eager to see how he would react to spotting this cover on the dollhouse when he entered the room.

---

[1] Clinicians are advised to stay sensitive to play therapy toys that are provided to children of diverse backgrounds and to always include multicultural toys in their collection (Gil & Drewes, 2006; Salazar, 2003).

On the eighth session, Wilson entered the room and immediately stopped. He grunted and pointed at the dollhouse—the most energy I had observed in this youngster. "You are grunting and pointing," I said to him, and he repeated what appeared to be his objection. "You are grunting and pointing again." He walked up to the dollhouse and literally yanked the blanket down, allowing it to fall on the floor in front of him. He then stood and stared at the dollhouse and at that moment, he bolted into action as he reached into the dollhouse and began to move the furniture around as well as pick dolls that would stay in the house and those that would go. This action signaled the beginning of his post-traumatic play. I will now chronicle how we arrived at this point in more detail.

CASE ILLUSTRATION OF SELF-DIRECTED TRAUMA PLAY

The Beginning: Setting the Stage

When Wilson arrived for his first appointment, I was surprised that he followed me to my office alone, without making any visible objection to his mother's request that he come with me. I considered that this could be consistent with the obedient behavior expected of Korean children by their parents. I asked the mother if she would like to come in and see the room where we would be, and she declined. She simply directed Wilson to follow me, and he did. When I first greeted Wilson (his mother insisted that he shake my hand, and he complied politely), I took the opportunity to set his mind at ease immediately by telling him that his mother had told me that he wasn't using his words right now. "I want you to know, Wilson, that it's okay with me if you don't use your words right now. There will be lots of toys and games and play activities that you can choose to do, and you won't need to speak any words to me at all!" I also told Wilson, "I work with lots of kids, and some of them don't like to talk at all, but they do like to do other things."

When we got to the play therapy office, I did what I do routinely: I showed Wilson around the room, making sure he could see all the toys and activities. I narrated, "As you can see, there are some puppets, an easel and paints and markers and pencils, some board games, lots of small toys on shelves, and a sand box." I always stop at the sand box to say, "This is a box filled with very smooth white sand." Wilson seemed to be listening and looking, but he also appeared less interested than most children his age are. As I moved the sand around with my hand, I said: "There are lots of ways to play with the sand. You can just touch it or move it around, doing whatever you like, or you can take as few or as many of these little toys and put them in the sand, making a little world, or anything you'd like to make." Silence. I then showed Wilson the dollhouse, as mentioned earlier.

I told Wilson that when we met in this room, he was in charge. "You can do whatever you would like to do, Wilson, this is your time and your space." I am here if you need anything. I also want to show you the clock. "We will be here for 50 minutes, and when this hand gets to this number, it will be time to go. I will see you once a week, on Mondays, at 2:30 P.M. each week."

This was a very atypical first session in that Wilson found a chair on which to sit and spent most of his time on it, looking around the room but making little effort to explore. Since children's natural response to any play therapy office is interest, curiosity, and exploration, I knew that being patient would likely yield some movement. I grabbed a little piece of clay, setting clay containers on the little table next to Wilson. I started rolling my clay into a ball, and eventually I merged some colors to make a small, colorful ball. As I focused my attention on this activity, I could spy Wilson beginning to look around with a hint of slight wonder in his eyes. The one very noticeable move that Wilson made in this session was that he chose to sit in one of three chairs—he sat in one chair first but moved to another. When he moved to his selected chair—a chair that would become his starting point of almost every early session—his back was to the dollhouse. I didn't really notice this for a few weeks, but then it became clear to me that his avoidance was being manifested in a very physical way.

Avoiding the Dollhouse

Wilson was literally avoiding looking at the dollhouse that I had showed him during our first meeting. I set it up each week for him because sometimes other children would come in, rearrange furniture, and leave things turned upside down (or very rigidly rearranged in some very unique way). I wanted to make sure that when Wilson turned his attention to the dollhouse (and I trusted that this would happen), all the tools he needed for his unique posttraumatic play would be available as he had seen them the first time. As described earlier, in the sixth session I decided to take some action to facilitate Wilson's use of posttraumatic play.

Tickling the Defenses

In the first five sessions Wilson had established a routine. He usually sat for a while in one of the small chairs, looking around the room and seeming to settle himself, and then he usually engaged in some kind of repetitive play: He took Lego pieces out, scattered them about, and returned them to their box. He kicked a ball from one side of the room to the other gingerly, he used cardboard building blocks and stacked them up, he took out different colored pieces of clay and rolled them into little long pieces (looking like worms), and sometimes he played with cars on the floor. When he did get on the floor and take his cars around the room, I noted that he avoided the entire wall where the dollhouse was. These early sessions were time well spent: Wilson learned that he could take me at my word—he really could decide how he would spend his time in the office. He also learned that I would not push for him to speak, and I didn't talk to him a lot except to make minimal comments, such as, "You're moving your cars to different parts of the room." Wilson also learned that there were few demands in this room, and he seemed to develop comfort with both the setting and me.

During our first visit, I had also put on some meditation music, which I often have available during play therapy sessions, but Wilson did not seem to notice the very faint background music. However, after our third meeting together, he began coming into the room and pushing the button to start the music. I took that as a sign that he was aware of, and possibly benefiting from, the rhythmic background music (Oldfield & Flower, 2008).

Although it was critical that I allow Wilson to work at his own pace and I didn't want to rush anything, I was also concerned that more and more time was going by (four months now total) since his brother's death, and it became apparent to me that Wilson's need to avoid and suppress this memory, likely etched in his mind with pinpoint accuracy, was becoming more and more entrenched (probably because his family was still participating in constructing and maintaining a world of silence). At the same time that Wilson was using considerable energies to avoid any semblance of his painful memory and subsequent feelings and thoughts, his symptoms remained unchanged: He was still waking twice or three nights a week in a sweat, he was unresponsive and distant with family members, and he was void of any of the optimistic, fun-loving personality traits that were prominent prior to his brother's death.

During this early stage of treatment, I concurrently made several attempts to assist the parents with their avoidance. I had talked with the parents' psychiatrist, and even though he was taking my lead and encouraging the parents to prepare some ways to approach their son, they persisted in their hesitancy and began to act out this hesitancy by missing appointments both with the psychiatrist and with myself. I felt concerned that the parents' denial and consistent hesitations would fuel Wilson's own ambivalence. I decided, therefore, to "move" something along by simply making explicit that which Wilson was showing me by everything he did and did not do; I chose to make explicit (and concrete) the family's defensive style. I brought a small child's blanket to the play therapy office and draped it on top of the dollhouse, sending Wilson the not-so-disguised message that he (and his parents) was drawing a curtain over the horrific memory he had witnessed with eyes wide open and that a "cover-up" was evident to me. I waited to see if Wilson would notice the obvious drape over the dollhouse. In essence, I offered him a metaphor for his own compartmentalized memory.

Wilson had habits in his sessions with me: He turned on the music, he sat in his chair for a few moments, then he stood in the center of the room, back to the dollhouse, and he selected where to go and what to do. I realized as soon as I observed his ritual beginning that he would not spot the dollhouse with the blanket on top because he had trained himself to avoid any sighting of this area. Interestingly, as he stood in the center of the room, he slowly turned, put his arm up with a pointed finger, and grunted "Humph." I calmly said to him, "You are pointing and grunting." He kept pointing and grunted twice. "You are still pointing and grunting twice now." He made a few alterations in the pitch and urgency of his grunt, which I dutifully noted, and he then walked over to the dollhouse, pulled down the blanket with purpose, and stood exposed to that which he seemed to have avoided so skillfully.

I waited to see what would happen next. To my delight, amazement, and wonder, he began to move objects around in the dollhouse, placing a woman with an ironing board in the top room, a woman in the kitchen, and three boys in the room with the washer and dryer. He likely worked for about 10–15 minutes doing this, and then he retreated and sat at his chair, as if starting his routine again. Next he played with some building blocks, this time stacking them and then kicking them with increased physical energy and intensity. This kicking gesture created a loud noise, and the cardboard blocks likewise made noise when they went flying here and there. "You're putting the boxes in a pile, you're kicking them with your foot, and the blocks are flying and filling this room with noise," I commented. I wanted to emphasize this incredible release, likely a matter-of-fact and innocuous act for any other child—

an abreactive event for Wilson. As he kicked, he let out breaths that were anemic and barely discernible, but breaths nevertheless. Wilson had found a way to quit holding his breath in this room. These are the moments that we play therapists wait for with great anticipation. This was a moment that allowed other important moments to follow.

The Middle: The Work Deepens and Moves

Wilson's routine changed from that day of the blanket provocation. My intuition told me to leave the blanket off, and as it turned out, Wilson did not appear to need it again. He came in, turned the music on, sat in his chair, stood in the center of the room, turned around and went to play with the dollhouse, arranging and rearranging the figures until he was satisfied (see Figure 5.1). Over the next three sessions, it seemed he arrived at how he wanted the miniature room to look, and it was very close to what he had done the very first time, with one exception: There were a number of sticks placed on top of the washer and dryer. He chose not to use the actual baseball bat that I had finally found for him in a miniature batter's hand (a keychain); instead he chose to line up a few sticks he had found in the play room with some other figures, and then he finally settled on one stick. It was interesting to note that one of the more challenging things to do with the little playmobile human miniatures that he had chosen to use was to stick the iron in the hand of the woman ironing. I think as he looked for sticks, he was also looking for

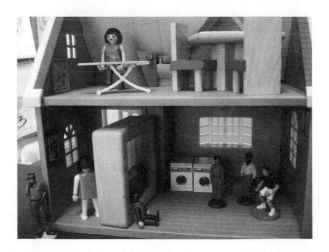

FIGURE 5.1. Everyone in his or her place.

something that might fit in the boy's hand. I noted that one of Wilson's earliest selections was a man holding a tennis racquet, which could have been his first attempt at having a weapon securely in place. He later opted to switch out the tennis player.

After Wilson set the stage for the play that would follow, I called his parents to see how he was doing at home. He had begun speaking phrases to them in the last few weeks, and they were happy for that. Ann told me that she had left a message with my assistant to tell me so but since my assistant was on vacation, I had not received this news. I told Ann that Wilson was beginning to engage in posttraumatic play (which I had described to her earlier), and that I felt it was a good time for us to meet. Ann said that her husband was currently traveling and that she would call as soon as he got back. One month after this phone call, I met with Steven and Ann to gauge the progress they had made in telling Wilson about the murder of his brother and the current location of his older brother. In the meantime, the next four sessions proved significant for Wilson.

The Beating Draws Blood

After the stage was set to his satisfaction, Wilson sat in front of the doll-house for quite some time, apparently making sure that he had everything he needed. I had long since become accustomed to Wilson's silent reflections on something he had completed. It is also possible that Wilson was honing the emotional and psychic energy he would need to both design and manage his trauma play.

Then the play really kicked into gear: He picked up one of the sticks, placed it carefully in the hand of one of the male figures, and began to hit the other figure. As he did this, he brought over the small boy miniature and placed him near the wall so that he was looking directly at what was happening on the washer/dryer (Figure 5.2). I had been intrigued by this boy's absence in all prior sessions in which Wilson had arranged the house briefly but then moved away. I didn't think he was as much forgotten as noticeably missing.

In the next two sessions, Wilson set up the scene quickly, now using most of his time not for observation but for doing. He reenacted the beating, at first with restraint, then toward the end of the sessions, with quite a bit of fervor. During these reenactments he expelled breaths, and his body seemed more fluid than before (Figure 5.3).

He also appeared to experience true emotions, although these registered only briefly on his face, his brows, the way he turned his mouth.

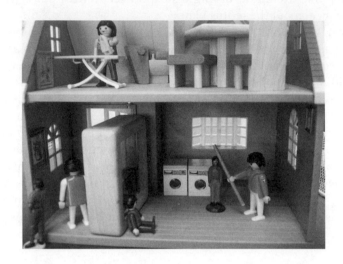

FIGURE 5.2. The weapon is fitted.

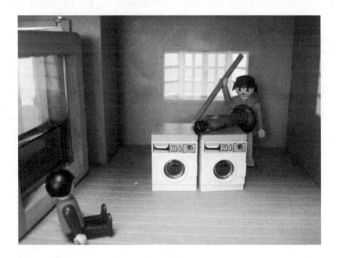

FIGURE 5.3. Hitting went from slight to vigorous.

He licked his lips quite a lot during these reenactments, and I began offering small cups of water, which he drank with gusto, at the end of these sessions. He always sat back in his chair at the end of a session, after the reenactments, and seemed to calm and center himself (while taking some sips of water) with his back to the scene in which he had just invested himself fully. I would always offer a behavioral description of what I saw him do, and he seemed to wait for these brief statements from me. As a matter of fact, it was as if the whole session had a natural rhythm of Wilson's careful design—an ebb and flow of our silent emotion and our silent witnessing.[2]

After these two sessions of reenacting the beating and discharging both breath and affect, Wilson took a departure from his play in our next appointment (session 18), and pointed again, this time at the paints. "You're pointing and grunting," I noted. His frustration was visible whenever I did not understand what he wanted. Finally, he took a stool, climbed a few steps, and pointed directly to the red paint bottle on the shelf. I brought it down for him without a clue of what he planned next.

The Blood Is Spilled

Wilson set up his toys and repeated the sequence of his play without any variation whatsoever. When he got to the hitting, however, he did something remarkable: He took the bottle of red paint and began to pour it on the figures on top of the washer–dryer. I leapt into action when I saw what he was going to do and quickly grabbed the bottle before he poured out all its contents. Both he and I were surprised by my atypical behavior—I could not explain to Wilson that these paint bottles often contained very watery paints that would jet out when the bottles were tilted. "I see you want to pour the red paint," I said, "Let me put some of the paint into a smaller container." I found a small bottle (used formerly as a glitter container) and handed the paint to him. To my surprise, this acrylic red paint was thick and painfully slow to pour. Serendipity. This paint consistency was perfect for what followed. Wilson managed this smaller bottle with greater ease, spilling a little paint, waiting, and spilling a little more. The amount of paint that he spilled seem tremen-

---

[2] It is often said that the therapist acts as a silent witness to a child's play work, yet I've often felt that both therapist and client alike become silent witnesses, bonded by this simple and profound act of seeing what is difficult to see, with unconditional acceptance.

dously important to him; I made a dropper available to him in case he wanted ultimate control of the paint. Indeed, how much of the paint he spilled and how close it got to the little boy sitting in the corner seemed to be of paramount importance. I watched as Wilson poured just the exact amount of paint to have it creep over to the boy in the corner, but he seemed hyperalert to ensuring that the boy was untouched by the paint. (I later read the police report and found that Wilson's play had exactly matched the sequence in the basement where the murder occurred: Blood had flowed onto the floor, which was somewhat tilted, and apparently rolled down toward Wilson, who was apparently in full freeze response and could not get up and run away.) Apparently the fact that blood had approached him slowly was one of the aspects of the trauma that most scared this young child. As happens in some traumatic events, children focus on some random idiosyncratic detail that diverts and holds their attention: For Wilson, it was the sight of the blood creeping toward him (see Figure 5.4).

As Wilson took this particular direction with his play, I wondered what would happen next. He continued to exercise great care to prevent the paint (which I now assumed was pretend blood) touching the small child, witness to violence and murder, hovered in the corner. After two more series of spilling and controlling the paint, Wilson turned away and made a beeline to the ambulance and hospital in the opposite corner of the room. He started rolling the ambulance (he had also avoided this larger car during his early play with cars) and began to mimic the

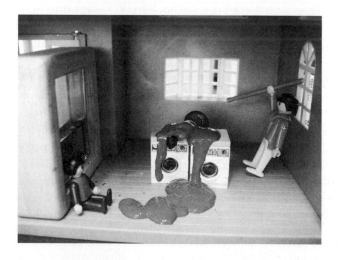

FIGURE 5.4. The spilling of the blood.

sound of the ambulance, which initially made circles and then made its way to the hospital. Nearly 5 months after this posttraumatic work had begun and 7 months since Sam was killed, Wilson was exposing himself gradually to the horrific trauma of his brother's murder, and he finally brought his voice, albeit in the sound of an ambulance siren, to our therapy room. He also had moved the posttraumatic play to its conclusion: The ambulance had arrived and taken the boy away (see Figure 5.5). This was the last time Wilson had seen his brother. I made the following statement, "The boy with the stick hit and hit the other boy. Lots of red paint fell on the floor and got pretty close to the boy who sat watching. The ambulance has now come to the house to pick up the boy and take him away to the hospital." Wilson offered no verbal response but his eyes yielded to my summary statement.

Resolution(s) Surface

And so it was that Wilson's play ignited a series of movements away from the dollhouse and into the rest of the play therapy room. First, the ambulance drew centering circles on the floor. The circles were drawn right in the center of the room, where Wilson usually stood prior to selecting what to do or where to go in the room. Once again, the ambulance drew its direction from first exploring the center, just as Wilson had done himself with the car play that had preceded this posttraumatic play. The ambulance then drove to the house, the doors opened, and the bloody

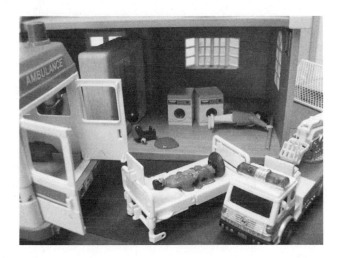

FIGURE 5.5. The ambulance arrives with a loud siren.

child was lifted and placed on the stretcher. Wilson used the dropper to ensure that some of the paint (blood) went with the boy on the ambulance. The ambulance then drove to the hospital and, as it did, Wilson's voice rose with the sound of the siren. "The ambulance is driving away from the house with the boy on the stretcher," I commented. "The siren is turned on and is sounding loudly." When I saw Wilson park the ambulance at the hospital, again I commented, "The ambulance has arrived at the hospital." After that, Wilson placed the boy on a hospital bed and doctors came to help him (see Figure 5.6).

Transitions Occur

Another 3 weeks passed as the play was repeated step by step. The only difference was that Wilson spent less time in the dollhouse play (beatings became almost perfunctory) and more time was spent in the hospital. Wilson had found medicines and an IV drip and many doctors to work on the small bloody figure now in a hospital bed (see Figure 5.7).

I watched very intently all aspects of the play. Had I not, I might have missed seeing Wilson take a small medicine bottle and place it in the sand box, out of sight. Within 2 weeks, his play had advanced to moving first the medicines and then the stretcher with the boy (his brother), placing him in the box (see Figure 5.8), and then pouring sand on him so that he could not be seen (see Figure 5.9).

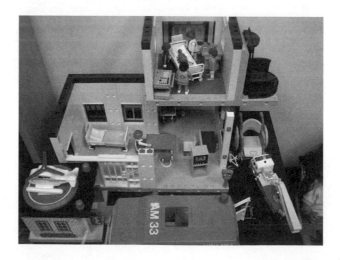

FIGURE 5.6. The boy surrounded by medics and medicine.

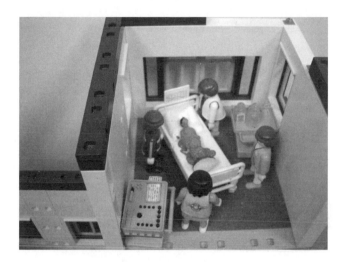

FIGURE 5.7. Attempts to help fall.

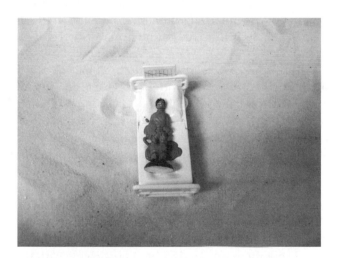

FIGURE 5.8. The boy is brought to the sand.

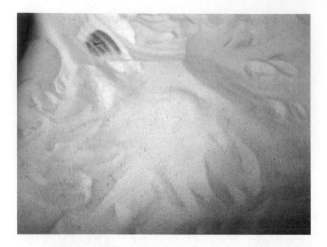

FIGURE 5.9. The boy is buried in the sand.

Finally, I had been successful in scheduling Wilson's parents to come to an appointment, and I hoped that they would not cancel it this time. I was interested (though not surprised) to learn that Wilson was now talking freely to many people and that he seemed to be sleeping through the night. Ann noted that sometimes she heard a whimper, and always got up to check on him, but found him resting comfortably most every time she checked. Once when he had a nightmare, she reported that she held him for a while and that he'd gone back to sleep. The parent's psychiatrist had done a good job of coaching the parents to be more physically responsive to this child (something the father objected to because, culturally, he had been taught that boys are not coddled).

Sensitive to keeping confidential Wilson's play therapy, I did not tell the parents exactly what he had done in our sessions, but I did tell them that he had used the play very well, that he was a good candidate for play therapy, and that he had engaged in posttraumatic play in which he was facing the memories of the afternoon and evening that his brother was killed. I asked the parents if they had found a way to speak to Wilson directly about the murder of their son as well as Clifton's incarceration; they had not. I kept them for nearly 2 hours reviewing with them how to talk with Wilson and why it was important. They were shocked to hear that he was still not speaking to me, and I responded that I had never asked him to do so.

We role-played many, many ways that they could tell Wilson about what had happened to his brothers, but in the end, the parents asked to come into session to do so. I told them that I would be happy to facilitate such a meeting, and we scheduled it for the following week. I told them to tell Wilson that they were going to be coming into the play therapy office with him so that he would be neither shocked nor alarmed. The parents told Wilson that they wanted to talk to him about some important things and they wanted my help in doing so. Wilson grabbed their hands in the waiting room and led them into the room.

The parents were a little surprised to see all the toys; they immediately took their seats in the center of the room, where I had made a circle with four chairs. Ann spoke first. "Today, dear, we need to talk to you about Sam's death." Even the word *death* seemed to stick in her throat and was said in a hush.

Wilson did yet another remarkable thing: He got up out of his chair and said, "No, Mom, come here, I show you about Sam." We opened up the circle of chairs and the parents pulled their chairs up as Wilson showed them his posttraumatic play, now a coherent trauma narrative with a distinct beginning, middle, and end. He used some of the red paint and dropper and put a little red paint on the stretcher, as was his custom. "No," Steven said, "don't dirty that." Wilson stopped abruptly and seemed to freeze for a minute, but then he looked at me and said, "It's okay, Dad, I decide what I do in here." I reassured Steven that this was so, and Wilson smiled. I smiled too and felt privileged to hear Wilson's sweet little voice for the first time.

The play took its usual course and eventually the ambulance arrived and Sam was taken to the hospital. "Quick, Mom, Sam has to get to the hospital fast." He made his siren noise and parked the ambulance at the hospital. "He needs an operation," Wilson exclaimed as he gathered the medicine and the doctors. After a while of watching this scenario, his mother's tears were flowing down her cheeks, and she furiously wiped them away so that Wilson did not notice. Wilson, of course, didn't miss anything! He stopped three times to go to Mom to hug her and be hugged by her. He then took the little boy from the hospital bed and put him in the sand box. At that point, he sat back in his chair and looked down.

"That's right, Son," said Steven in a soft voice, "your mother is sad, and I'm sad because the truth is that Sam is dead and he is now in heaven." "Will we ever see him again?" asked Wilson after a few seconds had elapsed. "No, we won't see him again." Wilson crawled into his mother's arms and both wept openly as she rocked him. "Never again?" he wanted to know. "No, honey, he is dead."

Then the harder questions came. "How come he died?" "Well," Steven said (the parents had decided ahead of time that the father would take the bulk of the conversation), "you know that your brother Cliff was hitting him on his head and, unfortunately, he hit him hard enough that he died." "His head cracked open," Wilson said. "Yes," said Steven. "His head cracked open." Wilson's voice hushed to a whisper as he said, "Lots of blood came out." Steven added, "Yes, it did. I'm sorry you had to see that. Were you scared?" "It was scary," Wilson said, then asked, "Were *you* scared, Daddy?" Steven was honest: "Yes, I was." Wilson concluded, "We were scared."

"How come Cliff hit Sam so hard like that?" "We don't know," said Ann. "We think that he might have taken some of that bad medicine that he used to take, and it made him do things that he didn't know he was doing." "Is he sorry?" asked Wilson. "He's very sorry," said Steven.

"Where is Sam now?" asked Wilson. "What did you do with him?" Ann answered quietly, "It's a little like what you did with the little boy who went to the hospital, Wilson, you put him in the sand." "That was Sam," Wilson said. "Yes," Ann responded. "I know that was Sam." "Our Sam is buried in the earth in a cemetery." "Can I go see him?" asked Wilson. "If Dr. Gil thinks it's okay for you to go visit Sam in the cemetery, we'll take you." He looked up at me, and I nodded in agreement.

Finally, Wilson asked. "Did Cliff die too?" "No," Steven said, "he didn't die." "Where is he?" Wilson said, sitting up erect. "He's in jail right now, Sweetie." "In jail? What's that?" The parents looked at me and signaled for me to answer. "Jail is a house where people live who have done things that weren't okay to do. Your brother Cliff hit your brother hard enough that he cracked his head, and that was wrong for him to do." "Can I go to jail to see him, Mom—please, Dad." The parents once again looked at me and then looked at Wilson, realizing that Wilson had thought that his brother Cliff had died as well. With all the strength Ann could gather, she said, "It will be hard for you to see your brother in jail because it's hard to see him locked up, but yes, Wilson, your dad and I will take you to visit as soon as we ask the judge for permission."

"Did you tell Mama Lilly that Cliff isn't dead?" Wilson asked. "Yes, Wilson, she knows." The parents could see that their child was coming back to them. They seemed relieved and startled at the same time.

I thanked them for coming, and I thanked Wilson for showing his parents the play work that he had been doing when he came to see me.

"Can I still come here to play, Mom?" he asked, looking my way. He was still unwilling to speak to me directly, perhaps nervous that doing so would alter our relationship. "Yes, Wilson, you can come for a little time longer." Indeed he came for another three sessions and then told his parents that he wanted them to come see me so that we could plan for visiting his brother. Not only did this child do his therapy, he sent his parents to me for a little more therapy designed to get them comfortable with his visiting the brother he adored.

Closure

In our last three sessions alone (I saw him a few times later on with his parents), Wilson developed a different routine. He no longer wanted to play with the dollhouse or the hospital. Instead, he wanted to make a series of pictures to leave for me, but as it turned out, after he finished each one, he wanted to take it to his mother, grandmother, or brother, and so he did. He continued to work in silence except in the family sessions. I opted to work with Wilson by coaching his parents. Rather than my reading him a book about people in jail, I had his parents read selected portions of the book to him (Gesme, 1999). Wilson was as ready as a youngster could be to visit his brother in jail, and the hardest part was hearing that there was a "no touching" rule. He also wanted to bring Cliff some of his favorite T-shirts and his grandmother's cookies, which Wilson loved. Wilson and his family had to develop lots of coping strategies to get through the 2-year period that Cliff lived away from home. In the long run, his crime was determined to be a result of his taking a mixture of street drugs; Cliff barely remembered the event, something his parents were grateful to know. He participated in a residential drug treatment program, a pivotal experience that helped shape him into a responsible, peaceful, sober, and productive individual, who later in his life became a drug counselor who worked with at-risk youth.

SUMMARY OF CLINICAL IMPRESSIONS AND FOLLOW-UP

Wilson had experienced an acute trauma as a result of witnessing his 17-year-old brother, Cliff, beat his 14-year-old brother, Sam, to death. Wilson's family, bereaved and despairing, opted to remove any reminders of both these boys and close up their bedrooms. The family entered a world of silence in which they were all grieving in isolation, unable to utilize each other as a support.

Wilson developed a number of symptomatic behaviors, the most obvious of which was a metaphor for his family's response to this horrifying tragedy: He entered a silent world with no words. Wilson's parents were misguided in their efforts to protect the only child they still had in their care. They opted to simply pretend that nothing had ever happened, even though it was clear that their whole world, as they knew it, would never be the same. Steven and Ann earnestly believed that Wilson would forget the horrible event that he had witnessed and that they would be making things worse by bringing it up to him. They found proof of their belief in the fact that Wilson had not asked about either of his brothers. That belief was challenged when Wilson stopped using his words, and friends and child care workers told the parents he needed help.

Wilson had seen and heard more than a child his age should ever be exposed to: the murder of his brother by his other sibling. He needed an opportunity to bring that event into his conscious awareness and establish a way to think about it, feel about it, and put it behind him. As it was, he had managed to suppress the material; he had found ways to simply avoid thinking and feeling anything about it. At the same time, there were periods when his defenses did not work fully, such as when he woke up in a sweat from a horrifying nightmare. It was critical for him to manage the memory without feeling overwhelmed.

Believing, as I do, in the tremendous healing potential of post-traumatic play (see Chapter 4, this volume), my primary objective was to establish a therapeutic relationship with him and then facilitate the play. I trust that children have the reparative capacities they require and that, given enough freedom, stimulation, and context, their natural inclinations to "play it out" will emerge.

In this case, it seemed clear that Wilson and his family were entrenched in avoidance of that which was intolerable to them: the death of their young son and brother. Enough time had gone by that Wilson had begun to rely on his defenses to avoid unbearable emotions. I opted to "tickle the defenses" by making explicit what he was doing: covering up what was painful and choosing to look away. When he saw the blanket draped over the dollhouse, with the depictions of the traumatic event inside, something stirred and rose to the surface in him: He chose to take down the blanket (lower his defenses) and to come face to face with that which he most dreaded—but in a way that he could make the pain smaller and more manageable.

The posttraumatic play that he utilized was nothing short of miraculous and leaves me once again reassured that children know what they need to do to initiate self-repair. This child played out the event, as he recalled it, with his whole body and mind, and in so doing, he went from a passive position (as a child who could not move) to an active position (as a child who could retell what he had seen without feeling a debilitating loss of control). As a matter of fact, when children play out and retell these stories, they are taking matters into their own hands (literally); toys allow them to physically manipulate the events, take new forms of action, and reveal some of what their difficulties might be. For Wilson, the fact that his brother's blood had trickled close to his feet was incredibly frightening. The fact that he was able to drop precisely the amount of red paint (blood) he wanted in a recreated scenario of the murder scene filled this child with mastery. The intent of posttraumatic play is mastery and, in this case, it fulfilled its potential more than I could have ever imagined. In this family, Wilson led the way not only of his own therapy but his parents' healing as well.

I am blessed to have witnessed this unforgettable process in this remarkable child and his family. As a result, a release and transformation ensued that served this family well as they coped with difficult and rewarding experiences in subsequent years.

REFERENCES

Association for Play Therapy. (2001) *Why Play Therapy?* Fresno, CA. Author.

Cohen, J. A., Mannarino, A. P., & Deblinger, E. (2006). *Treating trauma and traumatic grief in children and adolescents.* New York: Guilford Press.

Fiorini, J. J., & Mullen, J. A. (2006). *Counseling children and adolescents through grief and loss.* Champaign, IL: Research Press.

Gesme, C. (1999). *Help for kids: Understanding your feelings about having a parent in prison or jail.* Wayzata, MN: Pine Tree Press.

Gil, E., & Drewes, A. (Eds.). (2006). *Cultural issues in play therapy.* New York: Guilford Press.

Oldfield, A., & Flower, C. (2008). *Music therapy with children and their families.* Philadelphia: Jessica Kingsley.

Salazar, C. (Ed.). (2003). *Group work experts share their favorite multicultural activites: A guide to diversity-competent choosing, planning, conducting, and processing.* Alexandria, VA: Association for Specialists in Group Work, a division of the American Counseling Association.

Spasaro, S. A., & Schaefer, C. E. (1999). *Refusal to speak: Treatment of selective mutism in children.* New York: Aronson.

Webb, N. B. (Ed.). (2010). *Helping bereaved children* (3rd ed.). New York: Guilford Press.

CHAPTER 6

The Owner of a Broken Heart

The Cumulative Trauma of Surgery and Sexual Abuse

NICOLE ERIN JALAZO

Lewis and Steve were off to explore the woods for buried crystals and to fight the secret pirates who had created their forts just behind the biggest tree in the forest. Armed with a shovel and a makeshift spear fashioned out of a fallen tree branch, the two boys headed deep into the tall trees to discover new lands and fight off the evil pirates. For Lewis, up until now being special had meant being careful and fragile and that people always needed to look after him. There was nothing good about it. His pacemaker made it necessary to sit out the touch football games and the games of tag, and to be generally cautious of anything seemingly too playful. Watch out for magnets; they could mess up your pacemaker. Watch out for bullies; you can't afford a punch to the gut. Watch the ball; don't let it get too close to your chest. These were all variations of the same message: Be careful, you're vulnerable. But on this day, *special* meant something else.

Lewis was sure that Steve was the coolest kid in the neighborhood, and Steve had chosen Lewis alone for this adventure. Surely that meant that Steve felt Lewis was up for the battle and was strong enough to weather any enemy or foe that crossed their path. Being chosen by Steve for this adventure meant that Lewis was in store for an entire summer of capturing bad guys and fishing for sharks in the creek. Once they were alone and far enough into the woods, Steve's attention turned to his younger playmate who had followed him admiringly into the dangerous setting. Steve proclaimed to Lewis that he was indeed a special friend whom he intended to bring along on many more exploits into new lands. Steve told Lewis that there were other pursuits between special friends that Lewis would need to learn about and proceeded to act on these pursuits by kissing, fondling, and penetrating his younger friend. Lewis was confused and hurt by Steve's touches and intrusions into his body. He thought the two of them were off to invade and occupy new lands, and instead his body was being invaded and his mind was spinning. He felt powerless to stop what was happening to him. Was this what being special meant? How could he have been so stupid to think that Steve thought he was a worthy companion? Lewis heard himself tell Steve to stop—he was glad his voice had found its way back to his throat. It felt like it might never come back. Steve asked Lewis not to tell anyone what had happened deep in the woods, explaining that they needed to protect one another from the silly grownups who didn't understand their pursuits or conquests. Lewis felt like he owed it to Steve to keep quiet; after all, Steve had chosen Lewis out of all the other kids on the street, and the rest of the day had been adventurous and exciting. Plus, if his mom and dad found out about what had happened with Steve, they would worry even more and Lewis wouldn't have any freedom to play for the rest of the summer. Lewis knew that what Steve had done was wrong, but he also knew that he should have stopped it right away, especially because Steve had stopped when he had been able to tell him to do so. Lewis did not want to get in trouble, and he did not want Steve to get in trouble. He would just be sure not to let it happen again. All he had to do was stick with what he knew, keep his eye on Steve, and not head out into the woods again with Steve or anyone else.

CASE REFERRAL INFORMATION

I met Lewis's mother several months later for an intake appointment. A few weeks before our appointment—serendipity—she had decided it was a good time to sit down with Lewis to talk about inappropriate touching and keeping safe. She had gathered a few books on the subject from the library and had planned to have an open conversation about prevention, safety, and the regard one should hold for his or her body.

When Lewis's mother laid the books down on the table between them, Lewis thought his mother had read his mind. He thought she must know how hard he had been working to keep the day in the woods from ever happening again. He immediately disclosed the events of the day in the park with Steve.

Lewis's mom comforted him and assured him that he was not in trouble and that he was right to tell her. Inside she was reeling with anger and fear for her son. She called his father at work, and his dad was home within the hour. Lewis's dad had a difficult time understanding why he hadn't told them earlier and was angry that they had not been able to protect their son. Lewis's parents sat with Lewis again later that evening and relayed the appropriate messages to their son: that it was not his fault, that they would protect him, and that he was right to tell. A report was made to the police and an investigation was opened. Lewis worried about Steve getting into trouble but also felt a sense of relief in letting go of his secret.

Lewis's mother was a tall, well-put-together woman. In that first intake appointment, she recounted Lewis's history of multiple traumas to his body and heart. As she opened up about his struggles and fears, it became clear that this child was navigating the aftermath of cumulative trauma. Lewis's mother was matter-of-fact in her reporting of the details, dates, and specific conversations that she felt might be critical for me to understand her son. As she concluded her account of Lewis's life to date, she took a breath and the emotion that had been absent as she had recounted all the details of her son's life, began to seep into her face. Her expression was familiar to me. It asked, "Could I help her son?"

As an infant, Lewis had undergone open-heart surgery to repair a hole in his heart. Six years later he was back in the operating room for a second round of open-heart surgery. This time there were complications, and a third surgery was scheduled to implant a pacemaker. At 6 years of age, Lewis's chest was opened and a pacemaker was inserted and subsequently attached to his heart, to keep it beating at the right speed and to keep it from stopping.

With a pacemaker inside his body, Lewis had to become a more cautious child, being ever aware of the dangers that were possible if friends got too rowdy during a game of tag. An unintentional shove to the chest was much more serious than what would have otherwise been a few passing moments of having the wind knocked out of you. Lewis had to refrain from all contact sports to avoid the possibility of dislodging the pacemaker in such a small body.

Lewis had been present in several of the meetings with the cardiologists and surgeons. His mom and dad wondered to what extent he understood the dangers involved in these surgeries as well as his condition, in general. Later Lewis would tell me that he had overheard his doctors talk openly about the possibility that the pacemaker may not be the solution, that there might be a need for further surgeries and that he might not survive this surgery. Lewis was now forced to consider at the age of 7 the fact that he was more fragile than other children and that he might even die.

FORMULATION OF THE PROBLEM

Lewis had struggled for some time to manage his fears and emotions regarding his physical condition. The fall following the sexual abuse, Lewis's difficulties became more pervasive and heightened both at home and at school. Symptoms manifested as an attempt to hold things together, to survive, and to make sense of what seemed a very dangerous world. Lewis's teachers and counselors were in frequent contact with his mom and dad with reports of Lewis acting up, disrespecting adults, not doing as he was told, and being generally disruptive. Lewis had a low tolerance for change and was easily frustrated. At home his anxiety manifested in nightmares, stomachaches, sleep difficulties, inflexibility, irritability, and enduring fears. Mom and Dad both reported that these symptoms were amplified at times of transition. Lewis could not sleep alone in his room and often became so anxious that he would become physically sick and throw up. Dad saw Lewis as having an insatiable need for attention and had a difficult time understanding how to help, given that these episodes seemed to be triggered by seemingly minor events.

Mother reported that socially, Lewis was more of a loner and did not have many close friends. His social activities outside of school were limited to noncontact sports and activities that were not too physically rigorous. To engage with his peers meant being mindful at all times that if things got too rough, he would have to step out. Lewis's mother and father both admitted to frustrations as Lewis lost interest in activities he had once pushed for, including karate, Boy Scouts, and music lessons.

My formulation of the current problems was the following: Lewis was struggling with feelings of vulnerability and lack of personal control, further exacerbated by this recent interpersonal trauma at the hands of a trusted friend who had seduced him into feeling special and worthy of someone's friendship. This making of a friend in youth is a necessary step in developing a positive self-image (Berzoff, 1996), especially in Lewis's case, wherein medical vulnerability had left him feeling stigmatized and socially isolated. The sexual abuse also parodied experiences of physical intrusion he experienced during medical procedures. Steve's sadistic and exploitive behavior toward Lewis had increased Lewis's feelings of helplessness—which he sought to combat by developing compensatory aggression.

Lewis's parents had come to me to help them understand their son and to help him heal. The process that unfolded would at times be bumpy, misguided, and clumsy. Yet ultimately it would be extraordinary, significant, and beautiful, and a shift would occur that changed everything.

INVITATION TO PLAY THERAPY: THE FEARFUL EXPLORER AND WARRIOR

Lewis was 7 years old when his family brought him to see me for therapy. He was tall and thin with curly brown hair and big blue eyes. Lewis's shirt covered a raised pink scar that went down the center of his chest. In his tank top you could see the top of the scar peeking out, and you could almost sense the pain dwelling behind the scar. Lewis was a weary child who appeared to be taking in the details of all that was going on around him. He seemed small and fragile, although he presented with much bravado. Lewis wanted to let me know he was in charge and would decide how this all turned out. I wanted to help him.

In my first session with Lewis he asked me if I knew what had happened over the summer with his friend Steve. I told Lewis that I had met with his mother and father, and they had explained to me that Steve had touched and hurt his private parts. Lewis told me that he did not have any worries about Steve, and in fact, he did not worry about anything at all. Lewis had never met me before, and I imagine he wanted to impress upon me that he was okay and did not need me. In all the time Lewis spent proving to me that he was strong and in control, he didn't realize that I had seen and appreciated his strength before we had ever even met.

I showed Lewis around my office and told him that he could choose whatever he wanted to do while we met together. I pointed to the easel and paints, the sandbox and miniatures, puppets, board games, and other possible activities. As is my custom, I made no demands beyond ensuring that we both knew why he had come to therapy.

CASE ILLUSTRATION OF SELF-DIRECTED TRAUMA PLAY

The Beginning: Setting the Stage

The first couple of months were spent developing a relationship and a space that Lewis would be able to use to do the work he needed. I spent much of these months observing as Lewis fought violent battle after battle in the sand. Warriors were picked for each side, armed with swords and axes (Figure 6.1).

There was trickery and betrayal, and the warriors never knew whom to trust. Lewis was very much a part of the world he was creating in the sand tray. His sound effects mimicked the pain and suffering of the wounded as well as the anger and aggression of the warriors. Lewis shared that there was always war in his world. In these wars soldiers were stabbed, axed, and punctured. Large traps were erected in such a manner that the soldiers would walk over a hill and land on a large pile of swords and knives. When animals were introduced, their strength and power were determined by the sharpness of their teeth. Lewis showed me how sharp, intrusive, and penetrating the sword, scalpel, or hand could be.

Intermittently during this time, I introduced other play-based assessment tools to better understand this young boy and all that was going on inside of him. I used what I knew were helpful tools in understanding a child's world. For example, I asked Lewis to participate in

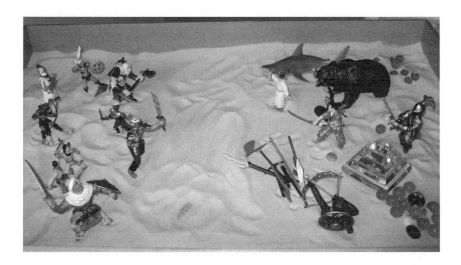

FIGURE 6.1. Warriors do battle.

making a "family play genogram" (McGoldrick & Gil, 2008), in which he could choose miniatures to show his thoughts and feelings about everyone in his family, including himself (Figure 6.2).

Each family member was depicted as a warrior. He created worlds in the sand that incorporated his family into battles over crystals that could keep people from ever dying and that saved all the babies in the world. Not surprisingly, these crystals (and their implied magical powers over life and death) became the cause of all the battles that followed.

Interested in the focused range of emotions that he was showing, I asked Lewis to participate in an art activity called "Color Your Feelings" (Hopkins, Huici, & Bermudez, 2005). In this activity, children are asked to make a list of the feelings they have "most of the time," then choose one color that best shows that feeling, and finally, to show the type and intensity of feelings they feel in their bodies in one or more than one situation.

Lewis identified and acknowledged feelings of weirdness, anger, worry, happiness, sadness, and confusion. Using color to represent each emotion, he showed me how much he felt these emotions and where in his body he felt them. I noted that he had a broad range of feelings that included, but were not limited to, anger (Figure 6.3).

While engaged in some play or expressive task, Lewis would occasionally look up at me with uncertainty and share some nugget of information before he turned back to his work. He began talking more

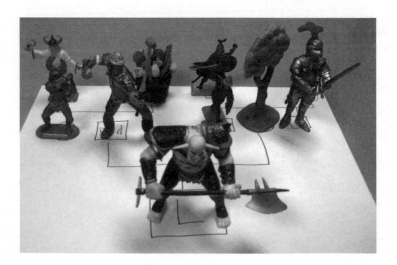

FIGURE 6.2. Family play genogram.

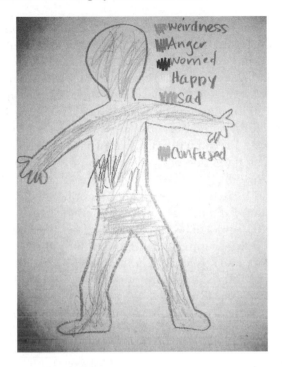

FIGURE 6.3. Color your feelings.

openly about his heart. He told me that he had to see his doctor every 6 months to make sure he was healthy. He spoke about the gel they put on his chest before doing an ultrasound and the bad videos that they offered him to keep him distracted. Lewis spoke with me about what he thought other children might need to know if they were going to have heart surgery. He thought it was important that they know that anesthesia stinks, that they can't eat 12 hours before surgery and that moms can help them remember that, that they will definitely feel scared, and that you will have scars—but scars can be cool. Lewis shared that kids needed to know that they could end up with a pacemaker, that it would later have to be replaced in another surgery, and that they are helpful but you have to be careful because the doctors will worry that the wires might break. Lewis informed me that other children would probably worry about dying, as he did, but that if they are healthy it shouldn't be a problem because he was healthy and he had survived.

   Lewis also began talking about the sexual abuse. Rather than talking directly about that day in the woods, he would bring in books about healthy sexual development and healthy touching. He would proudly show me his books and explore each page and chapter with me. Lewis began talking more about Steve and his worries that Steve was being held in some jail somewhere until he would tell the truth about what happened. Lewis worried that Steve wasn't getting enough food and that maybe he didn't have anything to do all day but sit in his room. Lewis spoke some about how his body and mind felt confused by Steve's attention to him and wondered out loud what that meant about him. As Lewis began talking about the sexual abuse, I began to introduce directive tasks to address it. Lewis typically engaged in these tasks and, although they addressed some of his needs, not much changed.

In these first few months Lewis shared with me a great deal through both his play and his spoken words. He and I were developing a relationship. Lewis was slowly beginning to trust that it might be all right to let me help him find a way to feel better, to feel safe again. Lewis became adept at talking to me about his surgeries, the sexual abuse, and the manifestations of all the feelings and worries somehow connected to these. Yet, even as we connected his thoughts, feelings, behaviors, and experiences, Lewis did not seem to get better. There was no shift in his experience of the world, no resolution, and no mastery. It was clear that he still felt that the world was a dangerous place, and he was still a very fragile boy. And while it was a challenge, I trusted that Lewis would show me in time what I was missing and what he needed. As the trust grew and our relationship became more valuable to him, he showed me his reparative process.

The Middle: The Work Deepens and Moves— Understanding the Brokenhearted

Lewis needed to work through what had happened to him: the loss of control over his body, the intrusiveness of the multiple penetrations to his chest and body, the fear of dying, and the loss of trust and safety. I felt like I needed to find a way to facilitate this work for him, but in reality I just needed to bear witness, to support him in finding his own way, and to be emotionally present. I also needed to create a predictable environment and a relationship of respect and trust—these had taken months to carefully construct.

Lewis expressed his dilemmas, fears, and internal conflicts in his anger, defiance, isolation, and anxieties. His anger was likely compensatory to experiences of helplessness in his early, formative years. Lewis was only an infant when doctors and surgeons opened up his tiny little

chest for the first time. Developmentally, children at this age are beginning to explore the world outside of their primary caretakers, prompted
by the novel experience of rolling, crawling, and eventually walking. I
have to imagine that Lewis's exploration may have been inhibited by
his fragile condition and by his considerably concerned and protective
parents. What was Lewis learning of the world outside of himself? And
what was he learning about the world inside of himself?

When Lewis turned 6, he was back in the operating room again,
with his chest opened up, his life at risk, and surgeons doing their job
to mend his heart with their hands and tools inside of him, working to
repair what was broken. Children rarely have to worry if their hearts
will keep on beating, if they will beat on time, and if they will grow in
tandem with their developing bodies. At an age when children are facing the developmental task of entering the social world and developing
a sense of industry (Erikson, 1963), and should be able to feel capable
and worthwhile, Lewis was learning he could not trust that his heart
would keep beating and that he would keep on living. Lewis and his
mom and dad met with the doctors regularly to check on the shape of
his heart and how he was healing. The doctors reported to all of them,
Lewis included, that Lewis did need a pacemaker. This pacemaker could
regulate his heart and keep him healthy. The doctors reported that this
pacemaker would have to be replaced again, and thus another surgery
was definite in Lewis's future. They also reported the possibility that the
pacemaker would not work and/or that the surgery would be too trying
on Lewis's little body. The doctors reported that Lewis could die, con-
firming this boy's and his parents' worst fears.

At 6 years of age, Lewis was learning that control over his body
was externally located, whether in the hands of doctors or the small
electrical mechanism lodged in his body to regulate his heart. Those in
control could be unreliable and even hurt him. Lewis had also learned
that he was vulnerable and fragile. It was necessary for him to be more
vigilant and on guard to ensure that his heart was safe and protected.
So as his social world began to widen with the start of school and group
play, he carried with him the knowledge that he was somehow different,
less secure and safe, and had to exercise extreme care.

The subsequent trauma of sexual abuse by a trusted and admired
friend awakened the familiar fears and conflicts inherent in this child's
early experiences. The sexual abuse served as an affective bridge to
Lewis's earlier experiences of intrusion, penetration, exposure, and loss
of control. The sexual abuse taught him that he was unsafe trusting others, and the medical traumas taught him he was unsafe trusting himself.

Together, these experiences solidified an internal working model of the world as a dangerous place.

Siegel and Hartzell (2003) (p. 148) explain the brain correlates of the internal working model:

> From a brain point of view, we can say that such a mental process is "ingrained" in patterns of neuronal firing in which past experiences and the adaptations that were generated in response to them create synaptic connections that are retained in memory. In the case of attachment, the model overlaps with a form of implicit memory: it is embedded early in our lives, is activated without a sense that something is being recalled, and directly influences our perceptions, emotions, behaviors, and bodily sensations. The mental models inherent in such learning are at the heart of what John Bowlby called "internal working models" of attachment.

Lewis's working through of the sexual abuse meant a working through of his cumulative medical traumas. Each trauma was connected to the other by the affective experience of helplessness and lack of control. They were no longer singular events but a web of experiences connected by common feelings of terror, powerlessness, confusion, and heartbreak. Each left him feeling vulnerable, afraid, and unsafe, and each was a violation of his mind and body that left him exposed and powerless. The work Lewis would do in therapy was an expression and a working through of a cumulative trauma. The swords and knives were the weapons of his battles for safety, for the safety of children and babies. This is what Lewis knew and what he had to work though.

"We Don't Want You to Freak Out"

Lewis and I were meeting once a week for therapy. A few months into our work together, Lewis attended a doctor's appointment with his cardiologist immediately prior to our session. When Lewis arrived that day, he told me that he liked his doctors and that they had taken good care of him. He brought in a book that the doctors had been giving out to all the pediatric cardiology patients that week. It was a simple book about the heart, what it looked like and how it worked. Lewis told me that he wasn't sure what his own heart looked like. He imagined it was different from healthy hearts, maybe misshaped or discolored. Lewis had undergone insertion of a heart catheter prior to his more recent surgeries, and he knew that the heart catheter had captured video and pictures of his heart. Lewis said that the doctors had not let him see the video or pictures because they thought it would freak him out. Lewis assumed that meant there was something very wrong with his heart that the doctors must have wanted to keep from him. He was curious about what the heart looked like, and what his own heart might look like. I began pulling up pictures on the Internet of children's hearts, both healthy and hurt. Lewis poured over these pictures at the beginning of our sessions, wondering out loud about the different shapes, sizes, and distinctions of each heart. Energy was stirring during these moments in our sessions. I could sense the wheels turning in Lewis's head and became more at ease with the idea that he would find his way.

Lewis arrived late one day to session and was frustrated at being thrown off schedule. He still did not do well with transitions or changes to plans. He asked if we could skip our usual routine and play a game for the remaining time. Out of the stack of nearly 20 different board games Lewis chose Operation, and for the remaining 25 minutes of our session Lewis and I played this game. For those who are not familiar with the Milton Bradley game, the board itself is an operating table lithographed with the naked body of "Sam Cavity," who has numerous openings on the surface of his body. Figuratively named ailments, such as "Butterflies in the Stomach," "Writer's Cramp," and "Broken Heart," are crafted into small white plastic pieces and are placed in each opening. Using a pair of tweezers, each player attempts to remove the ailment from the body on the operating table without touching the metal sides of the opening. If the tweezers touch the metal edge, the electrical circuit becomes closed, a loud buzzer sounds, Sam Cavity's lightbulb red nose lights up, and the player loses his or her turn.

The game itself wasn't all that remarkable to anyone else watching. Lewis became frustrated when his tweezers hit the metal. Each time the buzzer went off, the energy in the room seemed to amp up more and more. Lewis became angry at the operating board, claiming that it was lying and wrong about his failed attempts to remove the little white ailments. Eventually he stopped letting me take a turn and tried over and over to remove the little pieces without the shocking jump of the buzzer. When this didn't work Lewis became louder and more upset, shouting at Sam Cavity to "die, die, die." Lewis became determined to remove all the ailments and stopped paying any attention to the red lit-up nose or jarring buzzing. He became hurried and less precise, but every little white-pieced ailment ended up on the table in front of us and out of Sam Cavity's body. Lewis's urgency and intensity seemed motivated by a need to extract, a need to remove the toxin and the intruder, and a need to do it with surgical precision, without making a costly mistake.

When he was unable to do so successfully, he ignored the alarms and proceeded to give way to the possibility that even an error would not cause death.

This game was quite remarkable to me. In it the cumulative experience was tackled. The implications of the task of Operation suited both the sexual abuse and the more obvious surgeries. But the game I witnessed didn't distinguish between the two. It was not just removing the broken heart, the writer's cramp, or the butterflies in the stomach. It was expelling those things that had filled up the hollows of Sam Cavity's body. The work changed after this session—things were moving and mastery was in motion. Lewis was undertaking the job of opening his wounds to heal them and to have a different experience.

My agency's offices were moving and as our playrooms were getting packed up and ready to be put on the truck, Lewis's weekly session arrived. Rather than taking a break from therapy for a couple of weeks due to the move, Lewis and I met in the boardroom of our building. I brought in some art supplies and a few other items I thought we might use for an improvised play therapy session. Instead, Lewis directed his attention to our boardroom's large mobile electronic dry erase board. Lewis went immediately to it and quickly realized its special trick of printing out what was written on the board. At that board, with the dry erase marker in hand, Lewis transformed himself into a doctor leading a group of other doctors through a difficult surgery to assess the viability of a patient's heart. This imagined patient lay on the meeting table in our boardroom, and Lewis focused his attention on conferencing with the other doctors and mapping out the ailments of this patient's body on the electronic dry erase board. Lewis's voice was hushed as he acted out these scenes with the other doctors, and he covered his writings and illustrations. The patient and myself were left in the dark about what the doctors were seeing and saying—a very disempowered position, for sure. Every so often Lewis would move away from the board to allow me to peek at what he was mapping out. There was a small body drawn on the board with arrows pointing at, into, and around the head, with more arrows pointing to the heart and stomach as Lewis continued his conferencing. I marveled at his introduction of drama therapy at this point (and later on) and how it provided him with the mechanism for transitioning from a passive role (patient) to an active role (surgeon). Drama therapy has great potential as an expressive therapy technique in that it allows children to meet overwhelming challenges and express countless levels of conscious and unconscious material in productive and protected ways (James, Forrester, & Kim, 2005).

Eventually Lewis pushed "Print" and the details of the electronic dry erase board were magically transplanted onto a sheet of white paper. Lewis brought this piece of paper to me, reporting that he and a team of very smart doctors had discovered what was wrong with the patient. Lewis emphasized that they were very *smart* doctors and very good at what they did. He was letting me in on their secret. He told me that he knew that the patient was feeling very scared because of all the medical talk around him that he didn't understand, but that it was important that he not know what was going on. Lewis said in order to save him, the patient could not know what was going to happen. He showed me the multiple incision sites to which the arrows pointed on the patient's brain, chest, and stomach. Lewis added a small drawing to the printout from the dry erase board. It was a square table with a stick figure drawn in the center with little circles added to the end of each arm and leg. Lewis was moving quickly, then slowed down to turn and look at me. He told me that when he'd had his heart catheter inserted, they had to hold his hands and arms in place so that he would not move. He had to be entirely still as the catheter was inserted through his groin. I imagined this small child and the many moments he had now experienced in which he had been rendered helpless and immovable, with his hands and feet tied down, powerless to stop the pain and hurt. Lewis was not just detailing a single memory of a specific moment in time. Instead it seemed he was communicating collective memories and experiences of helplessness and lack of control over his own body.

Mending a Broken Heart

Lewis was navigating his way back, and I followed his lead. After the scenes in the boardroom I became keenly aware of the drive toward mastery in this little boy. This knowledge comforted me. I became more at ease and more trusting of the process that was unfolding. When we met again, it was in my agency's new home, and Lewis spent much of our first session in the new building exploring his new space. In his exploration, Lewis discovered the newly stocked art therapy room. He opened each cabinet, taking out the different materials and turning them in his hands before putting them back onto their shelves. He used the metal chair in the room as a ladder to reach the higher cabinets, where he found the molding clay that had just been purchased earlier that week. Lewis pulled the tub down from the shelf, opened it up, and began working the clay with his hands. It seemed he had found what he was looking for.

Lewis wanted to create a heart out of the clay. We collected the pictures of hearts, broken and whole, that we had cataloged together, and Lewis shaped the white clay into a heart. Along the way, Lewis invited me to join the process. He assigned me the task of creating arteries, by rolling the clay between my hands into a long hose, which I was then instructed to cut into smaller pieces that would be attached to the heart, at the site of the arteries. He seemed to trust that I would get it right and left me to my own devices. As he worked with his hands to create this heart, there was a great deal happening. Nervous, productive, and healing energies swirled around the room and kept pace with the thoughts racing through Lewis's mind and body. As Lewis shaped and molded this heart in his hands, he spoke to me about our next step: finding a pacemaker for his heart. We brainstormed different possibilities, things that looked like a pacemaker or were similar in size. Lewis even suggested that we check in with his doctors to see if they had any spares lying around.

The process of choosing the pacemaker was the first of several times in which the larger community would lend their hearts and minds to the healing of Lewis. I had brought the dilemma of choosing a pacemaker into supervision for a hearty dose of brainstorming when lo and behold, my supervisor and I were both incredibly moved by what followed.

She went home that same evening to further brainstorm with her husband, who happened to work in the electrical trade. The next day he went to his office, gathered his team, and posed to them the following question: Among their gadgets, wires, and electronics stored away in their toolboxes, what did they have that resembled a pacemaker? He briefly described to them that a child with a pacemaker was making a clay replica of his heart and now wanted to attach a fairly representational object that could serve as the pacemaker. By day's end, six electricians had gathered up their best trinkets and enthusiastically made their case for why their gadget should be selected over others. My supervisor came into the office the following morning and invited me into her room to see the pile of contraptions that her husband had brought home the night before. They had lights and wires, were square and round, big and small, of all shapes and sizes. I was so excited and so touched by the idea that busy electricians, who did not know this little boy, had taken time out of their busy schedules to find just the right piece for him. They wanted to help him, just as I did. That same week I placed all the gadgets on the table in front of Lewis and watched his eyes grow with curiosity, excitement, and wonder. Lewis asked where these gifts had come from, and I shared with him the story of their journey to our table. Lewis smiled quietly and slowly picked up each and every piece, studying it from all sides before making his selection. Most of the time Lewis seemed to be surrounded by a cloud of frenzied energy, so when there was a moment when he seemed to slow down, catch his breath, and look me in the eye, there was simply no missing it. Lewis's experience with the pacemakers was one of these times, and it had repaired something Lewis could not have repaired on his own.

As the centerpiece for his heart, Lewis chose a yellow transparent plastic box with some mechanical gadgetry inside and eight metal prongs mounted on top. He cut out a small hole in the center of the heart and worked the clay back with his hands as he pushed the box into the clay. With the yellow-boxed pacemaker in the center of the heart, it seemed finished—and indeed Lewis announced that the heart was complete. It was a beautiful heart (Figure 6.4).

That week we left the plastic covering off the heart for the first time, and it began to dry. This heart had been molded and cradled by the hands of this young boy, by my own, and by the inspiration of others that Lewis had never met. This heart was touched by many, and many aided in its repair. Steve had broken Lewis's heart by hurting and tricking him rather than loving him. The world had let Lewis down by not protecting him and by being an unsafe place for him to explore and master. The repair that had and would take place in the mending of this heart was

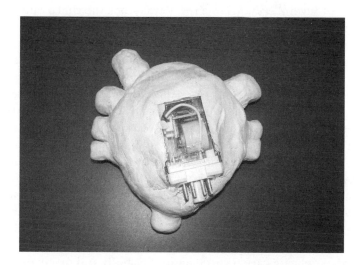

FIGURE 6.4. The pacemaker completes the heart!

repair on many different levels. It was repair of his emotions, his trust in others, his heart, and soul. It was an invitation to heal.

Body Building

Lewis kept moving forward, and I found myself at the art store picking up boxes of clay to bring back to our sessions so that he could begin crafting a body for the heart. It seemed the natural next step. Three reddish brown blocks of hard clay sat on a wooden plank in the center of the art room table. Lewis asked for my help, explaining that we were to fashion a head, shoulders, and a chest out of these three blocks of clay. At the end of each session we carefully wrapped up the clay in sheets of plastic and carried the wooden plank with the partially molded body down the hall from the art room to my office, storing it safely under my sofa. It became routine: Each week when Lewis came to his session, we pulled out the wooden plank and body from under the sofa, carried them on a makeshift stretcher to the art room, and worked at molding the clay into a body. I had found a set of clay modeling tools that I thought could be helpful for attaching eyes and creating textures in the clay. I somehow had overlooked their obvious resemblance to surgical tools, but Lewis had not. As this body was being built, it was also poked and prodded, opened and shut, punctured, invaded, and smoothed back over. As Lewis operated on this body, he told his story. This was the story of his heart surgery, but also the story of Steve and the aftermath of Steve. For several sessions in a row Lewis stuck the sharp end of each and every tool into the head of the body (Figure 6.5).

I could not help but notice the magnitude of these penetrations into this small body that had been molded by Lewis's own hands. I had become protective of this little body Lewis was building and felt pained by its recurring wounds. I felt compelled to shield this head from the sharp tools but stepped aside. This was a story of actual physical intrusion and the intrusion of thoughts, memories, and fears. Talking alone had not expelled the intruders. As Lewis was telling his story, working with his hands, he was healing his heart and he allowed me to be a part of, and now a witness to, this remarkable process (Sholt & Gavron, 2006). We pushed and hammered and rolled the clay as it came into form. When he needed to work on the back of the body or the shoulders, Lewis would ask that I gently lift the body so that he could reach. I found myself supporting the head as if it were a baby or a small infant that needed delicate care. I cared about this body and protecting it and nurturing it. Lewis saw that and mimicked it in his own care and han-

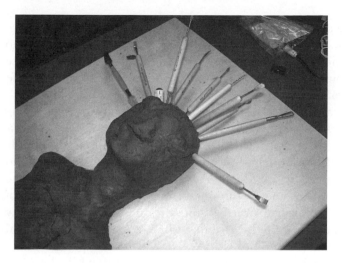

FIGURE 6.5. Scarring the clay head.

dling. It seemed that my nurturing and caring for this body gave him permission to do the same.

There were sessions in which Lewis needed to take a break from his clay body. He would check under the sofa to make sure all was in its place and then ask to play catch with a small soccer ball in my office or to play a game of Uno. Nevertheless, Lewis would always return to his clay body and create and shape just a little more. Large round eyes and a crooked nose were shaped from the round mound that was the head. A chin and lips forming a twisting smile slowly arose from the lower part of the face. Even a belly button was shaped out of a small poke hole to the lower belly. This was a very human little boy growing out of the three blocks of clay that had been put onto that table. The body was finished, and he was named Bob, and what Bob needed now was a heart.

Transitions Occur: Pass the Scalpel

In the weekly transfers on the stretcher between my office and the art room, the people at my agency came to know Bob. They looked forward to seeing him grow and develop as the weeks passed. They asked about him during the periods of time when he was resting under the sofa (when Lewis needed a break from him). As Bob was carried down the hall each week, staff couldn't help but notice his shoulders broadening, his hair coming in, and the two new eyes that sat squarely on his face.

Lewis seemed touched and surprised by the attention that Bob and he received. And although he rarely engaged in these conversations, the admiration he sensed seemed to bring a quiet smile to his face. Lewis was allowing in the warmth and care from others who were safe, which was clearly a sign of tremendous progress.

It was time for Bob to get his heart. Lewis was nervous on the day of the transplant. A great deal of planning took place beforehand, but it almost seemed as if the planning was a means of stalling rather than an actual tool to help figure out how and where Lewis wanted to put Bob's heart. The fear I sensed in the room was not Lewis's alone. I, too, felt the nervous energy running through my body and some apprehension about moving forward. I think the question on our minds was what would happen if the heart didn't work. What is interesting is that this was a heart made out of clay. The only concrete question was whether this already hardened heart would cause cracking in the still wet and malleable clay body. Although this was a real concern and an important one at that, the real question seemed much larger. Would Lewis be okay? The focus in the room that day seemed to be on the latter.

Lewis used the molding tool that looked most like a scalpel to trace the area he planned to cut out. It was a sizeable heart that would fill up the whole of Bob's chest. Lewis was thoughtful and precise in the steps he took to place the heart in the body. He started on his own, digging out the clay with the scalpel, little bit by little bit. I watched him as he pulled chunks of clay off the sharp end of the tool. A little while into the project he stopped to examine the selection of tools laid out next to Bob. He picked up a duplicate of the tool he was using and handed it to me, reminiscent of a surgeon and his or her surgical assistant. Slowly we carved out a large hole in Bob's chest. We had to be careful not to dig too far because the heart still needed a place to rest, and yet we needed to be sure to make enough room to hold the large heart and its pacemaker. When we stopped, we looked at this little body and its big empty hole in its chest. There was a pause for a few moments and then our energy was focused back into the surgery. What existed now was the simple knowledge that it was time to put in the heart.

Lewis gently lowered the heart into Bob's chest. He picked up the little pieces of clay he had carved out and pushed them into the spaces between the heart and the chest wall. I joined in as we carefully secured the heart in his chest. The solid white heart with its transparent yellow pacemaker stood out in contrast to the terra-cotta clay body (Figure 6.6). It was defined and pronounced, and one's eyes were drawn to it. Lewis found the bag with the spare pacemaker parts and chose some

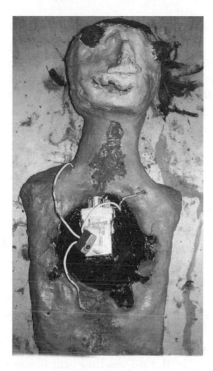

FIGURE 6.6. The body accommodates the pacemaker.

wires to connect the heart to his body. I watched as Lewis used a sharp
tool to make some deep marks in Bob's neck and stomach. These were
Bob's scars. At the end of session that day we didn't wrap Bob up before
putting him under the sofa. I found myself checking on him during the
week, pulling him out every so often to make sure that everything was
okay. During the time that Bob was drying, we pulled the stretcher out
from under the sofa and tended to any cracks or fissures with superglue,
clay, and water. Lewis and I took turns tenderly lifting up Bob's head
from the wooden plank to check for cracking on his back or shoulders.
If we needed to, we would gently turn him over, and I would hold Bob's
face in my hands so as not to smush or hurt his nose or eyes while Lewis
would work on the cracks that appeared in his back. Slowly Bob dried,
and all his cracks were tended to with care and love.

Lewis decided it was time to give Bob some color, so he started mixing different oranges, pinks, and browns to reach just the right peach
skin tone he wanted for Bob. Bob was given bright teal-blue eyes that
matched Lewis's own. His hair turned a shade of black and his lips had

a pinkish hue. The darker pink color pronounced the scars above and below the heart.

I had imagined that Lewis would choose a pink or red to color the actual heart. Instead he chose black, without any hesitation. I had a strong reaction to this choice; it didn't seem to fit with all that had been repaired and mastered in this room. I wanted it to be red or pink or even yellow, but of course I kept my feelings to myself. I made a mental note that the color black is often associated with death, darkness, and night-time. I consulted a book of symbols, which further defined black "as an absence of all light and colour. Black sucks in colour and does not return it. Above all, it suggests chaos, nothingness, night sky, night shadows on the ground, evil, anguish, sorrow, the unconscious, and death" (Chevalier & Gheerbrant, 1996, p. 95). I struggled to keep myself from questioning or even suggesting he choose another color. I realized how attached I had become to Bob and what he represented to me. I also saw that in some ways Bob represented more and something a shade different for Lewis. Bob carried the scars of this child, and maybe Bob carried the mark of pain so that Lewis himself did not have to bear it any longer.

As the last touches of paint were seen to, it was time to consider a proper goodbye to Bob. Before sending him home, though, I thought it would be important to sit with Lewis's mom and dad and to talk with them about their son and the incredible piece of work he had done. In my office that day Lewis's mom and dad got to know more about Bob, and I learned more about what Bob had done for Lewis. Lewis's parents saw changes in Lewis. He was sleeping through the night without any difficulties, and it had been months since the school had called with any complaints about his behaviors. Although he still liked to know what to expect, when plans changed it was not a trigger for the meltdown it used to be. Just as significant were the changes that were not linked to specific behaviors but were felt by Lewis, his mom, his dad, and myself. Things felt different for this child, and this child felt things differently.

I talked more with Lewis's parents about Bob and my plans for how to honor what Bob had become for Lewis and the relationships that we had all developed with him. It took a little explaining on my part for them to understand my plans for a fitting goodbye, but they went with it and became vital parts to its success. I am always grateful for moments when parents can reach back and connect to the parts of themselves that believe in the power of play and imagination. Lewis's mom and dad were both smart and thinking adults. They both loved their son very much and showed him much affection, patience, and kindness. I believe play therapy was a leap of faith for these great minds that might have been more comfortable with more planned and precise methods of addressing problems. I marvel at the trust some parents muster up in this process that can seem so far off and foreign to them. Lewis's parents let me spend months with their son creating a body out of clay. Along the way they chose to trust my assurances and explanations that this was real therapeutic work, and I believe that their trust in this process and me allowed for their son to trust as well.

Closure

At the time I met with Lewis's mom and dad I didn't know exactly what we were going to need to say goodbye to Bob, but I did know that they would need to be a part of it. This felt like an opportunity to connect all the pieces and to share warmth and love for this boy and his creation in a very safe way.

I spent some time thinking about what I wanted to do for Lewis and Bob to say goodbye, and it took some time for me to realize that it was not for me to decide. Lewis was the only one who knew what Bob needed to feel safe and cared for in his departure. I sensed that Bob was going to need to be taken care of and made to feel safe before he was ready to go home. I had been at the grocery store across from the office to pick up some lunch and thought that maybe I should grab some Band-Aids to bring into my session with Lewis later that day. I found it difficult picking up only Band-Aids and ended up with a basket filled with gauze pads, surgical masks, and medical tape. As I unloaded these supplies onto the little table in my office, my desire to fix Bob was evident to me and anyone else who stepped in to see the table spilling over with bandages.

When Lewis came in that day, he sorted through the supplies on the table and picked out a surgical mask, one gauze pad, and some tape. The rest of the pile sat there untouched. Maybe Bob did not need as much as I had thought. Lewis put the surgical mask on and took out the doctor's kit that was sitting on a shelf under the sand tray. Lewis acted as Bob's doctor and even took the name of his own surgeon. He used the plastic stethoscope to check out Bob's heart and brain and taped the small gauze bandage over one of his scars. I asked Dr. Lewis what Bob would need before he could be released from the hospital. As he checked Bob out, he relayed to me that Bob wasn't feeling any pain because he was still under anesthesia. Lewis turned to me and stated that Bob would need his therapist to take care of him before he could go home. Lewis told me that I would need to be sure that Bob could walk before he could leave. He said that I would need to let Bob sleep and that I would need to talk to him about the surgery and explain what had happened, but only if Bob wanted to talk or listen. I was to respect what Bob needed. Lewis said I would need to tell Bob that it was okay for him to ask questions and that I needed to be there to answer any questions he had. I was also tasked with teaching Bob about his heart, its capabilities and limitations, and what it meant to have a pacemaker. My own heart was touched by the responsibility I had been given. I took this job very seriously and in the week between this session and his last, I spoke with Bob in the quiet moments I had between sessions. In those moments I connected to Lewis and his changing experience of the world and the people in it.

Lewis had also outlined fairly clearly what kind of special foods Bob would want on his last day in the hospital, including Tootsie Rolls and Pixy Stix. I put together a little bag of treats and tied a helium balloon to it that read "Get Well Soon." The spirit of the session was cheerful and celebratory. We talked about Bob and took pictures. Lewis lay down beside him and made bunny ears behind his head (Figure 6.7).

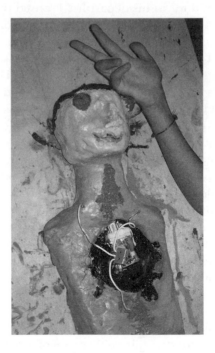

FIGURE 6.7. Playing with Bob.

We talked about what Bob would need when he got home from the hospital and who could help him. Lewis talked about plans he and his mom had made about where Bob would live in their home. Lewis's mom helped us load Bob into the do-it-yourself wheelchair I had fashioned out of a cardboard box, and together they carried him down the hall to the door. Different members of our staff who had become familiar with, and even attached to, Bob greeted them in the hall as they walked out, and wished Bob a speedy recovery.

I watched as Lewis and his mom loaded Bob into the car. I felt my own pangs of pride and loss as he left. I would miss Bob and the magic that he had created. As they drove away I was taken with the transformation that Bob had incurred in Lewis and us all. I didn't need to bandage Bob with my piles of gauze pads and tape; Lewis was strong enough on his own to take care of his body and heart. This capable young man could feel the warmth of others and the warmth in his own heart. And what a strong, kind heart it was.

SUMMARY OF CLINICAL IMPRESSIONS

Bob was a work of art. He brought life and healing to a boy, his family and his therapist. In creating Bob, Lewis told his story. The repair that ensued healed the wounds of many hurts. The sexual abuse had confirmed what Lewis's body and soul feared after so many surgeries: that the world was an unsafe place, that Lewis was disposed to pain, that he was powerless to prevent it, and that control of his mind and body lay outside his reach. To understand Lewis's story it must be understood that the traumas of his life were not singular events. The violations and intrusion of his body were affectively bridged to one another and became a cumulative experience of being in this world. And it was that experience that needed to be touched and transformed. Bob's creation was not a simple mastery of surgical procedures but rather the telling, shaping, and mending of a heartbreaking story and a heartbroken boy.

My initial attempts to sort through, process, and address the traumas of Lewis's life were helpful to him. He heard that the abuse was not his fault. He learned about loving and safe touches, how to breathe through his panic, and how to address his worries. But it was Lewis who showed me what he needed to do to transform his cumulative traumatic experiences into events that he could manage and overcome. Creating Bob allowed for the seeds of trust to be planted, the love and kindness of others to be accepted, and what was in the past to be honored and put away. Lewis was able to reclaim his body as his own and to take back control. Bob held on to the dark parts of Lewis's heart and, most likely, his fear of death and in doing so freed Lewis from them.

Lewis and Bob needed each other. Bob needed Lewis to give him life, and Lewis needed Bob to carry his fear of death and vulnerability, which had encroached on his ability to live life more fully.

REFERENCES

Berzoff, J. (1996). Psychosocial ego development: The theory of Erik Erikson. In J. Berzoff, L. Melano Flanagan, & P. Hertz (Eds.), *Inside out and outside in: Psychodynamic clinical theory and practice in contemporary multicultural contexts* (pp. 103–125). Northvale, NJ: Jason Aronson.

Chevalier, J., & Gheerbrant, A. (1996). *A dictionary of symbols* (J. Buchanan-Brown, Trans.). New York: Penguin Books.

Erikson, E. H. (1963). *Childhood and society* (2nd ed.). New York: Norton.

Hopins, S., Huici, V., & Bermudez, D. (2005). Therapeutic play with Hispanic clients. In E. Gil & A. Drewes (Eds.), *Cultural issues in play therapy* (pp.148–167). New York: Guilford Press.

James, M., Forrester, A.M., & Kim, K.C. (2005). Developmental transformations in the treatment of sexually abused children. In A. M. Weber & C. Haen (Eds.), *Clinical applications of drama therapy in child and adolescent treatment* (pp. 67–86). New York: Brunner-Routledge.

McGoldrick, M., & Gil, E. (2008). Family play genograms. In M. McGoldrick, R. Gerson, & S. Petry, *Genograms: Assessment and intervention* (3rd ed., pp. 257–274). New York: Norton.

Sholt, M., & Gavron, T. (2006). Therapeutic qualities of clay-work in art therapy and psychotherapy: A review. *Art Therapy: Journal of the American Art Therapy Association, 23*(2), pp. 66–72.

Siegel, D. J., & Hartzell, M. (2003). *Parenting from the inside out: How a deeper self-understanding can help you raise children who thrive.* New York: Tarcher/ Penguin.

CHAPTER 7

A Hero's Journey

A Boy Who Lost His Parents and Found Himself

VINCENT L. PASTORE

In recent years investigators have attempted to describe the psychology of boys and girls more accurately. Notable efforts have included *Reviving Ophelia* (Pipher, 1994), describing the transitions girls experience during early adolescence, and *Real Boys* (Pollack, 1998) and *Raising Cain* (Kindlon & Thompson, 1999), which addressed issues related to boys. These authors have rightly concluded that despite the great strides we have made as a culture concerning gender-related issues, youth still face great pressure to conform to old stereotypes and expectations.

In the case of boys, our culture stifles the development of an emotional language beyond anger and its expression through aggression, both directly and indirectly. Conformity to what Pollack (1998) and Kindlon and Thompson (1999) refer to as the "boy code" appears to peak during middle school. Icons, heroes, and myths that reinforce the image of men who deal with conflict through aggression, and often alone, are reflected to our boys through the modern story conveniences of television, cinema, and electronic games.

What our society fails to nurture with these images is the equally powerful alternative: the thinking, feeling, and intuitive aspects that many boys show in childhood. Like ballast on a boat, boys need these qualities if they are to negotiate their aggressive tendencies success-

117

fully. Campbell (1949), Jung (1989), and more recently Moore (2001), Johnson (1991), Moore and Gillette (1990), and Rise (1994) have demonstrated that all aspects of the mature adult must move toward balance and integration for the individual to continue the developmental process of individuation. When a culture denies its boys the opportunity to balance their aggressive aspects, it increases the possibility that that they will harness this aggression in destructive behaviors. Pollack (1998) and Kindlon and Thompson (1999) have demonstrated that one way we deny this integration is through the use of shame to control these aggressive tendencies.

A generally accepted tenet of child psychotherapy is that successful treatment must include working not only with clients but also with their families and within the environmental context. Through consultation, the teaching of parenting techniques, and family and individual therapy, the therapist can help facilitate the process of growth in children. Through individual therapy play therapists can provide children with verbal and nonverbal interventions that help them in this process. Nonverbal therapy is especially useful for boys, given that they frequently lack the expressive emotional language necessary to articulate what they are feeling. If children have also experienced trauma in their lives, as illustrated in the following case study, there is a strong possibility that neurochemical reactions in the brain related to the trauma will further impair their ability to express what they are thinking and feeling (van der Kolk, McFarlane, & Weisaeth, 2007).

This case study shows how the use of nondirective play therapy, specifically sandplay therapy, assisted one boy in his struggle with physical and sexual aggression. The sandplay approach used in this treatment process is based on the pioneering work of Dora Kalff (1980). Kalff developed sandplay therapy through a combination of her knowledge of Jungian psychology and the play techniques of Margaret Lowenfeld (Turner, 2005). (See Sharp, 1998, and Singer, 1972, for an in-depth discussion of Jungian theory and practice.)

Through the use of common objects and symbols of all types from all cultures, and sand trays, clients are given the opportunity to express themselves without words. Clients are instructed to use any miniatures in the sandplay collection to create a picture in one of the available sand trays. My office has three trays: one with wet sand, one with dry sand, and a third made of plastic suitable for water trays. The miniatures chosen by clients generally have some unconscious charge or meaning for them. In this manner, the unconscious of each individual is invited to express the inner conflicts with which it is struggling, without having to use words. I often describe the sandplay process as a "waking dream" subject to the same process of discussion and interpretation. The essential difference in sandplay is that the discussion piece does not occur until the clients' process is complete.

The process can be verbal or nonverbal depending on the needs of the client. As witness to their process, I record clients' pictures by drawing them and writing what they say about them. I then take a picture of the tray after the client has left the office. If clients say nothing about their tray, I will ask them if there is anything they would like to tell me about the picture and if they would like to give the tray a title; however, speaking about the tray is an option and not a requirement placed on clients.

CASE REFERRAL INFORMATION

Chris was referred to treatment at the age of 8. He lived with his 9-year-old half-brother, Alan, in a foster home where they had lived for 4 years. Chris's biological parents were Hispanic, whereas his foster parents were African American. Chris and Alan did fairly well in this faith-based home, though they historically had problems with fighting.

Chris was referred to treatment by his group therapists. He and Alan were in a group for sexually reactive and aggressive youth. They had molested a neighborhood girl. Chris had fondled her vagina on one occasion and had attempted intercourse. Alan had also been molesting Chris while wrestling. During these incidents Alan had been observed thrusting on Chris in a sexual manner. As a result, both boys had been referred to group therapy 6 months previously. The group therapists believed that Chris could benefit from collateral play therapy.

When Chris came into the first scheduled appointment, he was accompanied by his caseworker from the Department of Social Services. He entered the room without hesitation but appeared to be apprehensive, glancing around the room, quickly taking everything in, and attempting to "check me out" covertly. He was an attractive Hispanic boy of average height and build for his age. As he sat on the couch facing me, his eyes focused on the miniature toys on the shelves in front him. He smiled for the first time. Over the next hour I interviewed him and the social worker, together and separately. I was given an extensive history of the events that had led to his eventual removal from his mother. The only time he smiled was when he saw the toys in my sandplay collection.

Chris and Alan had lived with their mother, Suki, when they were younger. Chris's father had left the area with two of his older children from a previous marriage, leaving Chris behind with his mother. It was not clear where their father lived, although Chris was sure that he had moved "back east" to Chicago. Chris felt close to him, although he had never actually known his father. Suki had become a crack cocaine addict. The time sequence of these developments was unclear. Apparently she supported herself, her children, and her habit through prostitution. She would often leave the children alone while she worked. Alan was school-age and had missed a great deal of school. The boys had witnessed Suki being sexual on numerous occasions, as they usually lived in hotel rooms. There had been numerous investigations by the local Department of Social Services as a result of reports of neglect.

When Chris was 4 years old, his maternal uncle came to live with the family after being released from prison. Suki took advantage of his presence to go to work while he watched the children. The first time the uncle watched the boys, he brutally and repeatedly sodomized both of them in front of each other. Several days later, Chris was alone with Suki for the first time and told her about the molest. As a result of these events, both boys were removed and placed in their current foster home.

During Chris's portion of the interview he was nervous but honest, and he did not deny his sexualized behavior. He also briefly mentioned his own victimization. In addition to his pseudo-attachment to his absent father, he expressed strong positive emotions for his mother Suki and Alan, although his relationship with Alan was conflicted and often marred by fighting. He was loyal to Alan and Suki despite the adversity in their lives. He was depressed, but his mood was interlaced with humor and wit. His behavioral presentation was that of an older child, and at times he looked like an old man, carrying many years of emotional burden on his slumped shoulders.

Chris came to treatment from his previous therapist with a diagnosis of adjustment disorder with disturbance of mood and conduct. This diagnosis, while appropriate, did not fully describe Chris. The symptoms reported included depression, anxiety, and poor impulse control evidenced by aggressive behaviors, and difficulty following directions. Chris also clearly demonstrated symptoms consistent with a traumatic event, indicating a diagnosis of posttraumatic stress disorder (see Finkelhor & Browne, 1986, for an in-depth discussion of posttraumatic stress disorder in children).

Chris was a victim of sexual and physical abuse and parental neglect. He had changed schools multiple times and at one point had lived on the street with his mother and brother. The mother–child unity that Neumann (1973) discussed as being essential to the first year of life and subsequent development had been severely disrupted. According to Weinrib (1983) this disruption can create a poor foundation for the psyche. Chris was clearly experiencing this lack of foundation, especially in relation to the masculine and feminine archetypes (innate energies) and associated parental complexes (arising from the client's experience of his or her mother and father). Chris had also experienced a lack of good father energy in his early life. This lack of a good father who is prepared to receive a boy and lead him into adulthood can create a lifelong struggle of aggression, addiction, and emotional upheaval (Corneau, 1991).

INVITATION TO PLAY THERAPY

Chris was quickly drawn to the playroom. He was eager for the individual attention and demonstrated great intuitive skills. As a therapist and a father I could feel his cotransference[1] on both levels almost immediately. I knew at that moment that my own cotransference would revolve around the latter issue. He was a sensitive child and, at times, was still able to show his emotions. Alan, by contrast, was observed by his group therapists and in family therapy sessions to be more stoic and closed and as the more aggressive of the two boys.

During the course of 18 months of treatment, Chris created 17 trays. What follows is an accounting and interpretation of these trays. In addition to his work in the sand, he used other play modalities, including art, games, sword fighting, the dollhouse and puppets, storytelling, and singing, in addition to family therapy with his brother and mother as a part of their reunifcation plan. All of these interventions were client-directed. As his therapist I marked and protected the special time in the playroom from "normal life." By letting him guide this process, I took advantage of his intuitive senses and allowed his psyche to establish itself in the play and lead a path to healing from the horrific trauma he had experienced. In this way I functioned as his "ritual elder" for his "initiatory" experience into the energy of his psyche (for a detailed account of the similarities of the therapeutic experience with initiation, see Moore, 2001).

---

[1] *Cotransference* is a term used in Jungian sandplay therapy to designate the shared emotional field between the client and the therapist (Bradway & McCoard, p. 34, 1997).

This chapter tracks the masculine and feminine archetypes (innate energies) in Chris's work as the parental complexes (the client's experience of his or her personal mother and father, as distinguished from the client's experience of the mother and father archetypes) were reworked in his sandplay process. This reworking led to integration of previously nonintegrated material and assisted him in his journey from "victim" to "victor." His anger and aggression became more fully integrated and therefore more in his control through the use of the play process.

CASE ILLUSTRATION OF SELF-DIRECTED TRAUMA PLAY

The Beginning: Setting the Stage—A Hero's Journey

Upon creating his initial trays, Chris told me the following story:

> "A wizard king was trying to get all the bad people to come so he could make a blizzard. They were trying to destroy him. But he was too strong, and he made a blizzard that destroyed everything except the animals. But the lion took the wizard's crystal. The wizard turned the lion into a Chinese lantern. Then the blizzard came. The wizard was happy to destroy the lion. The castle was buried and the wizard had nowhere to go, but he used his power to uncover the castle. That's my story for now."

Chris worked diligently and talked about his tray as he created it. This would prove to be typical for him. He made three mounds in the tray and called them mountains. Later he stated: "The two princesses get the little mountains." The wizard was on the larger, central mountain. At the end of the process, realizing that I would take a photograph of the tray, he insisted that I take the first picture while he sprinkled sand over the tray to simulate a "sandstorm." Having to decide about taking the picture with him present was the first of many times he would ask me to confront my comfort zone in relation to my boundaries as a therapist. I followed his lead, making sure that just his hands were in the picture!

The dryness of the tray (Figure 7.1) is striking. The earth or sand appears to lack nurturing qualities. Both the outer two mounds are focused on a single main character, a silver princess, in each case surrounded by green dinosaur-like creatures. One of Chris's tasks in therapy emerged here as a need to reconnect with the watery and nurturing qualities of the feminine aspects of his psyche and to learn how to use

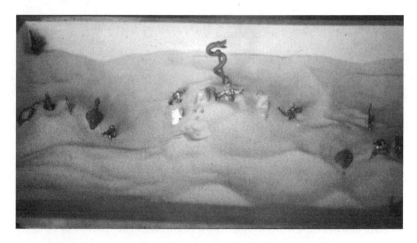

FIGURE 7.1. The wizard king.

their symbolic/healing/regenerative (and potentially destructive) qualities. At the same time the destructive aspects of the masculine energy
needed to be properly contained and channeled.

The presence of the caduceus with the wizard in the center of the
tray intimates that the therapy would be a healing process that is spiritual in nature. It hints at the possibility of a healing that could successfully unify opposites (Cooper, 1978). With this tray Chris had entered
the sandplay process quickly, by stating what the challenge ahead was
and what the solution might be. Like the wizard, he must know his own
energies and learn how to channel and contain this power (Moore &
Gillette, 1990). Moore and Gillette (1990) have presented four archetypal images of the masculine for consideration. They postulate that
these archetypes have opposing aspects and that the task of a developing male is to integrate all aspects of the archetype in its fullness.
They see this successful integration as the path to the development of
a mature, fully realized masculine that transcends the traditional, rule-
bound, and aggressive patriarchal male of today's Western culture. Failure to integrate these archetypes can lead to behaviors we have come to
view as destructive masculine elements.

Chris's story highlights both his struggle and possible healing in
this process. His selection of the wizard and a storm as inner representa-
tives reflects the masculine energy brought to this process. The wizard's
power is threatened by evil, and only with the use of his good power can
he defeat this evil. According to Moore and Gillette (1990) the wizard,

who is often seen as a mentor or a wizened old man, uses his power to assist others in the initiation process. The wizard represents the ritual elders so absent in our society that guide the internal and external process of transformation. In his shadowy aspects the wizard is prone to using his power not to guide others to their natural fulfillment but to manipulate others for his own ends. This theme is reminiscent of the abusive and manipulative power sexual predators use to groom and violate their victims. The wizard in this scene also represents the "healing technology" of the therapist and the therapeutic process, again intimating the cotransference relationship that appeared to begin at the first contact with this client.

The silver princesses and the use of the sand appear to reflect emerging feminine energy. On the left mound the princess is accompanied by a girl on a unicorn. The unicorn is seen as a lunar feminine principle symbolizing "perfect good" virtue and incorruptibility and is often associated with the "horn of salvation" (Cooper, 1992, p. 250). Similar to the wizard's powers, these elements can be dangerous, as expressed in this tray by (1) the dry and non-nurturing quality of the feminine aspects of the sands, (2) the lioness (which Chris incorrectly identified as a lion) who betrays the wizard to steal his power, and (3) in the destructive power of the sandstorm.

Chris told a detailed and elaborate story as he created his next tray.

> "One day the Russians wanted to fight the U.S.A., but the U.S.A. didn't want to fight. They were happy. The Russians threatened to destroy our country. They wanted to defeat the U.S.A., because they [the U.S.A.] had beat them five times. They [Russians] wanted revenge. But there were way more U.S.A. than Russians. It was a hard war. It went on for 1 month. Didn't stop fighting till one day a big U.S.A. tank came and shot the Russians. The Russian tank tried to fight back, but the tank was blown up. The Americans and Russians kept on sneaking up on each other. They got beat six times now. The Russians made the motorcycle be messed up and stole the motorcycle. The end."

While Chris told his story, I quietly sat nearby and wrote it down. When he was done, I asked if there was anything else he wanted to say about his creation. He indicated he did not, and I asked him to leave the picture so that I could take a picture of his tray after he left my office. I then invited him to explore the playroom and decide what else he might want to do that day.

When Chris began creating the scenario in the sandtray, he said that it was going to be the "army desert." He asked me if I would name the tray, which again stretched me out of my comfort zone. I resisted until he had decided on his own title (The Greatest War), at which point I named it "On the Battlefield." There are soldiers and tanks from two separate armies, one green in color and one brown, placed randomly throughout the tray, apparently simulating the naturally chaotic aspect of battle. Of special note are the two helicopters in diagonal corners elevated on mounds, as is the army ambulance. The only living creature, other than the soldiers, is a dog, which is apparently paired with one specific soldier to the left of the army motorcycles (which are in the center area of the tray). In this tray we have the emergence of the battle, typically seen in the trays of boys at this age. Here it appears to reflect Chris's need to come to terms with his aggressive masculine and feminine aspects. The battle is played out in a dry and arid place, where the forces of good and evil do battle. It is an elaboration of the first tray, where the masculine energy (in this case, the energy of the warrior) is grounded in the non-nurturing feminine aspect of the dry, arid earth. Without an appropriate relationship to the positive aspects of these energies, Chris lived in a world of chaos, battle, and aggression. His process appeared to have quickly deepened as he began his descent into the unconscious and into the depths of therapy.

The energy embodied in the two motorcycles (often associated with the masculine) is disabled through treachery. Much like the wizard of the first tray, the motorcycles' power is threatened through the treachery of an enemy (see his story description). In this scene, however, the mission is complete. The two motorcycles are victims of deceit and disabled, much like Chris and Alan were. This theme leads to the speculation that this scene embodies or recapitulates Chris's victimization by his uncle, his neglect and abandonment by his mother, and his betrayal by his brother.

The helicopters in diagonal corners appear to offer a possible solution or escape, representing a harnessed masculine energy that can rise above the situation, into the realm of the spiritual, and serve as a bridge to unite opposites. The helicopter has the ability to move between the earth, symbolically seen as mother and the source of nurturance, and the sky, symbolically seen as father and realm of the spirit. While the helicopters can serve as a bridge between these two aspects, in this tray the helicopters are still grounded in a non-nurturing mother earth, not yet able to ascend.

What can we make of the only other life form in the tray as represented by the dog accompanying the soldier? The dog is small and dwarfed by the surrounding scene, possibly representing the client's own untapped and underdeveloped instinctual life that may be activated through the play process. Dogs have been our companions and guardians for over 12,000 years. They guard us as we sleep at night and drift into the world of our dreams and the unconscious. This dog's presence in the tray further suggests that the client's play has gone deeper.

THE MIDDLE: THE WORK DEEPENS AND MOVES

Chris did not tell a story when he created his third tray. Initially he started working in the wet sand, then moved to the dry sand saying that it gave him "more space" to work with (even though both trays are the same size). When he finished the tray, he took some sand from the wet tray and sprinkled it over the scene. Then he did the same with some dry sand. He said, "The wet sand is like water and the dry sand is the wind."

Chris drew a line in the sand roughly down the middle of the tray. The left side of the tray he labeled "land" and placed shells on it. He said the right side was the sea. The scene clearly depicts the "aftermath of the storm," with boats and shells strewn about the land as a result. Chris was entering deeper into the sandplay process. Beneath the shells he carefully hid a naval "destroyer" (the shell is often seen as representing the containing aspect of the feminine principle), which was revealed as a result of the power of the storm (Figure 7.2). Chris appeared to be using the same power of the wizard (wind) present in his first tray to reveal his own fears of a destructive feminine element that must be addressed. (In tray 1 [Figure 7.1] he portrayed this element using the lioness who betrays the wizard).

In general Chris appeared to be closely in touch with his thinking and intuitive aspects. Given that he often played the role of sensitive, intuitive younger brother to his much more aggressive older brother, it is ironic that he could only hint at it in his trays. This sensitive aspect of his personality had been ripped away (or more accurately, hidden), possibly because of his past abuse. He expressed sadness and destruction in his trays and aggression in his outer world. His suppression of the nurturing feminine element was apparently related to the aggressive

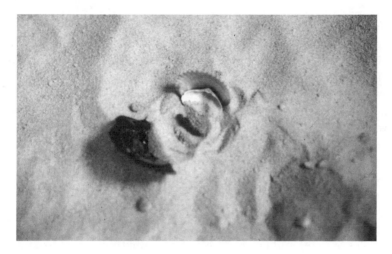

FIGURE 7.2. Aftermath of the storm.

masculine energy he had been exhibiting. He denied this element even further when he equated the dry sand with a masculine energy (wind).

However, in creating this expression as an "aftermath" of the storm, he was touching the deepest wounding of his past and, as a result, his repression was beginning to lift. Here we see what Jung (1969b) referred to as the moment of complete abandonment and loneliness. Chris was beginning to approach that aspect of the feminine that is negatively charged (the destructive aspect of the feminine). He had to confront and reintegrate it in a healthier or reframed manner if he was to free his masculine energy from its destructive/aggressive expression. This process reveals several key aspects in working with boys. In order for boys to have a healthy relationship to their own full masculine energy, they must first have that relationship to their own feminine energies. Chris was able to do this, almost in silence, using his psyche and instincts as his guide. As his therapist I was holding the space for him and making sure that his work could proceed in safety and be witnessed with compassion.

When creating his fourth tray, Chris stated that he had selected the dry tray because "it's gonna be winter." In explaining this comment, he indicated that the dry sand looked like snow to him. He tried to partially cover some of the figures with sand, as if they were buried in the snow. He said nothing else about the tray.

This tray intimated a turning point in Chris's sandplay process. No longer was he mired in the dry, arid earth. Instead he had moved into the watery, nurturing mounds of the snow and trees, with cars and planes in various positions around the tray, some buried. He was possibly rising above the conflict to find the positive aspects of the masculine and feminine principles.

Although the conflict continued in a chaotic fashion and planes remained grounded, they were grounded in the life-giving waters of the snow. Here the wizard reemerged in the tray as a guide in his journey in the guise of the wizened old man. He is surrounded by dogs and joined by a bird in the tree (seen as a messenger of the spirit and as an aspect of the wizard); all are guiding Chris on this instinctual path of healing.

A cooling down is occurring, symbolically represented by the appearance of snow, greenery, and animals. Chris introduced animal and plant life, again representing the renewing aspects of the feminine principles of water and earth. This was also the third scene in which he included weather in his description of a tray, this time in the form of snow. These watery feminine symbols represented the potential to both nurture and modify his aggressiveness.

The tree introduced a potentially unifying symbol in this tray. The tree, rooted in the earth as it stretches up to the sky, is often seen as a symbol of life (e.g., the tree of life), the *axis mundi* (cosmic axis; center of the world) representing the entirety of manifestation and unifying heaven, earth, and water. The *axis mundi* belongs to a coherent body of myths, images, and symbols intimately associated with the creation of humans and of many religions. It is the center of absolute beginning, where the sacred entered our universe and creation began. Passing through the middle of the three cosmic zones—air, earth, and underworld—the tree is seen as connecting us to all things (Cook, 1974).

In one of the trees to the left of the center of the tray is a yellow bird. The presence of the bird represents the transcendent function and is an aspect of the divine power descending to the tree of life (Cooper, 1978). The bird, like the dog, frequently accompanies the hero on his quest, and at times has represented the wizard's or shaman's ascent into the heavens. It appears to be a conduit and mediator of the spiritual aspects of the father archetype in this process, as well as a guardian/guide in mediating instinctive energies.

For his fifth tray Chris told a lengthy and detailed story:

"One day there was a castle with lots of houses around it, but the houses were forbidden to be near the castle. One day a Chinese man built a house by the castle. A series of attempts were made to knock the house down. Guards from the castle tried, a dragon tried, a soldier shot an arrow at the house but it came back at him. The dragon tried to burn it. Then two Chinese guards came and said: 'Leave our house alone.' The two guards beat up everyone. They carried the house back to the country, and the guards are always there to protect the home. But the dragon came back and shot fire, and the guard used his shield to bounce the fire back at the dragon, and it died. Then they ate the dragon. One guard stands by the house to guard it. The other one went to the top of the castle to watch for other enemies. The people were happy because the great castle was mean."

Chris came to this session agitated and complaining that he had been grounded for a week for breaking a house rule at the foster home: telling family business to someone outside the home. As he created this tray, he told his story and acted it out in the sand. The final scene is the result of this dynamic sandplay sequence.

In this scene Chris chose another culture to express his conflict (Figure 7.9). According to Kalff (1980), when clients are deep in their process, they will often move to deep imagery of an opposite culture. It is this image of the "other" that cannot be manipulated as easily by the psyche as images that are more common to our everyday experiences. Here, the conflict of the moment—telling family business—and

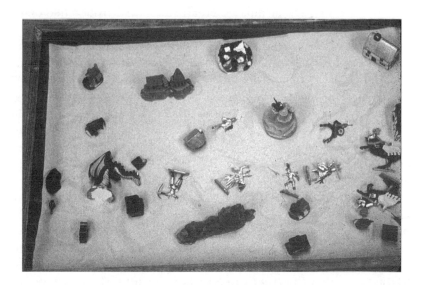

FIGURE 7.3. "Leave our house alone!"

the reality of the past—telling of the molestation he suffered, merge as a "hero" fights back against perceived injustice.

In Chris's story, the hero is moving from victim to victor. He uses elements of trickery in his battle with the enemy. The shadowy, aggressive element of an "evil king" comes into direct conflict with its opposite: a masculine energy that has a strong sense of self and purpose, who is able to stand up for what he believes in. Chris is finding his own inner hero, with a sense of the trickster, which can help him contain his shadow and at the same time respect it, remaining eternally watchful of its power (in the form of the guards standing watch).

Robert Johnson (1991) has indicated that the true outcome of the battle with the shadow is not its defeat but recognizing its existence and power, containing it, and remaining respectful and vigilant of its presence. The dragon, which is sometimes associated with shadow and evil, guards the treasure that the hero must claim by defeating it. In the tray, the defeated dragon is returned to the earth, bringing its energy (treasure) to the healing aspects of the feminine (sand). This is the positive aspect of the dragon's energy that must be honored and that can be harnessed with the help of the life-giving feminine.

As the reunification with Suki was getting closer, Chris's sixth tray demonstrates a deep descent into the depths of the unconscious and the watery feminine principle. The scene was set in a plastic water tray half filled with water. On top of the water float soldiers and planes on a raft. Below, in the water, are various sea creatures. A turtle is perched on the edge of the tray looking over the scene.

There is a clearer separation of masculine and feminine energies as this part of the descent appears complete. Chris was beginning to marshal the warrior energy of the masculine and aspire to the spiritual. At the same time he was also beginning to separate the positive and negative elements of the feminine he had associated with the mother archetype. The journey he was on continued under the vigilance of a guiding and protective spiritual presence (the green sea turtle overlooking the scene). The sea turtle is a symbol of creation and unites the masculine and the feminine principles as well as sky, earth, and water.

Chris did not tell a full story about this next tray, but he did make many comments about the scene as he created it (Figure 7.4). He called the figures to the left of the wet strip near the center of the tray "good guys' army" and the group to the right "bad guys' army." He indicated that the water strip was "lava" from a volcano. "One of the bad guys fell into the lava and his partner came looking for him. He fell in too, but the good guys rescued him and he became good." At the end of this

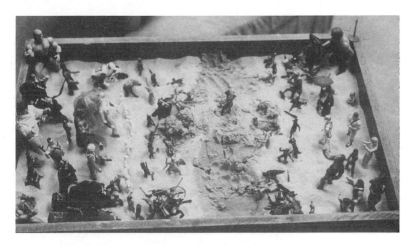

FIGURE 7.4. The good guys' and the bad guys' armies.

process, he said, "All of this was caused by a little man" (the wizard from the first tray), and then he turned to me, cautioning, "But don't tell no one . . . it's a secret!" Overnight visits with his mother had commenced, and Chris's sister, who had been removed from Suki at birth, had just been reunited with her.

In tray 7 Chris moved the process along to what had to occur next. As the opposites had emerged and been separated, the potential for healing and integration also had to be present. For Chris this healing came in the recognition that the evil or shadow elements in his life had a purpose that was potentially positive for his full development. In this tray Chris built a bridge on the secrets of his past (the land bridge is built on top of the three monkey miniatures—hear/speak/see no evil) and used the energy of the aggression associated with this injury, and its denial, as a catalyst for healing.

Signs of integration on several levels were emerging as Chris began to come to terms with his own anger and violence. This energy was now moving between "goodness" and "evil" as it assisted in the healing battle. The deep spiritual aspect of the masculine energy (the wizard he referred to as the "little man") continued to lead and protect his new-found energies as well as beckoning across the great divide to the more primitive, uncontrolled aggressive energies that had to be relativized and integrated.

Clearly Chris was in the throes of a battle in an attempt to contain, relativize, and integrate the dark forces of his psyche. The healing powers came in the form of lava as the "bad guys" fell in and remerged as "good." Hot and destructive, lava moves like water as it ultimately creates new land that forms a bridge between good and evil (see Rise, 1994, for a detailed discussion of the battle of good and evil in initiation rites).

According to Kay Bradway (1985), the emergence of a bridge indicates that the transcendent function is at work. Jung (1969a) described this function as the psyche's movement to transcend its own deep divisions and, in the process, join what previously appeared to be irreconcilable differences. Bradway indicates that this reconciliation leads to new attitudes that transcend old ones. In Chris's case he had to reconcile that his monster/destroyer/victimizer was a part of him, and that it had to be relativized as he moved to a more respectful and contained relationship with this energy. Of special note is that good and evil forces in this tray contain both masculine and feminine images, another indication that integration was occurring.

As Chris created his eighth tray, reunification with his mother had occurred. Chris told a lengthy story related to the tray, detailing the return of Dorothy to Oz, reunification with her friends who have lost the use of their gifts, and discovery of the treasure (hidden pearls). The tale he told reflected how masculine (wind, football players) and feminine energies (Dorothy, good witch, ballerinas) represented in the tray defeated the wicked witch and found their treasures. The story ended with a ritual baptism and the marriage of opposites (football players and ballerinas).

Once again Chris told his story as he created the scene, and he also told me to take the picture looking at the scene sideways (Figure 7.5). He commented that snakes are powerful and balloons last forever. He said that Dorothy would want to live in Oz forever. As in his first tray, he asked me to take a picture of the tray as he sifted sand over the scene.

In this tray Chris provided us with a story that was alive on many levels. On the surface we see that the emergence of the large snake came when he was reuniting with his mother. Many colleagues viewing this tray voiced concern about Chris's emotional safety as a result of the reunification. Chris worked hard at creating a fairy tale ending in which everyone lived together in safety and happiness; he also created a great wind that uncovered a treasure of hidden pearls. This process appeared to be guided by the masculine (football players, the wind, and Dorothy's companions) and feminine energies (Dorothy, the ballerinas, the crone figures, and the snake that devours the witch) embodied in the scene, which was replete with heroines and crones who guided the integration and movement in this tray.

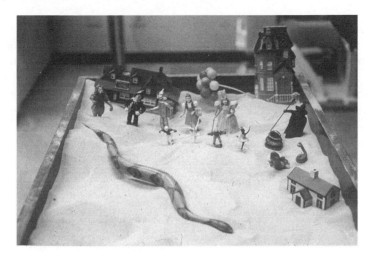

FIGURE 7.5. Return to Oz.

The presence of the snake in this tray implies movement and is portrayed as that which devours evil. Chris said that the snake had great power, as did the balloons. In this way elements of earth and sky, the innate energies of mother and father, again appear to be the vehicles he used to tell his story of healing. The snake could well reflect the energy that was released in the previous trays, now moving forward in an attempt to reconcile and integrate and yet potentially devour. The balloons, in particular, appear to reflect this movement. In the previous trays the wind brought danger and destruction. Here it functions more as a spiritual or godly element that Chris said "will last forever." The balloons have allowed the feminine principle to rise above the fray and return home in search of family and to restore the gifts that the great wizard had bestowed on the psyche.

In tray 3 (Figure 7.2), the winds brought a storm that revealed a destroyer hidden in empty shells. In tray 8, the wind uncovered a hidden treasure of pearls. The pearl is the true treasure of the shell. It is seen as a lunar symbol, the essence of the moon and its control of the tides. It represents the embryo of cosmic life and the Great Mother archetype. In the past, pearls were thought to be caused by lightning penetrating the shell of the oyster and are therefore regarded as a union of fire and water (Cooper, 1978).

Edinger (1994) pointed out that such a symbol reflects a union of opposites. This can also be seen in the configuration of football players and ballerinas, joined together, black and white "married," united in the common cause of defeating the wicked witch and retrieving the treasure. Thus, Chris advanced the theme of moving from victim to victor guided by reordered masculine and feminine principles. Like a rebirth, Chris said that all the characters would take a bath, cleaning, renewing and being reborn as he apparently began to develop his own sense of a collective, or a sense of belonging to a community larger than the self.

Chris was fairly quiet when making tray 9 (Figure 7.6). He had reported low-level conflict at home. As he finished creating this tray, he stated, "The plane is going to Chicago . . . there's a cloud over the plane . . . there is a thunderstorm." He then sprinkled water over the cloud and the plane and said, "It's raining."

This tray reflects both sadness and movement for Chris. On an everyday level he was expressing unhappiness with his home life now that he had returned to live with his mother. His sadness seemed to be one of reconciliation with the realities of living with his mother and his expectations in anticipation of this move. She did not nurture in a way he understood.

Tray 9 shows that Chris's masculine energy, in the form of the airplane, was indeed ungrounded and moving, moving away from the moon, or lunar principle, through yet another storm to "Chicago." During our very first meeting Chris had told me that he believed his father

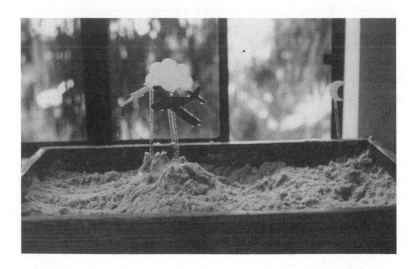

FIGURE 7.6. Return to Father.

lived in Chicago. The airplane was also pointed directly at where I was sitting during the session. Chris was moving away from his actual mother to his imagined father in search of understanding. He was also using the light of his lunar Great Mother (moon) as a guide on this journey to the masculine.

This was the first time that Chris had used a wet sand tray. He sprinkled water on the figures, creating a sense of rain or dew descending. Edinger (1994) points out that the cloud symbolizes the presence of Yahweh, and the rain or dew it brings revives the "dead" body. The Great Father (Sky) and Great Mother (earth) are present in this tray in a regenerative relationship. They stand freely, yet as supportive and related guides, as Chris moves to the next level. These appear to be signs that an integration of opposites is occurring.

After creating tray 9 Chris turned to me and wanted to talk more about home. He moved sideways so that the empty dry sand tray was on his right; his seat positioned him just at the lower edge of the tray. As he talked to me he moved his hands through the sand, creating the image seen in the tray 10 (Figure 7.7). He talked about his sadness and anger at his mother. Chris had earned some money working for a neighbor, but his mother had taken his money to pay for food and diapers for his

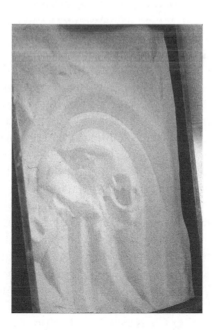

FIGURE 7.7. The god of light.

baby sister. He became tearful as he communicated feelings of power-lessness in his life. However, unlike the past, when these feelings had often led to acting out, this time he gave voice to his sadness and sense of helplessness.

The creation in tray 10 appeared to come completely out of Chris's unconscious mind. Chris was unaware of what he had created in the sand. When placed sideways, we see the tray from Chris's perspective from where he was sitting. Of the many colleagues who have seen this tray, all have been taken by its simple beauty. Some have seen the hat of the wizard in Chris's first tray, whereas others have seen a bird of some type, usually a bird of prey. Still others have speculated that it looks like Quezalcoatl, the plumed serpent.

The airplane in the previous tray, which he had created the same day, was pointing directly at his creation. Often in the sandplay process of boys I see a tray that is remarkable for its starkness and the pres-ence of a single large figure that is invariably an animal of some type. I have come to understand this as that moment in the process when the boy finds his secret name/self/power (much like that seen in initiation rites). A sense of healing and movement usually accompany these trays.

That some colleagues see the wizard's hat and others a bird is logical given that both of these symbols have acted as guides in this cli-ent's journey; they have served as messengers and conduits of his spirit and power. The imagery also leads to speculation on the connection to Quezalcoatl, a mythical figure from Mexico, the country of Chris's ances-tors. Quezalcoatl is a representation of the *hombre/Dios:* half-man, half-god and worldly king. In one version of the myth, after encountering his own dark shadow, Quezalcoatl abandons his kingdom, wandering the land and being pursued by enemies. He is ultimately transformed into a god of light in a manner that resembles the Christ story. As a god of light he represents renewal and sustenance. There are many incarnations and stories of Quezalcoatl that include mastery of the wind, and one in which he avenges his father's death, which casts him as the "heroic" child (Baldwin, 1998).

I believe that at this point in treatment, Chris had begun to capture his own light as he moved from his literal mother to the unknown world of the symbolic father. As Chris avenged the losses and traumas of his life, he had to face secret names and dangerous journeys. It is the lunar/feminine energy of the previous tray that has led him to this place of the deep masculine.

At the next meeting Chris asked me to draw with him in the sand. He drew two lines in the sand, creating a cross and four separate quad-rants, and asked that we each draw two pictures. On the upper left he asked me to draw a picture of a sad moment in my life and in the lower left a happy moment in my life. Chris then drew a happy time in the upper-right quadrant depicting him and his mother being reunited. In the lower-right quadrant he first drew a picture of him being taken from his mother by the Department of Social Services as his sad time. He then erased this and drew a picture showing him getting hit by a rock. While drawing this, he stated, "It didn't even hurt . . . I didn't know I got hit, but there was blood everywhere."

Chris then asked what scenes I had drawn. Being true to his process I had chosen to participate in, I indicated that my sad time was the day my father died in a car accident and my happy moment depicted the day my son was born. At the end of the process both our happy and sad times were diagonal to each other.

Chris's insistence that we both depict happy and sad moments in the sand created what felt like a confessional and spirit-filled moment. As a therapist, it pushed me into considering a direction that would affect the cotransference relationship. Being relatively new to sandplay, my first reaction was to resist his request, but then, because of his intensity, I understood that he intuitively knew something I had not yet fully grasped as a therapist. Chris instinctively knew what the destination of the therapy process was for him and how to get there. I was becoming increasingly aware of my role: to witness, contain, protect, and hold the therapeutic space while he did the work he needed to do to heal his deep childhood wounds. This lesson would inform my life as a child therapist.

So, Chris brought us to the crossroads by literally creating a cross in the sand: a place in time and space where opposites were united. It was also a dangerous and magical place. The crossroads is seen as a sacred place and in many cultures is symbolic of the tree of life. For Native Americans it is the place of the four winds: the North is all powerful and intelligent, the East is the heart and source of life and love, the South is the place of fire and passion, and the West is the gentle wind from the spirit land (Cooper, 1978). In Mexican culture the cross is often associated with Quezalcoatl as a symbol of fertility. In Christianity it is often seen as the acceptance of death or suffering, as a passage to redemption and atonement. It was a symbolic representation of all the work to that point in treatment.

For Chris, it was the moment when he had to come to terms with the personal pain and suffering he had experienced in his past with a trusted mentor/elder. On a symbolic level, Chris was reconciling the great powers of the deep archetypes and the negative experiences that had been attached to them through his life experience (complexes). If his psyche could realize this distinction, then his "redemption" from his abuse and atonement for his own aggressive behaviors could proceed.

Weinrib (1996) has indicated that the cross can represent the "rites of passage." Chris had come to the crossroads as he began to reconcile the great pain and loss in his life with the hope of the "birth" to follow. Each of us quietly drew pictures of loss and birth without conscious awareness of this, representing a passage from one level to the next and the inextricable relationship between these two forces of nature. In this moment, Chris and I seem to be have been working at the same unconscious level, perhaps communicating to each other about the relationship of father and son at an archetypal, age-old level, as well as at present-day and personal (cotransferential) level.

However, Chris was not yet ready to openly express the pain of the loss of his mother. Perhaps it still loomed as a future option in his mind despite their reunification. Instead he gave us a literal injury as a symbolic representation, and then said: "My head was hurt . . . but it didn't even hurt . . . I knew I was hurt because there was blood everywhere." This is probably how Chris, as a 4-year-old, would have processed the loss of his mother and his own sexual abuse.

At the next session Chris was in a very relaxed mood. He began the session by creating a picture in the sand (Figure 7.8). He said that the picture was of Jesus. After completing the picture he asked to sword

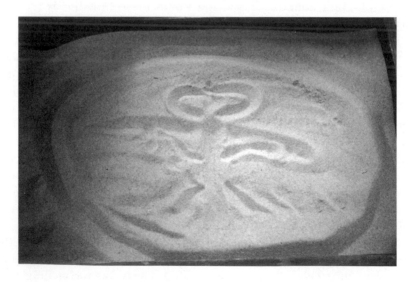

FIGURE 7.8. Jesus inside a circle.

fight using the plastic swords, which he did vigorously. We then sat down to rest for awhile. Chris began speaking about the bus ride to school and how he had made friends with a girl who was in the grade above him. She sang made-up songs on the bus. Chris was now also "learning" these songs and creating his own as well. He sang several of these songs about family, feelings, separation from his mother, and other life themes. He then sang a song about me, his therapist. In his song he described his therapist as being someone who trusted him and cared, no matter what he did, even when he lied. When he lied, he continued, I would "help him in his lie to see the truth."

With a smile (and a song) on his face Chris drew "Jesus inside a circle." His drawing and the moment were numinous, from deep within his spirit. Kalff (1980) describes the circle as a manifestation of the self and a symbol of wholeness. Jung (1956) characterizes the circle as a symbol of perfection and of the perfect being, and as an expression of heaven, sun, God, and the ideal of human and soul. It clearly represents a constellation of Chris's wholeness and unity.

Two and a half months then elapsed between this tray and the next one. Chris had been out of treatment for most of that time because of his mother's lack of cooperation with the Department of Social Services. As he was drawing the face in the sand, he said, "This is God, his eyes and his mustache." As he finished the tray, he stated, "It feels like Jesus Christ is with me. This is nice, ha? . . . Jesus with Mary . . . they were like husband and wife?" In this scene Chris placed three crosses, two of Jesus crucified and the third made by the lit candles. The risen Christ figure and the ascending Mary figure completed the tray above the "eyes of God" he drew in the sand. Following a constellation of the self in the previous tray, Chris had now set about reworking his traumatic past.

Weinrib (1996) indicated that in her experience the cross often emerges well into the sandplay process, when a strong center has coagulated and some constellation of the self has occurred. At this point the ego can feel supported and sufficiently developed to withstand tension between powerful personal values or the creation of a powerful polarity that needs resolution. In this way the unacceptable aspects of the self (shadow material) can be incorporated.

Chris's tray presents two aspects of Jesus: the victimized, betrayed, misunderstood human son of God dying on the cross, and the risen Jesus, numinous and at one with his father. The death or ending of one aspect of life leads to rebirth and the revealing of another, opposite aspect. In Chris's tray the polarity that is being resolved relates to his victimization and victimizing behavior and his movement to a victor position, as reflected so well in the images he chose for the scene. The lit candles, in particular, allude to the possibility that Chris had captured the chaos of the storms in his previous trays and had harnessed this into a life-giving energy.

At the end of this process Chris revealed his lack of direct knowledge about religion by speculating that Jesus and Mary were married. Actually, they appeared to represent another set of opposite energies Chris had been struggling to understand and integrate: strong masculine and feminine principles that now appeared to sit on their own, but also in positive relation to each other.

Chris and his brother were brought to the next session by a Department of Social Services case aide. Their mother was supposed to accompany them for family session but did not come when the boys were picked up. Both boys were seen individually instead. During the first part of the session Chris was complaining about being unfairly treated at home by his mother. He felt that his mother favored his older brother and seemed to be badly in need of attention to these feelings.

Chris then created tray 14 (Figure 7.9), which, in some ways, was an elaboration of the previous tray. With a birth scene depicted, he was moving forward in his process as he and his newly relativized ego could take their proper place in his psyche. When placing a pregnant woman

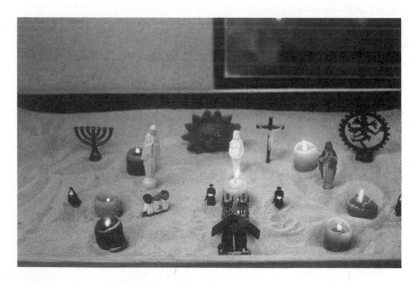

FIGURE 7.9. "This is a religious place."

in the sand, Chris said, "This is pregnant Mary," and then added, "This is a religious place." As he was creating the scene, he began to sing, "Ding dong, the witch is dead." When he finished, he knelt in front of the tray, made a sign of the cross, and quietly prayed to himself. The death of the evil/destructive aspects of the personal mother was being subsumed into this larger, equivalent presentation of the psyche.

In this tray the light was now captured in the eternal menorah. The stem of the menorah is often seen as the tree of life, and in this tray it finds its place with the cross, again capturing recurring symbols and themes in Chris's process: death/endings and rebirths/beginnings. This holding of the tension in harmony is also captured by the symbol of Shiva, the god of destruction and creation.

Chris's social worker had been in touch with me and the group therapist frequently during the previous month. The placement at Suki's home appeared to be deteriorating. Chris had come to a recent session dirty and with a black eye. He reported that Suki allowed Alan and him to stay up as late as they wanted. Chris related that Suki had been spending a great deal of time at the other house on the property, where the man who owned the property lived. The boys referred to him as "Grandpa." Chris said that his mother was over at Grandpa's a lot, "organizing."

Chris's description of Suki and her behavior indicated that she was exhibiting escalating symptoms consistent with depression, partially related to treatment. During the previous family session, both boys had given Suki details of the molestation by her brother. Her own victim issues also surfaced. In addition, I was planning a trip that Chris was aware of; however, he did not know that I was going out of state to a job interview.

When Chris showed up for the next family session, he appeared agitated. His mother was a no-show for the session again. Chris reported that he had gotten into a fight at school. He had been problem-free at school for some time, but recent developments at home had activated his behavior problems.

Given the circumstances and my own issues of cotransference, I suggested that Chris work in the sand that day. Giving this suggestion was contrary to everything I had learned and practiced in sandplay therapy. Chris had not done a tray in 4 months. Often this incubation period is necessary for appropriate processing, and I have found since then that younger children often stay in this "dormant" phase of the process longer than older teenagers and adults. However, Chris was under a great deal of stress, and in the back of my mind I feared that he would not be able to finish his process, either because of the mounting problems in his own home or my possible departure from the state. These considerations led me to commit what I believe was a therapeutic error. I was no longer letting Chris lead this process; instead I allowed my own issues, including fear, to get in the way of his work.

This gentle nudge into performing versus leading the therapy process at the client's own pace engendered some regression in the two trays created during the session. Old themes of good versus evil reemerged as Chris created one tray and directed me in creating a second tray.

The scenes created during this session carried many elements of Chris's anger and frustration. He was angry for many reasons, and my maneuvering him to do this tray appeared to be the focal point of this anger, at least at the surface level. Chris was reacting to the many fears that were facing him at this moment in his life. I have since wondered if he intuitively suspected that I might be considering a change that would directly affect him.

In looking at the battle in these trays, Chris had clearly made a statement. He selected figures for both trays and gave me the ones he wanted in the tray he was directing me to construct. He referred to the figures in my tray as the "enemy." It is populated by more solar, modern-day soldiers, including the villainous Hitler figure. He referred to the soldiers as cowboys (the Indians' victimizers in these trays). Of special note in this tray is the wounded soldier.

The symbols of the Indians appear to reflect Chris's growing identification with his own ethnicity, instincts, and increasing connection to nature. The knight on horseback guarding the tray is also important. According to Cooper (1978), the knight on horseback symbolizes the spirit guiding the body, and his quest represents the soul's journey through the world which presents temptations, trials obstacles proving of character, and his evolution to perfection, in effect the hero's journey.

Chris's tray also contained three "wise people." The first of these was the silver wizard who had appeared in other trays, including tray 1. This wise man continued to guard him, as he was strategically placed over the battle scene in a position of protection. The second wise man was tied to a tree, captured by the enemy (the therapist, and perhaps the client, being trapped into making these trays). The third wise man was actually a female Indian, although Chris did not realize this. Chris was extremely clear about her: "He must be protected. If he dies, then all hope is lost." Chris had clearly come to unconsciously recognize his own strong and wise feminine energies, which had been suffocated as a result of his many negative life experiences. This figure sat almost squarely in the center of the tray and was well guarded.

Closure

Chris's last tray (Figure 7.10) came 3 months after his previous tray. At this point he was aware that treatment with me would be ending because of my pending departure from the state. Three subsequent sessions would take place focused on termination and transfer back to his original group therapist. Chris had been engaged in some truth or dare play the previous week. There was "kissing" among all the participants, one of whom was his brother. No other touching or fondling took place. The treatment team believed that these behaviors were more in keeping with his peer group than with aberrant sexualized behavior. Chris's home life had calmed down, and as a result, so had his acting out.

Chris was appropriately expressing sadness at the pending termination and fears and concerns about his future treatment. These issues were addressed by and for the client through the termination process. Chris's mother Suki was not involved in this termination process, although she was invited. A transition session with the group therapist was also provided for Chris.

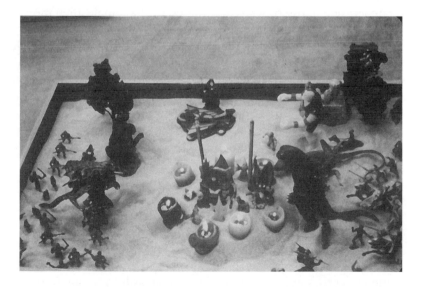

FIGURE 7.10. Good guys versus bad guys.

Upon creating tray 17 Chris again labeled this a "good guy" versus "bad guy" scene. The bad guys are on the left side of tray and the
good group is on the right side. He called the gorilla "King Kong" as he
placed it in the tray. When he placed the female warrior/dragon figure
in the tray, he said that it was the wizard's son, who killed the dragon."
Upon realizing the figure was female, he indicated that "she was helping
the wounded dragon."

Chris counted both sides to ensure that they were relatively equal.
As he placed the king with the dragon in the center of the tray, he said:
"This is the wizard on the throne, and these four wizards are his helpers. . . . One of them [the silver wizard in several of the previous trays]
is the brother of the wizard on the throne." When he finished the scene,
he asked for the pencil I had been using to draw and jot notes and then
placed it in the tray. He then asked for a second pencil and also placed
it in the tray.

At this point, Chris's process in the sand is clearly incomplete. A
basic analysis of this tray quickly reveals the internal tension and dialogue that was continuing as he attempted to reconcile and integrate
the concepts of good and evil and the relationship they occupy in the
self. However, the energy he put into equalizing the elements in this tray
indicated that Chris had achieved a balance point and was returning to
the more ordinary aspects of his life.

The left side of the tray was dominated by the female alien monster
from the movie trilogy *Alien*. The right side of the tray was dominated by
the more masculine figure from the movie *Godzilla*. I have seen this pairing in battle in the trays of many boys, preteens, and teenagers. Usually
these boys have been through some type of parental abuse or neglect
and are attempting to reconcile masculine and feminine archetypes.
These figures share some common aspects. They both represent raw,
primitive, and instinctual power. They are both perceived as dangerous,
when in reality their dangerous behavior is simply an attempt to survive.
This metaphor is most appropriate for children who are attempting to
deal with unusual and out-of-the-ordinary life experiences. They adapt
as they are able, and we as professionals label the adaptive behavior as
maladaptive, which it is in many ways. This labeling often causes us to
lose sight of the fact that the child is trying to cope with a situation that
cannot be "coped" with.

Chris was telling me that these aspects still existed within him; for
the time being they appeared to be in balance as he attempted to reenter the real world. This theme of balanced tension was furthered by the
use of the female warrior figure. She stood over a fallen dragon at the

top center of the tray. At first Chris mistakenly identified her as a "him" and implied that he had vanquished the dragon, the role of the warrior. This was the third time Chris had misidentified a female figure as a male (see tray 1 and 15). This time, however, his budding identification and integration of his feminine aspect became conscious as he realized that "he" really is a "she."

What Chris did next with this realization is most important. He said that she was trying to help the fallen dragon, as a healer or shaman would. With one figure he provided two views of his developing integration: warrior and healer. These assertive and intuitive aspects had been a part of Chris all along; through the sandplay process they had been expressed in all their light and dark aspects and allowed to coalesce into a more peaceful coexistence.

The final statement of balance came in the center of the tray. In fact, Chris had actually centered this tray and in this center was a place of great power (the place of king energy). It brought back several of the figures from tray 1: the silver wizard, the maiden, and the female riding the unicorn. In tray 1 each of these figures occupied a separate mound of the tray. In this final tray they were together in the place of the king/wizard, surrounded by other wizards, making this a place of power and magic. In many ways it was a representation of the great themes of Chris's developing self.

The silver wizard, which had apparently functioned as a transferential representation of me as his therapist/guardian/elder, was now identified as the brother of the king/wizard, which clearly appears to be a representation of Chris's own emerging masculine power. We are connected, psychic brothers, and Chris has internalized this therapeutic representation as his own, perhaps as his own wizard archetype began to be activated (and, he is the king and in charge as I am his servant brother).

As the session came to an end, Chris asked for two of my pencils and placed them inside the centered circle, like two pillars. My pencil had been my tool throughout our relationship as I documented this boy's journey, and with it perhaps Chris was reassuring us both that he could continue to write the story we had started together on his own.

SUMMARY OF CLINICAL IMPRESSIONS

Chris entered treatment as an 8-year-old struggling with many issues. He was a victim of sexual abuse and parental neglect who was removed from his home and placed in foster care. For 4 years he had attempted to behave and comply; however, his early childhood experiences had created an emotionally delayed boy who did not have the appropriate social and interpersonal skills for his age. He developed in the context of how he was treated, and his resultant manner of relating to his environment was aggressive and impulsive.

This attempt to cope clearly caused Chris many problems, both at his foster home and at school. It also represented a short-term solution that was ill-fitted to his basic nature, which was more thoughtful and empathic. The stifling of this part of his personality only further stagnated his psychic development. Without the appropriate tools at hand, Chris could not come to terms with his aggressive nature—an essential aspect of the development of all children, especially for boys with histories of violence.

Chris was immediately drawn to working in the sand tray with the miniatures he had gazed at on their shelves the first day we met. Sandplay afforded Chris an opportunity to work on his trauma-related issues at a deeper level. For boys who have been aggressive, especially sexually, cognitive-behavioral therapy has proven to be very successful. My experience indicated that the boys who benefit most from this treatment are those who also have the opportunity to do less structured, in-depth work.

In Chris's case the nonverbal depth work of sandplay therapy gave him the opportunity to lead and heal. He was able to nurture and reclaim his lost feminine principle as he reconciled the negative and aggressive experiences attached to feminine and masculine archetypes. By doing so he was able to begin to contain his aggressive nature and respect it while not allowing it to take over. Accessing personal power in a full yet contained manner permits this delicate arrangement, which can facilitate the discovery and utilization of self-control.

The sandplay process allowed Chris to move from being victim and victimizer to being an ordinary 10-year-old with the potential to be a vital, contributing member of society. This potential was reflected by the fact that, at the time of termination from treatment, Chris had successfully completed his treatment for his sexually aggressive behavior. He was doing fairly well at school, had developed appropriate social skills, and, except for an isolated fighting incident, had engaged in no further physically or sexually aggressive episodes.

Chris's work was clearly unfinished. During the creation of his last tray, Chris had stabilized, but with this tray he appeared poised to reenter and move to the next level of this process. He had managed to capture and contain his aggressive energy; continued work could allow this energy to be transformed into a catalyst for further integration and psychic development. Chris's relationship to the collective/archetypal mother and father appeared to be reworked, but his relationship to his personal mother and father would most likely continue to present a challenge to him in his life. Hopefully, he would have access to continued therapy as he coped with this challenge.

Chris would also need assistance to continue the development of his nurturing and creative aspects as he defined himself in relationship to his own power. In terms of archetypes, Chris would continue to need help in developing the feminine and masculine aspects so powerfully demonstrated in his final tray.

Eventually, Chris's mother Suki relapsed, and her children were again removed from her home. Chris and his older brother Alan were returned to the foster home they had been in when I had worked with him. Alan's behavior became increasingly unmanageable, and he was placed in residential treatment. From all reports, Chris remained at his foster home, free of any significant physically or sexually aggressive behaviors, doing well in school, and moving toward independence.

REFERENCES

Baldwin, N., (1998). *Legends of the plumed serpent.* New York: Public Affairs.

Bradway, K., (1985). *Sandplay bridges and the transcendent function.* San Francisco: C. G. Jung Institute.

Bradway, K., & McCoard, B., (1997). *Sandplay: Silent workshop of the psyche.* New York: Routledge.

Campbell, J., (1949). *The hero with a thousand faces.* Princeton, NJ: Princeton University Press.

Cook, R., (1974). *The Tree of life: Images for the cosmos.* London: Thames & Hudson.

Cooper, J. C. (1978). *An illustrated encyclopedia of traditional symbols.* London: Thames & Hudson.

Cooper, J. C. (1992). *Dictionary of symbolic and mythological animals.* San Francisco: Thorsons.

Corneau, G. (1991). *Absent fathers, lost sons.* Boston: Shambhala.

Edinger, E. F. (1994). *The mystery of the coniunctio: Alchemical image of individuation.* Toronto: Inner City Books.

Finkelhor, D., and Browne, A. (1986). Initial and long term effects: A conceptual framework. In D. Finkelhor (Ed.), *A sourcebook on child sexual abuse* (pp. 180–198). Newbury Park, CA: Sage.

Johnson, R. (1991). *Owning your own shadow: Understanding the dark side of the psyche.* San Francisco: Harper.

Jung, C. G. (1956). *The collected works of C. G. Jung. Vol. 5. Symbols of transformation.* Princeton, NJ: Princeton University Press.

Jung, C. G. (1969a). *The collected works of C. G. Gung. Vol. 8. Structure and dynamics of the psyche.* Princeton, NJ: Princeton University Press:

Jung, C. G. (1969b). *The collected works of C. G. Jung. Vol. 11. Psychology and religion: West and east. Princeton, NJ: Princeton University Press.*

Jung, C. G. (1989). *Aspects of the masculine.* Princeton, NJ: Princeton University Press.

Kalff, D. (1980). *Sandplay: A psychotherapeutic approach to the psyche.* Boston: Sigo Press.

Kindlon, D., & Thompson, M. (1999). *Raising Cain.* New York: Ballantine Books.

Moore, R. (2001). *The archetype of initiation.* San Francisco: XLibris.

Moore, R., & Gillette, D. (1990). *King, magician, warrior, lover: Rediscovering the archetypes of the mature masculine.* San Francisco: Harper.

Neumann, E. (1973). *The child.* Boston: Shambhala.

Pipher, M. (1994). *Reviving Ophelia.* New York: Grosset/Putnam.

Pollack, W. (1998). *Real boys.* New York: Holt.

Rise, C. (1994). Men's violence in sandplay. *Journal of Sandplay Therapy, 4*(1), 19–35.

Sharp, D. (1998). *Jungian psychology unplugged: My life as an elephant.* Toronto: Inner City Books.

Singer, J. (1972). *Boundaries of the soul.* New York: Doubleday.

Turner, B. (2005). *The handbook of sandplay therapy.* Cloverdale, CA: Teneros Press.

van der Kolk, B. A., McFarlane, A. C., & Weisaeth, L. (Eds.). (2007). *Traumatic Stress.* New York: Guilford Press.

Weinrib, E. (1983). *Images of the self: The sandplay therapy process.* Boston: Sigo Press.

Weinrib, E. (1996). The shadow and the cross. *Journal of Sandplay Therapy, 1*(2), 22–29.

CHAPTER 8

A Tornado Disrupts the Wedding, to the Relief of the Unwilling Bride

A Girl's Quest for Healing after Sexual Abuse

MYRIAM L. GOLDIN

CASE REFERRAL INFORMATION

Lillian is a 9-year-old African American girl who was referred by Child Protective Services for an extended play-based developmental assessment (Gil, 2006). She was sexually molested by her second cousin, Frank, a 16-year-old boy who was a trusted member of her family. Lillian was the youngest of three sisters and lived with her mother, Gloria, as did Neima, 12, and Celeste, 10. They lived in an apartment located in a safe neighborhood.

Lillian's mother and Frank's mother had maintained a supportive relationship both before and after the abuse. Prior to this incident, both families had spent weekends and holidays together and had allowed their children to have sleepovers in both homes on numerous occasions. It was during these visits that the abuse occurred at Frank's house.

Gloria had responded with disbelief and shock when she first heard about Lillian's abuse and reported feeling confused and hurt. She had loved Frank like a son, and his actions were hard for her to comprehend. The abuse came to light after Lillian shared with an older female cousin that Frank had touched her private parts while she was sleeping over at his house. Gloria and a group of trusted relatives, after discussing Lillian's disclosure, decided to call the authorities. Multiple agencies got involved in Frank's case and as part of the intervention plan, Lillian was referred to therapy.

Gloria attended our initial meeting. She was a warm and soft-spoken woman in her mid-30s. She shared relevant aspects of her family history and specific concerns regarding Lillian's overall psychoemotional development. Gloria had divorced Lillian's father 7 years ago. She noted that Lillian had limited contact with her father and that she seemed well adjusted to his absence. Gloria spoke honestly about her initial response to Lillian's traumatic experience. She was clear about both her disappointment for having been unable to protect her little girl from harm and her desire for Lillian to "grow healthy."

Gloria talked about Lillian's overall development, her strengths, and her areas of concern. Lillian was described as a jovial and assertive girl. Being the youngest of three sisters, Lillian had learned to be independent and to readily compromise with those she loved. Mom noted that Lillian had strong coping skills, and she was hopeful that her family's spiritual faith would guide them through this adversity with compassion and kindness.

After the disclosure Lillian and her mom had not addressed the subject again. Mom had tried to help Lillian cope with the events by maintaining a predictable routine and by focusing on day-to-day activities. Lillian hadn't volunteered to talk about what had happened to her, and Mom hadn't pressured her to do otherwise.

FORMULATION OF THE PROBLEM

Lillian entered counseling showing a few signs of distress. She had maintained expectable behaviors at home and at school for the most part. I asked Gloria if she had noticed any changes in Lillian since the occurrence of the abuse. She noted that Lillian had developed more defiant and aggressive behaviors at home and also mentioned that Lillian didn't like talking about what had happened. Aside from her defiant attitude and constricted affect, Lillian seemed to have been minimally affected by the abusive experience.

Lillian's engagement in therapy was initiated mostly as a preventive measure. Lillian's mom had decided to follow up with the recommendations from Child Protective Services to have Lillian undergo an assessment to determine her overall functioning. During this assessment, clinicians pay keen attention to the child's expressive play, internal and environmental resources, and symptomatic and/or problematic behaviors. In other words, the clinician identifies the traumatic impact of the abuse, if any, through observation of the child's symbolic play, by asking the child to engage in specific play-based assessment activities, and by having parents complete a number of assessment instruments (Gil, 2006). The clinician then develops recommendations that meet the specific needs of that child and his or her family.

The initial goal of the extended play-based developmental assessment was to assess Lillian's unique functioning, identify her problem areas, rule clinical symptoms in or out, understand her perceptions of her important relationships, and subsequently develop recommendations that met her specific needs. After completing the assessment with Lillian, the specific treatment goals were (1) to assist her in processing the abuse and (2) to provide her with psychoeducation regarding safety and prevention.

INVITATION TO PLAY THERAPY

Lillian waited for me patiently in the waiting room. She was immaculately dressed and her hair was nicely done. I invited her to follow me, and she quietly complied. Once in the playroom she seemed attentive and curious. I introduced her to the different toys, the miniatures, the sand tray, and art corner. She moved around cautiously, observing my movements as much as, or even more than, her surrounding environment. I asked her to tell me about her understanding of why she had come to see me, but she did not respond. I clarified to her what my role as a therapist was, briefly describing to her that I have worked with children who had been touched in their private parts or have been asked to touch others in their private parts. I also clarified to her that these actions may have been done by a parent, a relative, an adult or teenager, a friend or a stranger, and that it was my understanding that a teenage relative had touched her private parts. Lillian looked at me intensely but did not utter a word.

I also told Lillian that she was free to talk as much or as little as she wanted. She seemed to embrace this comment giving her permission to talk as *little* as she wanted. From that day on until the day she completed her treatment 5 months later, Lillian communicated mostly through nonverbal play. She rarely spoke directly about the abuse, and on the few occasions when I felt compelled to ask her to verbalize aspects of her play, she voiced her confusion about my inability to decode her language. Lillian would say, "I don't get you . . . I just told you."

It is important to note that when Lillian started treatment, I felt honored to have been entrusted with the mission to help her heal from her traumatic experience. I envisioned a process in which I was going to listen to her story, and I was going to provide her with the necessary psychoeducational and cognitive-behavioral tools to help her heal. I somehow thought that assisting her to verbalize what had happened, listening to her story, and processing it with her would be the most effective way to intervene. Little did I know that Lillian had selected to share and process her story, her fears, and her sense of mastery in her own unique way.

Carl Jung (1928) once said, "Learn your theories well but set them aside when you meet the miracle of a living soul" (p. 361). I was grateful to have learned the theories of client-centered play therapy as well as cognitive-behavioral approaches, so I felt confident in shifting and following the client's lead. The mostly nondirective approach seemed the *right treatment match* for working with Lillian. Throughout our work together I encouraged her to externalize her internal thoughts, perceptions, and feelings by providing her with a variety of nonverbal methods to access and utilize symbolic language as well as spontaneous verbal communication. Lillian allowed me to witness her inner world through her dynamic posttraumatic play.

This type of work is not employed by every child in treatment. Many children seem willing and ready to engage in their recovery process through verbal means. However, others such as Lillian appear less interested in verbal communication and seem to welcome the opportunity to be heard in a nonverbal communication style. As I am writing this case today, I realize that there was much about her symbolic play that I missed, misinterpreted, or misunderstood during the course of her treatment. It has also been remarkable to me how little impact my lack of full awareness may have had on Lillian's resilient ability to care for her own injuries. This point emphasizes the fact that it is the client's understanding and processing of his or her own work that is much more relevant and useful than the clinician's full understanding of the child's work at the moment.

CASE ILLUSTRATION OF SELF-DIRECTED TRAUMA PLAY

The Beginning: Setting the Stage

During the first few sessions, I observed Lillian's mode of communication. As mentioned earlier, she appeared uncomfortable talking directly to me, favoring the use of play to express her needs. Lillian also seemed to enjoy the structure and consistency of her sessions. During the first 2 weeks, Lillian chose all her activities; however, after those 2 weeks and as part of her assessment, Lillian had the option to complete a weekly task before and/or after her free-play time. Often, Lillian chose to complete the structured activity first. She liked calling the activity "homework," noting that she had to finish it before she could play.

Lillian moved freely around the room during her first visits. She enjoyed coloring, playing doctor, and creating miniaturized scenarios in the sand tray. As Gil (2006) suggests, I showed Lillian around the room and when I showed her the sand tray and shelves full of miniatures, I told her that she could use as few or as many miniatures and build a world in the sand tray or simply make anything that she liked.

Lillian liked coloring with chalk, and she often drew heart pictures and inscribed them with the words "I love my mommy." She also created portraits of people with eyes and noses, but not ears or mouths. Lillian played doctor often, directing me to become either her patient or the mother of a doll patient who presented some ailment that required surgery or vaccinations. Her doctor play became repetitive. On one occasion, Lillian, acting as an assertive, "in control" doctor, guided me to be the parent of a doll she named "Yolanda Goldin." Lillian created a doctor's note specifying Yolanda's need for services. She then directed me to make Yolanda cry or not cry. Lillian often switched in her role from assertive to aggressive. She carried out intrusive procedures with big pointy needles. She talked to the doll in a rough manner, ordering her to stay quiet. After the medical procedures were completed, Lillian would become less demanding and more empathic toward Yolanda. She placed bandages on the doll's body and guided me to nurture Baby Yolanda. She also instructed me not to make the baby cry, and she ordered me not to cry either. Once the doctor–patient sessions ended, Lillian acted appropriately toward me; her demeanor was respectful and cooperative.

Lillian's initial play suggested several important issues. For one, she seemed concerned with the reception and expression of emotions: Her drawings suggested people who could see and smell but could not hear or talk. Furthermore, her doctor play appeared to hold various meanings, all of which seemed to have facilitated Lillian's processing of her unspoken feelings. Lillian's spontaneous choice of playing doctor may have had a reparative component. Doctors, for the most part, help us to feel better. They are also figures of authority that often children can't question. However, in this game she was in control. Lillian directed every action for me to take in my role as a parent or in my role as the baby's spokesperson. Somehow Lillian got to role-play various parts. She was the person in charge of the suffering and the healing, and, at the same time, she put herself in the role of the vulnerable child and/or the disempowered parent. This doctor was invasive, and Baby Yolanda and her mom had no say on how intrusive the procedures were. Gradually, Lillian would allow the baby doll to express her pain, to cry. She would also allow herself to comfort Yolanda by placing bandages where the medical procedures had occurred. In this play, Lillian acted out the roles of feeling ill and in pain, asking for help, allowing someone to help her, experiencing aggression from a purported healer, and then reclaiming personal control. In essence, Lillian seemed to be nurturing the part of herself that had been injured. Her doctor game may have also suggested how she felt about keeping the abuse quiet for some time. The initial repetitive aspects of her game appeared to be reenactments of situations in which her cry was stifled and she was forced to keep still. However, her themes shifted as she changed the sequence of her game, making the doctor acknowledge Yolanda's pain and respond to her in a comforting and nurturing manner.

When Lillian finished playing doctor, she directed her attention to the sand tray. Her interaction with the sand evolved throughout the sessions. Her initial encounters were explorative in nature; she touched the sand, made hand prints on it, and funneled the sand back and forth. She seemed calm and in control while playing this way. At some point Lillian started creating spontaneous sand worlds in a meticulous manner. She would scan the miniatures on the shelves, carefully observing the attributes of each. She would pick up each miniature, scan it, and either select it by placing it on a pile or put it back on the shelf. Lillian worked in silence. Sometimes she reflected out loud on whatever was in her mind. She did not seem to need my feedback and rarely included me in her sand play. Once Lillian made all her miniature selections, she devoted herself to the creation of her worlds.

Lillian's first sand world reflected the life of a community in which there was a volcano at the center (Figure 8.1). In the surrounding area there were young children playing and an older (miniature) boy next to the little children. There were also animals in a pasture. The young children were placed deep in the sand with their legs mostly covered and one baby figure showing only its head. All the animals (cows, a pig, and a dog) were facing away from the volcano. The largest cow was the closest one to the volcano; it was keeping its head in the sand. There was a church not far from where the children were playing. When Lillian fin-

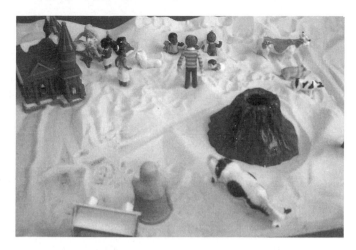

FIGURE 8.1. The volcano in the center.

ished arranging the miniatures, I asked her to tell me about her world. She noted that the older boy was taking care of the younger children. The children's mothers were not there, and the older boy pretended to be nice. I invited Lillian to verbally explore more about her world, but she did not appear interested in adding more verbal comments. As I reflect back on Lillian's first sand world, I realize how much she had told me already!

Lillian chose to place a volcano at the center of her world. This selection may be suggestive of what she experienced as the presence of a potentially explosive danger threatening the calmness of her world. Lillian seemed to reflect on the vulnerability of the little children playing so close to the volcano. She noted that potentially protective adults were not there and that there was danger around them. Lillian explicitly stated that the older boy who was accompanying the little children seemed nice but was not! She positioned the cows and the pig looking away, suggesting that the animals may have had some apprehension about facing the volcano. The presence of a church may be suggestive of Lillian's faith and also her sense that even having a church close by could not change the reality of the events. In this scenario, however, she placed both a sign of danger (volcano) and a potential sign of repair or resource (church) within the same world, signaling her ability to acknowledge both threat and rescue.

I pondered different reasons for why Lillian may have placed the cows and the pig in the way that she did. Was it her sense that adults, though in the vicinity, had not been able to see what was really going on—or had looked the other way? Was the larger cow's hiding of its head symbolic of not facing the events? Was Lillian somehow externalizing observations she had made about her mom expressing difficulty in dealing with the whole issue? Were the cows a symbol of how Lillian and her sisters had stopped seeing Frank? The list was endless and, in reality, only Lillian knew why her selection of miniatures and placement had meaning. It was possible she already knew as she manipulated these small toy figures, and it was possible that the embedded meaning would reveal itself over time. However, my full understanding of how the symbols told the story was not as important as how Lillian had found a vehicle with which to convey, in a cohesive manner, what had happened to her. She narrated her story noting both danger and vulnerability.

Lillian's subsequent work illustrates how, with great courage, she worked through her initial sense of vulnerability to become empowered and in control. Lillian created her second sand scenario following the same pattern as before. She selected many miniatures similar to those in her previous sand world and added a few new ones (Figure 8.2). Lillian created what she called a "Halloween scene" (Figure 8.2). She talked out loud as she worked. Her scenario took place somewhere outdoors. In it there was an emergency room in one corner of the tray. On top of the emergency room she placed a rescue helicopter that had a face drawn

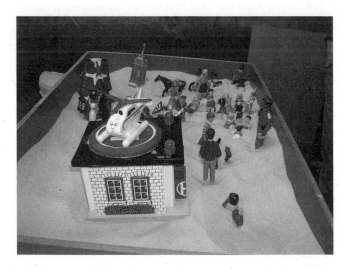

FIGURE 8.2. Lillian's Halloween scene.

on it. The helicopter's face was not looking at the large crowd dispersed all over the sand tray.

Lillian's world contained younger and older children, policemen, ghost horses, couples, and fairies. She made a policeman figure talk to the same older boy figure that was present in her previous sand tray scenario. In this one, "the older boy was being bad," but the policeman could not arrest him because he was only a pretend officer (reminiscent of her first sand tray in which the boy was also pretending). Lillian played a lot with all the characters. She moved them around, making them fight and befriend each other repeatedly. She said that this was a "pretend world," and people were pretending to be bad. Lillian also noted that in her world "only goodness gets in," and that she was "protecting her world from bad things."

Lillian seemed to continue to struggle with her sense of being fully protected by the adults and authority figures present in her sand world. Her sense of disguise may be also suggestive of how she perceived that people may not have been what they say they were. Frank had faked being nice, and the adults around him had somehow been unable to see what was really happening to her. Lillian's decision to state that this was a Halloween scene seems to have given her permission to take control of the situation by declaring that it was all pretend and that in her world, this new construct, only good things could happen. Also, her emphasis on a pretend world may suggest her own difficulty with holding and processing ambivalent feelings she may have had toward Frank. The presence of community helpers such as the emergency room and the paramedic helicopter may be seen as a resource to be accessed at some point or as a protective factor for her new recreated world.

The Middle: The Work Deepens and Moves

Although Lillian shared a few spontaneous smiles with me as her treatment continued, for the most part she remained emotionally flat in her affect. I often wondered how she was truly feeling. One activity that seemed to help Lillian identify, process, and express her emotions was the "Color Your Feelings task" (Drewes, 2001; Gil, 2006). In a self-expressive and nonthreatening manner, Lillian identified an array of feelings when thinking about different situations. She responded to my inquiry to first identify feelings she felt most of the time, then find a color that best matched each feeling. I then provided her with two figures of people (gingerbread figures) that she could color using her affective color code. One figure represented her on any given day

(Figure 8.3), and the second was her when Frank was touching her private parts (Figure 8.4).

She was able to identify feeling happy (yellow), sad (blue), and mad (red) when thinking about her everyday life, and feeling mad, hurtful, and sad when thinking about what Frank had done to her. It was after completing this activity that Lillian took the initiative to express in more depth how she felt about disclosing the abuse.

She asked me if she could color one more gingerbread figure and instructed me to write: "Feelings I feel after I shared what Frank did to me and he got in trouble." Seconds after she stated her sentence, she asked me to scratch the word *Frank* and to write *somebody* instead (Figure 8.5). Lillian took over writing and coloring her feelings with a degree of energy I had not witnessed before. She identified feeling excited, amazed, and really, *really* happy!

Lillian added the spontaneous comment that she did not have to worry now that her cousin had gotten in trouble. Lillian expressed the multiple feelings she felt toward Frank as if talking to herself. I just happened to be a fortunate witness at that time, benefiting from her decision to say out loud what she seemed to have felt inside all along. Whenever she volunteered information, I usually asked her to verbally

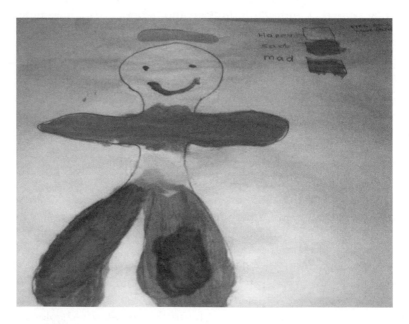

FIGURE 8.3. Lillian's Color Your Feelings drawing for an ordinary day.

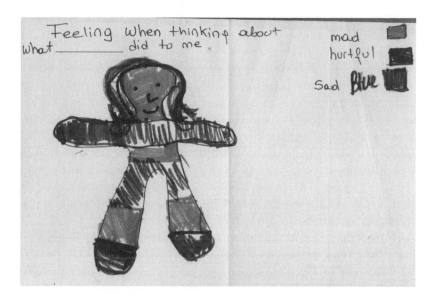

FIGURE 8.4. "My feelings when Frank touched my privates."

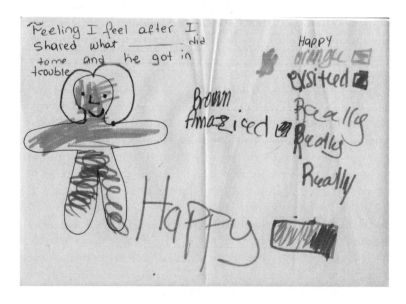

FIGURE 8.5. "Feeling happy after I told and Frank got in trouble."

elaborate more about her experience. Her response to me, once she realized that I was asking her to directly address the issue, was often the same: She did not like to talk about that subject.

Lillian seemed to have a lot to say, yet she still seemed uncomfortable about saying the offender's name out loud. Her discomfort around directly verbalizing his name suggests a possible lack of readiness to face what happened to her, without the support of symbolic buffers. Lillian's desire to switch Frank's name to *somebody* may also suggest her natural reparative ability to regulate her exposure to her trauma gradually. Asking Lillian to participate in the Color Your Feelings technique gave her the opportunity to process and express previously guarded feelings. Lillian's affect changed following that session; she acted more relaxed and cheerful. On occasions she voiced her preference for playing certain recreational board games after she had done her tasks.

During one session, Lillian created another sand tray in response to my directive to create two scenarios in the sand, one about how she felt "before she told" and another to show how she felt "after she told." She worked silently dividing the sand tray into two halves. She created a densely packed forest scene filled with trees and big birds. The trees in this forest were extremely close to each other and the birds had large wings and big beaks. The other half of her scene was an open space, just sand. Lillian identified the forest scene as her world before she told and the spacious sand area as her world after she told. She did not make additional comments.

During that same session, she directed her attention toward the miniature replica of a courtroom, made out of wood, including wooden, painted figures that have one emotional expression on one side and a different emotion on the back side. Lillian arranged the court participants as if a jury session were taking place. She placed the wooden figures where she imagined they needed to be sitting. She put a male figure in the witness chair, a female figure in the defendant's seat, a judge at the bench, and a group of jurors in their jury seats. Lillian turned all the wooden figures' faces to show sad expressions and then announced that she had finished (Figure 8.6). Her demeanor was calm and resolute.

This time Lillian's sand tray conveyed a clear picture of how she felt about what had happened to her. While she was being abused, she seemed to have felt oppressed and trapped. The scenery was of a compacted forest with big scary birds roaming around. Her description of her world "after she told" conveyed a sense of space and openness. What

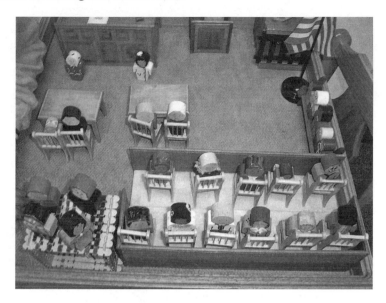

FIGURE 8.6. Frank faces the judge and jury.

was most evident was the stark contrast between these two worlds in the sand tray: One half was crowded and constricted; the other half was extremely open. Lillian's transition from her sand tray work to her play with the court set may have been suggestive of how she viewed the process of bringing justice to her case and how much sadness the sexual abuse had caused her and her family.

Resolutions Surface

Lillian's spontaneous play gained momentum in her subsequent sessions, more understanding, meaning, and resolution added to her narrative. She utilized a hospital dollhouse in the play therapy office. She started playing and talking out loud while she played. She chose a male figure and started making this figure walk around. Then she played out a scene in which a shooting took place. She noted that the boy was being bad in the streets and that it was for that reason that he got shot. She proceeded to take the boy to the hospital, where he underwent surgery. The boy remained in the hospital while nurses and doctors took care of him. Lillian then left the boy scene and directed her attention to some babies that were also at the hospital.

She noted that the hospital needed doors to protect the babies from harm. Lillian added that the boy's mother was also at the hospital and that she could not help her son but that she was worried about him. Lillian wrapped up her play by adding walls to the babies' rooms and by making the boy roll on a wheelchair around the hospital. She made sure that the boy did not get close to the babies. Lillian then made the boy start walking again. She also made his mom feel recovered. As noted previously, Lillian played without including me in her games. When she finished, I told her that she could tell me about her story, to which she responded, "I just did."

Lillian's choice of characters and setting reflected her thoughts and feelings about what had happened to her and how she felt was still vulnerable but would be able to heal and repair the pain she had felt and the pain that people she loved had also felt. In addition, Lillian seemed to express empathy toward her offender and designated him as ill, in need of help himself to get better. Lillian endowed the boys' mother with strength so that she might take better care of him.

Lillian's story took place in a hospital, a place where people who are injured seek attention. She noted that the boy had been doing things he was not supposed to do, and because of that he had gotten hurt and needed some repair work. Lillian's performance of his surgery, followed by the boy needing to use a wheelchair, may suggest Lillian's view that Frank needed major interventions to get better and that he also needed time to heal. Interestingly enough, Frank had been court ordered to receive treatment, and this may have been the manner in which Lillian assured herself that he would get the help that he needed.

Lillian's story was inclusive. It identified a whole group of people needing help, from the character that was acting out of control, to his mom, and to the little children who were vulnerable and needed nurturance and protection. Lillian's comment about the lack of doors may suggest her interest in stronger boundaries that could have helped her to feel less vulnerable and exposed to Frank's nocturnal intrusions. It may also reflect a built-in sense of mastery as she altered the initial hospital scene to provide the safety that she needs. In other words, she noticed what was needed to make the hospital safer and she mobilized her resources to bring change.

Lillian's story seems to elaborate on what happened to her and on her need to explain and make sense of why her cousin Frank had done this to her. It appears that her narrative moves from being thrilled that he got caught and in trouble, to feeling empathic toward him and noticing that he was ill and needed some help. It is also possible that she overheard adult family conversations in which Frank's status (and the need for him to participate in therapy) was discussed. In the end, Lillian's story provides each character with whatever they seem to need to feel better.

Lillian's affect became more expressive during subsequent sessions. Her play continued to evolve and deepen into what appeared to be her way to develop reparative trauma work. She smiled more and started making more spontaneous verbal comments and engaged in more verbal interactions with me. In addition, she explored areas of the playroom in which she had not shown interest before. She started to cook elaborate meals with a toy kitchen and pretend food. She also began to create puppet shows. Lillian liked to dress up with big butterfly wings and wear oversize glitzy sunglasses. With this costume on, she created puppet shows in which policemen and animal detectives would look for bad animals that were getting in trouble. Once they were caught, the policemen would lecture them on being nice to each other. The mischievous characters would respond by becoming submissive and kind.

Lillian repeated this play many sessions. The plot always stressed someone doing something wrong and rescue figures stepping forward. On one occasion Lillian and her mom created a puppet story together. I had invited her mother to join some of our later sessions once it was clear that Lillian's posttraumatic play had positive outcomes and once Lillian was more comfortable having her mother be present during sessions. Mom chose a puppet that had reading glasses and white hair, which displayed an aura of wisdom. Lillian chose a wolf and a monkey. The theme of their story centered around a concern for safety; the wolf had not been treating the monkey well, and the wise-man puppet seemed to want to facilitate the dialogue between them. The wise-man puppet noted that the monkey was in a bad mood all the time and asked him what was bothering him. The monkey responded that it wanted to be left alone, and the wise-man puppet noted that he wanted to help him. The wolf puppet asked to be forgiven for his nagging behavior, and the monkey decided to forgive him.

At one point, after they played the puppet show for me, I addressed the monkey puppet and reflected on his statement of being angry all the time. The monkey noted that he felt other feelings but that he did not tell others how he felt. The wise-man puppet advised forgiveness for the monkey for having acted crabbily, and for the wolf that had also annoyed the monkey. Wolf and monkey made amends, the wolf apolo-

gized to the monkey, and the monkey apologized to the wise-man puppet. In the end, they were all friends.

Lillian's puppet stories, at first, appeared to address her need to
have the misbehaving characters be disciplined. However, as her play
and storytelling deepened, she also seemed interested in exploring
the possibility of establishing a dialogue between the offender and the
victim. Lillian's joint puppet story with her mom culminated with the
resolution of the conflict between the wolf and the monkey, just as the
hospital story ended in a nurturing manner after acknowledging and
expressing other feelings. Lillian's polarized puppet selection also indicates her attempts to master the affect that the abuse provoked in her.
On one hand, Lillian chose a monkey, an animal that, for the most part,
is seen as playful, active, and nonaggressive. On the other hand, Lillian
also selected a wolf, a clever animal that can be deceptive and predatory toward other animals. Her theme was consistent and relevant to
her real-life situation: She had been a playful and trusting girl who had
been taken advantage of by someone whom she and her family thought
was honest and trustworthy. She became moody after the abuse and
struggled with expressing her emotions. Lillian appeared empowered
by the wolf's acknowledgment of his mistakes and by his apology toward
the monkey. In this puppet story, the issue of forgiveness seemed to have
been driven by Mom's character; however, Lillian seemed to embrace
the story's ending. Lillian welcomed the opportunity to make the wolf
apologize to the monkey and also to make the monkey acknowledge his
bad-tempered behavior toward the wise man and the other animals.
Mom's puppet behaved empathically toward the monkey and the wolf,
offering comfort to both animals.

Transitions Occur

Lillian continued to use her nonverbal approach to her own healing,
and I continued to struggle to validate my interventions and impact on
her recovery process at times. During one session, I asked Lillian to create a sand world that reflected her experience of coming to therapy,
and how she felt "coming to therapy" had been for her. In other words,
I asked her to create a world keeping in mind the following questions:
Why do you think you came to see me? And what has been "helpful or
not" to you about coming to therapy?

Lillian set to work quietly, placing a wooden jail in the center of the
sand tray. Inside the jail were marbles and jewels. In one corner of the

sand tray Lillian placed a fence, behind which she placed people and horses. In another corner of the tray, Lillian created an elaborate wedding scene where a number of adult figures were surrounding bride and groom miniatures (Figure 8.7).

The rest of the sand tray initially held parked ambulances, fire trucks, police cars, and helicopters. At some point during her creation Lillian asked me if we could walk to the art room because she needed to get something; there she selected a group of fuzzy pipe cleaners and brought them back to the playroom. She started twisting the pipe cleaners until they all looked like a thick mass measuring approximately 2 inches. Lillian started talking out loud while she interacted with her chosen miniatures. She did not speak directly to me, but engaged in a self-dialogue.

Lillian talked about a world where people and jewels were trapped in jails and places were they could not escape. She noted that the small bride and groom figures were Frank and her. Lillian stated that she was being asked to marry Frank because only married people do "those things." To the little bride figures she said, "What if you have to marry him?" And the figure would respond, "Oh, no. . . . " And as she talked she moved her figures from one place to another. Then she grabbed the

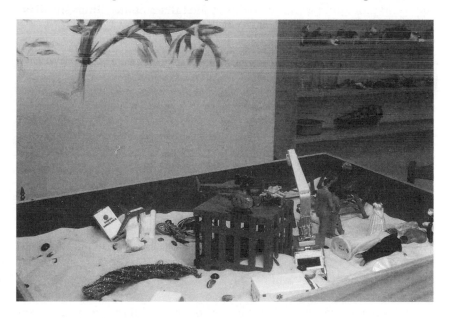

FIGURE 8.7. A wedding with an unwilling bride.

pipe cleaner design and voiced that a tornado had hit this world of a possible wedding between a groom and an unwilling bride.

Lillian made the tornado twirl around her sand world, destroying everything in its path. In the mist of a devastated scene, Lillian made her rescue force come into action. She mobilized the police cars, fire trucks, and helicopters, making them drive through the sand, surrounding the wooden jail. She shook the jail structure, freeing the marbles and some of the jewels. After what looked like a fierce battle between the tornado and the rescue squad, the tornado seemed defeated, lying motionless on the sand. Lillian noted that the police and her "special therapy" had come to her rescue.

Lillian's affect seemed attuned with the sequence of events that was occurring in her play scene. She worked meticulously and calmly while setting the scene. Her energy level increased when the tornado hit her world, and her dynamism peaked when she mobilized her rescue crew. Lillian appeared in command of her emotions, fighting that tornado with intense determination. At the end of the encounter, Lillian seemed relieved and pleased with herself. My sense is that she had interrupted the "wedding," that is, the abuse. She'd had an experience of mastery and control that elated and strengthened her. Afterward she asked if she could paint, and while she painted she talked about things she liked and things she feared. This time she talked to me, acknowledging my presence.

Lillian's sand world (and everything that preceded the making of this sand world) was a detailed and organized recounting of her trauma narrative. Her sense of entrapment seems to have been exemplified by her selection of the jail and long fences that, in her words, "kept people and jewels trapped." Lillian's creation of the wedding scene suggests that, in her mind, she felt that Frank had trespassed her personal boundaries, and one way to make sense of what had happened to her was to infer that she was getting married to him. Her choice of a tornado suggested that the whole experience had swept her off her feet in a manner that she could not initially control. However, her response to her overwhelming threat revealed that she could bravely manage to access her inner resources (and free her trapped jewels, likely her innocence and goodness) to fight against the tornado in an inspiring manner. Lillian seemed to have felt that her family's response, the agencies and designated professionals who were involved in her case, and her therapy sessions had helped her in her journey. Lillian's story appeared to evolve from her role as victim to survivor to conqueror.

Closure

Lillian continued to attend treatment for a few more weeks. After building her tornado sand tray, she seemed more relaxed and chatty during the sessions. She expressed her feelings more openly and acknowledged still feeling angry toward Frank at times. I reflected on her sand tray work and thanked her for the courage she had exhibited in creating her tornado sand tray. She noted that she did not like to talk about "that" and casually mentioned that she had left the tornado pipe cleaner somewhere in her house, as if the tornado did not carry much value for her any more.

As the focus of treatment moved toward increasing awareness of her safety, Lillian seemed more receptive to objectively discussing appropriate and inappropriate touches. She felt comfortable commenting on her reactions to situations that we had read in books or watched in psychoeducational movies. She empathized with a particular movie character who had experienced bullying and abuse by an older boy. She noted that what this character went through was not fair and that it had not been the young boy's fault. Toward the last sessions, in a surprisingly expressive manner, Lillian started spontaneously singing a preventive song she had heard in one of the movies we had seen. A turtle and a clam sing a song about what to do, "What Tadoo," when children find themselves in sexually uncomfortable situations. These two characters explore ways in which children could safely respond to the unwelcome situations (Mitchell, 1995). Lillian sang that song openly while playing and/or painting. I often wondered if her singing was somehow her style of telling me that she got it, her way of telling me that now she knew "what to do, " or another expressive way of emphasizing her current mastery experience by lifting her voice in song.

Lillian appeared to have woven together all the elements of her treatment by setting her own pace and finding her own balance of nondirective and (compliance with) directive therapy. At our celebratory final session, Lillian, her family, and I enjoyed chocolate cup cakes, juice, and a great sense of accomplishment.

SUMMARY OF CLINICAL IMPRESSIONS

Lillian was a solemn young girl who had come to therapy after she had been sexually abused by her male adolescent cousin. She and her family had been very close to this young man and his mother, and the whole situation had provoked great anguish and shock in both families. Lillian presented few signs of overt distress or measurable symptoms upon her referral. She behaved as expected at home and at school with the exception that at home she acted in a more defiant and grumpy manner. Recognizing these signs, her mother decided to follow through with the recommendation by Child Protective Services and voluntarily brought Lillian to participate in assessment and subsequent treatment.

The implementation of the extended play-based developmental assessment led Lillian to externalize her initial feelings of anger and vulnerability as she engaged in multiple expressive play activities. Lillian worked through her sense of exposure by expressively creating different play scenarios in which she felt in control of what happened to her characters. She added endings to her stories that reflected her ability to integrate all the aspects of her abuse. Lillian's healing outcomes in her stories attest to her amazing coping skills and resiliency.

Lillian's play during her treatment held some of the characteristics of what has been described by Gil as dynamic posttraumatic play (Gil, 2006). She crafted a natural way of self-imposed exposure to her traumatic experience in a gradual manner. She created play situations that symbolized the important characters (victim, victimizer, and rescuer) who experienced feelings of vulnerability as they were exposed to dangerous situations. Progressively, Lillian added elements to her play that indicated that she felt gradually more in control of difficult situations. Her affect became more available, and her interactions with her play and with me became more fluid. Her initial gravitation toward playing doctor in a rigid manner changed as her roughness shifted toward an assertive but nurturing style. Lillian's initial doctor's play also seemed to have helped her reenact some of the constricted feelings she may have experienced as she was being abused. As her level of comfort increased, Lillian's play reflected her efforts to venture out to experiment with a self-created gradual exposure to the abusive experience and its initial and current meaning and impact.

Lillian's sand trays also captured movement in her play themes. Her initial sand trays reflected a preoccupation with a degree of danger that somehow no one had noticed except her. She also seemed concerned with the manner in which people could betray others by pretending to be something they were not and by getting away with behaviors that were hurtful to others. Lillian's play evolved by adding new elements and compensatory endings to her stories. She seemed to incorporate healthier and more adaptive responses as she created her sand trays and her hospital and puppet stories. Lillian managed to decrease her characters' sense of vulnerability by introducing community resources and healers.

She also seemed to process some of the offender's behaviors. She appeared to design situations in which the misbehaving characters were caught and brought to justice. She seemed pleased to be able to offer them an alternative and/or remedy for their problems. Lillian's scenarios in her sand trays, as well as her puppet and hospital stories, captured her need to restore a sense of safety not only for herself but also for those around her.

The most consistent theme of her work was the presence of a character that has misbehaved, as well as the presence of an opposite force that took control of the wrongdoer. Her play seemed to validate a reality in which someone had been impacted by the harm and that help was available not only for the injured, vulnerable characters, but also for the transgressor. Furthermore, Lillian added creative ways to protect the vulnerable characters. She seemed to want to avoid further damage as she strongly voiced the need to build doors at the hospital to protect the babies. Lillian's affect seemed more and more relaxed after her play sessions, indicating a release of affect that seemed beneficial to her.

As I noted earlier, Lillian embraced the nondirective (mostly nonverbal) approach. She seemed much more naturally assertive than I was in the process of trusting this therapeutic modality. She understood that there was no urgency to verbalize what she was feeling and/or thinking in order for her to process her painful experiences. Most importantly, Lillian knew how to access her own resources to restore her sense of confidence and safety. I am thankful to Lillian that she, as most children do, understood the language of play. Lillian's treatment started with my invitation for her to play. She mastered my invitation, and I became the learner and she became the teacher. Lillian guided me through her emotional maze. Our mutual nurturance, respect, and emotional connection created an environment in which Lillian successfully designed her reparative motif. In this particular case, I simply followed Lillian's need, since she seemed to know best how and when to address relevant issues related to her interpersonal trauma. Her mother's support and help were invaluable, and likely Lillian's reparative capacity was greatly anchored in her mother's substantive capacity to be of assistance as well as her great love for her daughter.

REFERENCES

Drewes, A. A. (2001). The gingerbread person feelings map. In C. E. Schaefer & H. Kaduson (Eds.), *101 more favorite play therapeutic techniques* (pp. 92–97). Northvale, NJ: Jason Aronson.

Gil, E. (2006). *Helping abused and traumatized children.* New York: Guilford Press.

Jung, C. (1928). *Contributions to analytical psychology* (p. 361). London: Hesperides Press.

Mitchell, J. G. (1995). *"What tadoo": Child abuse prevention.* Sabastopol, CA: Mitchell Film Company.

CHAPTER 9

Finding the Treasure Within

Spontaneous Storytelling and the Sandplay
Journey of an Emotionally Despairing Girl

ROSALIND L. HEIKO

Silence. In the best of therapeutic circumstances, it sustains the spiraling descent of the inward journey, the longed-for and most difficult part of any self-exploration. The dictionary gives four meanings of silence: the absence of sound or noise; the practice of keeping secrets or maintaining concealment; the ending of life; or the verb compelling or reducing to silence.

All of the definitions of silence come into play in the case of Stella. My work with her, primarily using sandplay, taught me much about active listening. She also taught me about silence—and the depths and the joys and pain inherent in it. There are so many verbal ways to examine and interpret our work with our clients. What stands out with Stella is the joyful *non*sound—so different from the raucous noises of her home and siblings—of contemplation and intensity of feeling.

CASE REFERRAL INFORMATION

Stella, 6 years old, was initially referred by her father's insurance company. Her dad stated in his initial phone message that Stella was "show-

171

ing signs of depression," and he wanted help for her. Both parents were concerned about Stella's difficulties with decision making, her behavioral problems at school, her time-outs at home that seemed "deliberately" designed to get her into trouble, her noticeable lack of interest in any peer relationships, as well as her increasingly escalating temper tantrums (e.g., "She makes big issues out of little things").

Stella's parents worked a split shift of the same job. The only day the whole family was together was on Sundays. After church came an exhausting round of cleaning, chores, grocery shopping, etc. Mom worked 2 full days a week; Dad was home with the children while she worked. Of interest to me was that mom's voice was hoarse and shaky, as was her handwriting, and it intrigued me to learn that in her professional life she helped people breathe more easily.

Stella was the oldest of three children. Her middle sister was 3 at the time of referral, a very sturdy and assertive child. Her younger brother was a toddler, also a very boisterous and active child. They moved to the area from another state about a year ago. Stella "lost" her best friend in the move away from her home state, as well as her beloved cat, who wandered away 3 days before the move. According to Mom, Stella was a "mommy's girl" who needed private time, and was very serious and very advanced for her age. She was not coping well at home or school, saying things like, "I don't want to grow up" to her teacher, or "I don't want you to leave me" to her mother.

Stella appeared very angry and hurt by the birth of her other siblings, particularly her sister. In fact, when her sister was born, Stella told her mother, "You ruined my life." After 3 weeks, Stella wanted to throw the baby in the bushes, saying, "I'm sick of all this baby crap!" Dad's sister lived in the area, but the relationship proved very disappointing to Mom, as her sister-in-law pleaded frequent headaches and was unavailable much of the time to relieve Mom in child care. Mom also appeared very depressed and weepy; she told me that her feelings alternated between emotional abandonment and anger at being nastily criticized by her own mother. Stella's mother brought in many examples of notes by and to Stella, emphasizing Stella's aloneness and insecurities, her desire for her parents to physically punish her, and her depression.

At the first parent meeting, we decided that I would administer IQ testing so that the school could evaluate Stella for the academically gifted program. Stella was reporting that the school day "drags on forever," and her parents believed that the work wasn't challenging enough for her. Stella's teacher didn't give the impression that she believed Stella was a gifted child. Stella's private Christian preschool did tell the parents that they believed she should enter an academically gifted program in first grade. My assessment of Stella indicated an IQ above the 99th percentile in relation to her peers. She was extraordinarily efficient at processing verbal material, and both her verbal and nonverbal abilities were relatively similar.

In terms of projective testing, the Rorschach Inkblot Test, using the Exner scoring system protocol, indicated that Stella was experiencing noticeable distress and was significantly depressed. Under the stress of taking the test, and the chronic overload, she tended to become more impulsive and disorganized—appearing similarly to a child exhibiting attention-deficit/hyperactivity disorder (ADHD) symptoms. Stella was an intuitive child who depended on her feelings to work through situations. However, she had become a child with negative and angry feelings who was beginning to feel hopeless about feeling better. She regarded herself more negatively when comparing herself to peers. The protocol also suggested that she was experiencing frequent difficulties interacting with others, particularly authority figures, and that her relationships tended to be more superficial and less easily sustained, causing her considerable internal anguish.

Stella's school placed her in their academically gifted (AG)/gifted and talented program approximately 2 months after the assessment results interpretation meeting with parents and the school. School officials told Stella's parents that they had never had a child that bright in the system. Stella's school brought in an AG consultant from the middle school to work with her and her teacher. At her parents' urging, the school found another child of similar academic interests and abilities, and the consultant worked with them at the same time, fostering a peer relationship.

I had a very useful talk with Stella's teacher, who believed that Stella was "lazy" and "very manipulative." She seemed astonished by the results of my testing. The teacher's major complaints were that Stella "behaves more like my peer" and would get off task with very immature behaviors and a smirk on her face, with "no remorse." The teacher agreed to work on giving Stella more challenging work and also to meet for lunch once or twice with Stella alone over the course of the next few weeks. Stella loved the attention and began to settle down in class and "allowed" the teacher to be the dominant authority over the course of the next several months.

FORMULATION OF THE PROBLEM

The theme of Stella's work is the indestructibility of love and of the human spirit. Children are often brought to therapy when either they or their parents feel in crisis, in fear, with loss of confidence and self-care issues, manifesting in reactivity through stress, anger, and anxiety. Stella's overall task was to face her fears of mother loss and abandonment and come again to believe that she was deserving and capable of inner nurturance and love. "Finding the treasure within"—to recover the belief that love is inextinguishable, both as a gift to herself and a promise of hope—was our goal during therapy. In particular, Stella needed to begin to separate out intergenerational issues of abandonment and sibling displacement, replace her demonstrations of anger and sullen withdrawal with a more balanced expression of feelings and communication, and learn to embrace both the masculine and feminine aspects of herself.

My sandplay journey map (Figure 9.1) is based upon previous formulations of the sandplay process by two sandplay teaching members—Betty Jackson (2008) and Donna Johnson (1999). The hero's journey was, of course, originally mapped by Joseph Campbell (1949). Jean and Wallace Clift (1988, p. 15) elaborated on the journey's keys more fully. The sandplay journey map conceptualizes a spiral journey into four quadrants plus a midjourney centering. Quadrant 1 includes the initial stage of the inner journey in which the client "answers the call" to the process and makes the decision to work on the issues confronting him or her. Quadrant 2 involves both discriminating and facing internal and external potentially traumatic shadow material and the tension of the opposites. The *shadow* refers to that internal material that we either don't yet want to face, aren't ready to know about ourselves, or aren't yet capable of understanding and integrating. It doesn't have to do with concepts of evil, really, just those darker denied aspects of ourselves to which we aren't yet reconciled. The term *tension of the opposites* refers to the dynamic and often ambivalent strain between two aspects of our nature, our yearnings, our needs—such as love and hate or a belief in one's essential goodness versus one's feelings of worthlessness or inadequacy.

The centering midpoint of the journey, between Quadrants 2 and 3 in Figure 9.1, is characterized by constellation-of-the-self trays—trays that show the beauty and metaphorical light within the client in a centered, numinous way. Quadrant 3 is characterized by trays that reconcile the struggle of the tension of the opposites and that work through

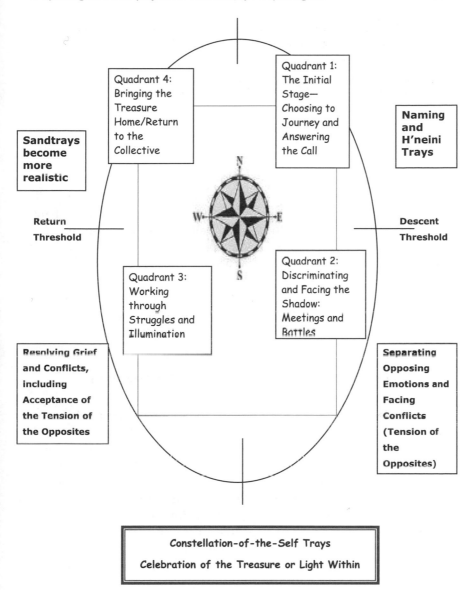

FIGURE 9.1. Map of the stages of the sandplay journey by Rosalind L. Heiko, PhD, ISST. Copyright 2006. Reprinted by permission.

the psychological conflicts manifested in Quadrant 2. In Quadrant 4, the client metaphorically "brings the treasure home" by integrating the psychological material and the struggles, and this integration is manifested in more realistic sandtrays that represent a return to everyday life and naturalistic settings.

INVITATION TO PLAY THERAPY

When I walked into the waiting room to meet Stella for the first time, I was unsure who she was. I saw a rambunctious toddler; a large, prettily dressed girl skipping around the room; and a child with a Prince Valiant-styled haircut reading intently, a book concealing her face as she ignored the loud, happy screams of the other two children. I came forward and said that I was looking for Stella; the seated child looked up at me with a scowl on her face. This scowl was to remain in place for the next several months. Everything was imperfect and yucky, and my toys and manner appeared to irritate her hugely. Stella's vocabulary was excellent, and she picked her words carefully and precisely when she spoke.

CASE ILLUSTRATION OF SELF-DIRECTED TRAUMA PLAY

Stella made use of many play therapy modalities during her sessions, although sandplay was the focus of her work. She also used the doll-house; painted extensively; created rituals (she'd say, "as we always do") of eating a snack with me at the beginning of many sessions and at ending times; brought in materials for a dreamcatcher, which we made together from items she brought and shells I'd found at special places; and worked with clay. We spent hours in the initial sessions playing hiding games in the sand, using gem "treasures" and miniature pigs and wolves, etc. Stella also had access to a library of children's books that included books about anger and loss, passive–aggressive behavior, moving and losing friends, and the crisis of the loss of self-confidence and generativity. Stella brought me two gifts during the course of our work together: a book called *The Forgotten Filly* (Dickerson, 1993), and a special mug (to be discussed later). Accepting these gifts gave me great joy, but it was her excitement in sharing her choices and her affection that told me how well she was doing.

I worked with Stella for about 1 year, during which time she created 26 sand trays. I met with her weekly during the first 9 months of therapy (except for 4 weeks when I was away studying sandplay in Switzerland), then bimonthly for the last 3 months. She created two sand trays during the latter period. I have selected 10 sandplay pictures from different phases of her work to illustrate her journey.

The Beginning: Setting the Stage

Stella entered the therapy room eagerly, separating easily from her family. She immediately began burying colorful fish in the dry sand tray, and then exclaimed over finding them again. She created a jungle scene. In response to my question of what she might call this place, she softly said, "A jungle of Africa, 'cause I kind of like Africa some," followed quickly by, "I'm going to change it to a cat scene, instead." She immediately took everything out of the tray, including the foliage. It was impossible for me to ask for permission to photograph that first tray. In fact I believe she was not ready to keep that scene in active memory.

Stella selected many symbols in this first tray that were strongly feminine. The snakes, spiders, and the spider web all bring forth images of the dark goddess. The placement of wild animal families (mostly in threes) could point to her enmeshed connection in the triangulated relationships between Mother, Grandmother, and self, or to the three children in her family. The fierce predators and the jungle may symbolize her uneasy and frightened relationship to her unconscious. These huge, potentially freeing instinctual energies seemed to rear up out of her unconscious, without real boundaries or control. In order to contain these energies, Stella may have understandably needed to get them out of the tray as quickly as they had arisen. Her perfectionism, guilt, and neediness made mastery and control important developmental issues for this little girl. From the beginning, Stella also brought in the masculine and spiritual side of herself by placing two palm trees in the tray. According to Walker (1988, p. 469), palms and their branches represent the sacred as well as masculine virility.

When creating her next tray immediately after the first (Figure 9.2), Stella placed foliage leaves, then cats. She then wanted to draw a picture of a Dalmatian after rearranging (but not playing with) the dollhouse. She said quietly and assertively, "I'm a good artist." When compared with her earlier scene of the same day, this tray is startling in terms of its sparse quality. Although seemingly organized, it conveys depression. The path doesn't lead anywhere. I felt her sadness as she finished it. However, this tray also points the way for the possible direction of the therapeutic work: the process of finding her way back "home" to

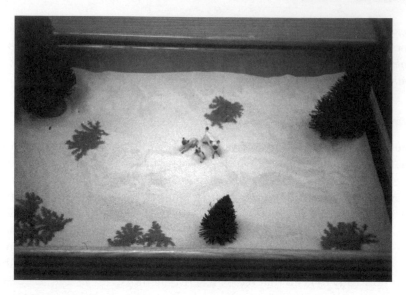

FIGURE 9.2. A forest with some cats lost in it. *Description of the tray:* An adult cat and two smaller cats stand in the middle of the tray all facing the front. There are three large, medium, and small pine trees in the tray with some greenery scattered about. The sand has lots of indistinct pathways and churned-up sand.

herself and her family. When I saw this tray, I thought about what wasn't there: food, resources, a map, directionality, hope.

These initial trays can be taken together as suggestive of Stella's problem statement and of a potential path for her journey. The three cats lost in a forest could be a female and her kittens, or three small kittens of varying sizes. There are three fir trees in this tray. Two are fairly large in proportion. They are possibly the representation of her original nuclear family: mother, father and herself as child. The two larger, stronger trees could be the parental representations, albeit disconnected from each other. Walker (1988, p. 464) suggests, "Evergreens in general were powerful symbols of ongoing life or immortality, because they seemed to keep themselves alive when everything else died during the winter." The triangular nature of her tree and cat placement and the repetition of three symbols in both Figures 9.2 and 9.3 appear significant. Walker (1988, p. 34) has referred to this trinity both in terms of Christian symbology and goddess mythology of virgin, mother, and crone.

What fascinated me about Stella's name for the scene ("A forest with some cats lost in it") is that she so completely ignored the biological fact that cats don't get lost—they generally have an unerring sense of knowing how to get back home. Apocryphal stories abound about cats that have moved across the country and still managed to return to their original home. Thus she immediately tells me nonverbally: "I am lost." Whether this is representative of her mother's difficulty—and her own—with individuation or her unforgiving and angry wish to punish herself and her parents for having two more children does not change her problem of not knowing where to go or what to do next. She is lost, so to speak, in the landscape of the unconscious. It seems as if Stella is asking herself in my presence: "How did I manage to get so out of touch with that instinctual part of my nature? Where is that part of me that always manages to find my way back to center? How do I find my way back?"

Cotransference issues are crucial to understanding the relationship between therapist and client in the sandplay process. Sandplay therapists have coined this phrase to mean that the therapeutic bond is a mutual relational one. There is a give and take, a mutuality, which cannot be translated into the more hierarchical meanings of *transference* and *countertransference*. In regard to this issue, Stella did something very significant at the first session. She began the process of bonding with me on a very deep but nonverbal level. In this tray, as well as in Figure 9.6 (below), she chose objects (of which there are very few) that I had brought from my childhood to place on my shelves: the three porcelain cats and, later, the black and white pony. As I have stated earlier, it was hard to get close to Stella. She did not talk very much but she did scowl and complain about the imperfections in my room after the first session. However, from the very first she did look directly at me. And through her symbol choices, she connected to that part of me that admires and enjoys the spirited loner, the feisty and "difficult" oldest child in the family that we both are.

At our next session, Stella began drawing a Dalmatian when she first entered the playroom. She had noticed a book I had placed out on the table, *Nobody Has Time for Me* (Skutina, 1991) and asked me to read the whole book to her several times. She then wanted to do a sand tray, adding that she liked the idea of not having to clean up. (Children usually enjoy not having to clean up. Sandplay therapists and play therapists generally clean up the trays for many reasons: so the children leave the room with their tray intact, not taken apart in front of them; so there is some control over which miniature symbols are placed on the shelves;

and so that children feel few demands or expectations.) Stella placed three trees, then smoothed the sand for a while. She mentioned her mother, aunt, and father while constructing the tray ("I bet Mom would be very interested in these horses, because she likes horses," and "My Aunt Gloria likes pigs—she would like these," and "My dad would like the soldiers here," the latter two comments referring to shelved minia-tures). She found the horses and scattered them in the tray. She then found the larger pony ("Here's a bigger one") but put it back on the shelf, only to use it in a later sand tray.

During the next month, Stella played hide-and-seek games in the sand with the wolf from the Little Red Riding Hood set and a beauti-ful set of painted pigs: a female and three little pigs. The predator wolf was set up to be rescued by the little pigs, but often he chased and bur-ied them as well. Whenever Stella became too anxious about this play, she would bring in the mother pig to rescue the piggies and chase the wolf away. Stella's hiding, finding, and rescuing games may have to do with her handling her anxiety and concerns over the more masculine energy (the predatory wolf) "harassing" and being in conflict with the feminine, represented by the pigs. Piglets must find their way to the sow's teats; the sow does not help the piglets suckle. Additionally, sows can unknowingly kill their young by sitting or rolling over on them; special pens are typically constructed to prevent this from happening. Stella's mother is unaware, on a certain level, of just how bright and sen-sitive her daughter is, and of how to "feed" her emotionally. Stella found that she could not yet rely on her mother to sustain her in this arena. I wanted to gently emphasize my awareness of this need. Thus, I found several books on this topic and left them out on the table. She appeared to enjoy being read to and understood in this way.

The presence of three fir trees appears to be very grounding for Stella. She continued to use them throughout the first part of her pro-cess. In her next tray, eight smaller horses are all moving in a different direction. It would appear that energy is beginning to come forth in preparation for the journey. She called that tray "Gathering the energy." Water is again present in this tray, underscoring the potential for emo-tional expression and making available literal sustenance for the horses. A pond appears on the left side of the tray and seems an unconscious expression of her growing need to connect emotionally with her inner self. Additionally, there is an expressed desire to strengthen the connec-tion with her mother (through her reference to her mother and aunt) and father. The slender thread of holding her parents in her thoughts as she draws on the energy she will need for the journey is present here.

One of the many wonderful things about Stella is that she has such a clear, lively intelligence. She tells me often, through her process, just where to direct my attention, just in case I miss the point.

The Middle: The Work Deepens and Moves

Stella's fifth sand tray (Figure 9.3) marks her decision to commit to a heroine's journey. Here she enters the second quadrant in the sandplay journey map. The choice of a beautiful, large pony I had carried with me from adolescence further heightened the sense of a growing connection between us. I believe that the black-and-white pony is an important early self-symbol for Stella. Later, she will use a black stone and white sea star, and even later, the Dalmatian—black and white back in animal form.

Stella believes she is abandoned; the archetype of the orphan child captures her loneliness. The struggle to integrate the dark and light aspects of the feminine has vital meaning for her. She repudiates both the archetypal and the personal mother's gentler and more compas-

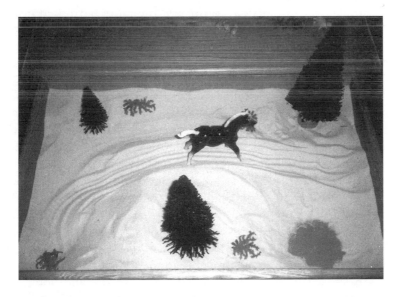

FIGURE 9.3. Beginning on the path. *Description of the tray:* A large pony faces the right side and is set firmly in the middle of the path in this dry tray. The same three pine trees are set into the sand, with only three pieces of greenery. There is a small pond (made out of sand pushed aside to reveal the paint at the bottom of the tray) at the right front of the tray facing the client.

sionate side for the wild, aggressive, and fierce dark mother aspect. The path she chooses for the pony is clearly set from left to right, possibly signifying a path from the unconscious to the conscious. Additionally, on the hero's/heroine's journey, she must go alone at first. Stella chooses an oversized horse figure—possibly representing very powerful and focused energy—to meet her challenges. This consolidation makes clear that she's going to bring more of herself to this process, although the path is still wispy.

A pond appears this time on the right side of the tray, possibly balancing both aspects of unconscious and conscious needs for a constructive emotional outlet. Of course, the water may also represent the depth of the emotional wounding in her family. The pony is set on the path outward, and the water is what she encounters next on her journey. A source of nourishment for the archetypal heroine is available at the start of this journey. When she states that she doesn't think she "can make up *this* story," I believe that Stella is beginning to step outside of herself and observe the journey's process. This is an extremely important step in dealing with her depression and understanding herself. I felt very hopeful when viewing this tray.

As Stella draws Dalmatians on paper, the more harnessed instinctual energy, as represented by the dogs, is beginning to be tapped by her unconscious. However, what is most needed at this point is for her to identify, contain, and then reconcile the opposites of her conflict before she can go further.

In her next sand tray, Stella mounds the sand and places tiger cubs atop the mound, a representation of the "wilder cat." Harnessing the ferocity and power of these jungle cats can be a fearsome business. Stella was unable to place wolves in the tray earlier; now she may be able to present her anger and aggression in the form of these animal cubs and leave them in the tray. Baby tigers play aggressively, and this positive young aggressive energy comes into the tray. However, not only does Stella constrict the energies of the tigers by keeping them as cubs, but she also cages them and denies them access to the water as well.

As I watched Stella create this tray, I wondered what she was saying about her resistance to committing to the journey and her sadness. What was she saying about her restlessness at school and home? Did doubling the cubs in the cage possibly represent her aggressive feelings toward her mother and her need to separate from her? Did that part of her really feel "locked up"? She places the locked cage on the top of the mound, creating heightened perspective. She uses both solar (represented by the tiger cubs) and lunar (more feminine mounding) aspects of the whole in this tray but restricts the expression of the solar energies. It is a huge challenge for this child to use her intelligence, aggression, and sensitivity in the service of healthy growth.

In her next tray Stella molded the sand up in the back of the tray and put in three handprints and one footprint. She then put fences and a bridge in the tray, and finally water and water animals. She again worked silently. It remains Stella's challenge to hold the hope that she will get the love she needs to survive and grow. This time there is a delineated path in an east–west orientation, leading to, or away from, the water. It is still not clear where the path is going. I could see the outlines of another, less delineated path as well. But white garden fencing and a bridge covered with sand mark the path. There is still a feeling of barrenness to the tray, but there is also access to the watery element and sustenance, in stark contrast to her second tray. Stella grounds the imprint of her hands and feet in this tray. In the Judaic tradition, God comforted Moses by saying, "*H'neini*," "I am here," after seeing the burning bush. Moses was frightened. After hearing God call to him twice, finally Moses called out "*H'neini*" ("Here I am"). What is so poignant about this story, and about our clients' journeys in the sand, is that there is so much resistance to answering the call. Moses argued with the Lord that he could represent the people, since he was "slow of speech," and then he hid himself with shame. The story illustrates the need to take responsibility for oneself and one's needs, to pay attention, and to be present to ourselves. When children make this kind of tray, they usually place one or both hands, and sometimes a foot, into the tray itself as a way of giving themselves a name in the world of the archetypal passage. Stella now makes this commitment. With children, there are two types of trays that manifest in the first quadrant: naming trays and "*H'neini*" trays. The naming trays are literally about writing their name in the sand or using colored pebbles, tiles, or treasured objects to create their name in the sand.

Stella began to work with wet sand in her next tray, becoming more comfortable with the messiness (and affective component) of the added water, and she spent a long time mounding and patting the sand. She placed cages again, symmetrical to the mound, locking the baby tigers in securely. What struck me first about this tray was the central breast-like mounding. Her feelings of grief and abandonment are very great, and she allowed them expression here.

For the first time she moved to the wet sand and did not contain the water to a certain area. This wet realm holds the shadow material of the negative mother, particularly immense pain and feelings of abandonment and separation. The tiger cubs are separated in their cages. They do not have access to the mother's breast, to her comfort or her nurturance. This tray appears to reflect Stella's past hurts. For the first time as well, there is some differentiation here: The two cubs occupy separate cages. In previous trays there were two large pines on either side of the tray in those places. The central mounding here corresponds to the place in the earlier tray where she placed the lost cats. Children carry the pain for their parents at times, just as Stella appears to have done with her mother's past hurts at the hands of her maternal grandmother. I believe that Stella calls this place "A desert" for that reason. Stella's mother experienced her life with her own mother as an emotional desert. Whereas some nurturance emerges for Stella, little remains for Stella's own mother. This is a shared issue for both of them: the despair that there will be no love and no sustenance, and the hope that somehow they will find what they need. In this tray Stella may be saying that although they do share this problem, they are still separate people.

In a positive sense, the creation of this huge mound may foreshadow creative energy that may come "bubbling up" from a very deep place inside Stella. Furthermore, the aggressive but caged energies face the left side of the tray. Perhaps they point to an inner direction—a turn of the path that Stella must take now to regain a sense of wholeness and security. Sachiko Reece (1995) speaks of the mound as "the holy place, the healing center," a place that helps to activate the feminine principle.

After Stella completed this tray, she drew a lion and then an Easter egg. The lion, a solar symbol, is associated with the masculine principle. Cirlot (1995) noted that the egg, as a symbol, represents "potentiality, the seed of generation, the mystery of life. . . . The Easter-time custom of the 'dancing egg,' which is placed in the jet of a fountain, owes its origin . . . to the belief that at that time of the year the sun is dancing in the heavens" (p. 94). These were very hopeful and expressive signs that Stella was deepening her inner journeying.

Stella began her next session by ritualistically hiding Dalmatians in the dry sand. She then asked to use the basin. She put the female Dalmatian on top of the pyrite (fool's gold) in the back, right-hand corner of the basin. Then she began exploring my basket of minerals and semiprecious stones. As she floated all the dogs (mother and two puppies) in the basin, which was filled halfway with water, she breathed very heavily through her mouth (Figure 9.4).

Several important issues came to the fore in this session. From a cotransference perspective, Stella had come to trust our relationship

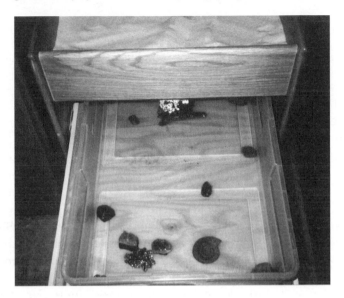

FIGURE 9.4. Navigating feeling waters. *Description of the tray:* A mother Dalmatian and her puppies stand on a large rock, peering out from under the overhang of a dry tray above the flooded tray. Dark rocks and amethyst and pyrite stones as well as a trilobite and several "logs" (i.e., pieces of petrified wood) are scattered throughout the flooded tray.

and the relational field as a safe container of shadow material (i.e., that part of ourselves that we'd rather not accept or examine). Additionally, she referred to the "log stopper," a piece of petrified wood, twice during the creation of the tray. I believe that this wood transforms into the bone she creates later in her process—and which transmutes into the white and gold ceramic bead treasure at the end of her process. I will speak later about the significance of the bone; for now, I believe that this tray is a representation, after the session with her mother, of her quest for ever-present love.

The work that Stella now begins to do in the sand comes from a deep level in her psyche. She chooses several self-objects throughout her process, one of which is the Dalmatian. Woloy (1990) quotes Boris Levinson as saying the following:

> The dog can act as a transitional object. A dog lives in a natural way unless it has been abused by humans. Therefore, interaction with a dog allows children a way of responding to and accepting certain instincts, such as sexual feelings, sibling rivalry, dealing with aggression, and the natural-

ness of bowel habits. As children develop tolerance of the dog's difficulties, they develop tolerances of their own inabilities. A dog can be a mirror in which children may see themselves loved, not for what they should be or should have been, but for what they are. Acceptance is total. (p. 17)

The Dalmatian is a rescue dog, bright and resourceful. The dog's coat color also reflects the balance of light and dark through its spots. The story "101 Dalmatians" tells of the adoption of Dalmatian pups by very kind and loving human and dog parents, their subsequent kidnapping, and the trials by which they are recovered by their animal friends and family. This theme plays a strong part in the positive resolution of the orphan child myth that is invoked by images of helpless puppies.

I believe that this tray expresses how difficult it feels to Stella to navigate "feeling waters." In the previous session, Stella watched her mother weep when she talked of her own feelings of abandonment by her mother. Stella hardly ever let herself cry, instead holding in many feelings she needed to release. This tray seems to show a greater comfort level with the feeling aspect of Stella's existence. An initially playful scene turns serious for the three Dalmatians, mother and pups. One of the pups can only float, hanging out "without a clue," without direction. However, for the first time, Stella allows herself to get in touch with her inner resources and has the mother Dalmatian rescue the helpless pup. Does she make reference here to the rescue of her own "inner child"? There are no overt monsters in Stella's tray. The implied threat is one of emotionality, when the pup does not know what to do or where to go at first. Depression can be a miasma within which there are no solutions, no hope. But with the rescue, there is evidence of dynamic vitality in this tray.

Jung (1968) states, "The 'treasure hard to attain' lies hidden in the ocean of the unconscious, and only the brave can reach it. I conjecture that the treasure is also the 'companion,' the one who goes through life at our side. . . . I conjecture further that the treasure in the sea, the companion, and the garden with the fountain are all one and the same thing: the self" (p. 177). Stella's Dalmatians in the basin peek out from under the overhang of the sandtray above, almost as if in an underground grotto. She insisted that we leave the basin inside the cabinet, although she took it out and laid it on the floor in a subsequent session. According to Jung, "The purpose of the descent as universally exemplified in the myth of the hero is to show that only in the region of danger (watery abyss, cavern, forest, island, castle, etc.) can one find the 'treasure hard to attain' (jewel, virgin, life-potion, victory over death)" (1968, p. 335).

Knowing about her fears of losing connection, literally and figuratively, with her mother, I talked with Stella about there being an invisible but strong cord, from her heart to her mother's heart, that works even when her mother goes away. We mused quietly about its shape and color, and then Stella turned to the wet sand tray and worked in a concentrated manner while constructing it. This tray shows the beginning of Stella's centering process (Figure 9.5). There is an outer ring containing an egg shape with a hole inside it to the bottom.

Using the wet tray seems to hold great significance for Stella. Something now has "opened up" and is being held within the tray at the same time. The water seems to be holding the hole (the sadness) in her heart. It is a tray that seems to explore and accept her femaleness as well as her longing for her mother's attention.

After constructing this tray, Stella created a "bone," as she called it, of white clay, about a quarter inch in length. She took her time in finding just the right basket in which to put the bone. She said, "The Dalmatian has the basket with the treasure sometimes," referring to the bone she'd made as a "treasure."

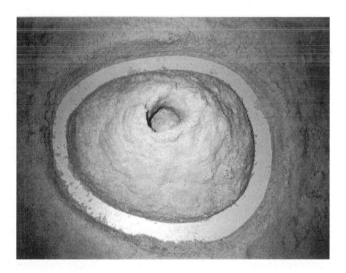

FIGURE 9.5. Opening up. *Description of the tray:* A large mound with a hole dug out of it was made by the client in wet sand, encircled by a ring formed by the bottom of the tray.

In creating the next tray, Stella flooded her tray with as much water as it could hold. I felt that she was very deep in her psyche at this point. Stella has delineated a clear path to the "treasure" through the water this time. The Dalmatian must retrieve the treasure and keep it safe in the basket. The emptiness and loss that the hole in the previous tray may have represented can now be filled with internal treasure. This tray was almost all black in choice of symbols, except for three things: the black-and-white Dalmatian, a sea star, and triangular-shaped gold (pyrite), which continues the themes of the nuclear family and of the sacred.

The bone making and the quest to retrieve the bone remind me of the story of La Huesera, Bone Woman,or the name to which she is also referred, La Loba, Wolf Woman. Estes tells of the old woman who "sings over the bones" of the desert creatures, particularly her favorites, the wolves. She prowls the arroyos looking for bones and assembles an entire skeleton. When she gathers enough inner knowing about which song will bring out the life of that particular creature, she sings out. As she sings, the skeleton comes alive. When it runs away, it transforms into a laughing woman whose breath and spirit infuse the desert land (1996, pp. 27–28).

Cirlot refers to the bone as

> a symbol of life as seen in the character of a seed. The Hebrew word *luz* stands for the mandorla, embracing both the tree and its inner, hidden and inviolable heart. But according to Jewish tradition, it also refers to an indestructible, corporeal particle, represented by a piece of very hard bone . . . and is comparable with the symbol of the chrysalis from which the butterfly emerges. (1995, p. 31).

Townsley-Murray (1995) also speaks of the permanency of the bone. In Stella's creation of the bone may be seen the manifestation of her belief in the indestructibility of the human heart.

Another self-symbol emerges in this tray: the sea star or starfish. The lore on this symbol of wholeness is fascinating. Biologically, this small sea animal with a hard, spiny covering has five arms arranged like the points of a star. It is a tenacious predator that can regenerate lost or damaged parts of itself. Metaphorically, it is the "light in the water."

Stella, arming herself with a prickly exterior, may yearn for the healing ability of this creature. The five arms are the number of members in her family. She longs to again be the "star of the show" and stand out in her family. Stella Maris, star of the sea, is one of the names of Mary and of the mother goddesses who rose from the sea: Isis, Ishtar, Aphrodite, Venus. The symbol represents divine love and the inextinguishable power of love, as well as "the grace of God, not quenched in the sea of sin" (retrieved from *Encyclopedia Mythica, www.pantheon.org*). The starfish contains polarity even in its name, being of both sky and sea.

The shell laid on the sea star is a poignant self-symbol in Stella's quest for reintegration. It is treasure placed on top of the archetypal human shape. For a constrained child without secure connections to adults or other children, the use of animal symbols is an excellent choice to express what is closest to her heart. The Dalmatian in this tray points to the star, that essence of the feminine self.

At our next meeting, in the waiting room, Stella's mom urged both her daughter and me to help Stella work on "self-esteem" issues, making suggestions about what we might read together. Stella chose another book to read instead. Then she worked on a tray without comment and next went to get the basin to fill it with water. Stella continued to work silently as she put all sorts of natural marine objects (e.g., shells, rocks) into the flooded basin.

If I could have redone a part of therapy in hindsight, I would have said strongly to Mom that although I appreciated her suggestions, Stella and I were working on these issues as Stella directed, and that I trusted Stella's ability to know what was best for her to do and when. I also would have made a separate appointment with Stella's mom and dad to talk about their daughter's progress and their input and concerns. Because Stella had such difficulty finding her own internal and external space, I would have better protected her natural tendency to know how to heal herself, and I would have recognized that she was quite capable of doing so. But I was a much less secure therapist 15 years ago, from the vantage point of 25 years' perspective.

Two other symbols used in Stella's later process appear for the first time here. One is a "stone mountain," with a flat surface, that I picked up at a pet store. Walker describes many traditions as worshipping stones as representations "particularly [of] the spirits of female ancestors or Goddesses" (1988, p. 523). The empty walnut shell has special significance in Stella's later trays as the holder of a white and gold ceramic bead treasure. Walnut trees were often held to be sacred to the goddess.

At our next session, Stella took down the basket of balloons and said, "I've never gone exploring on the top shelf before . . . we're going to have quite the little birthday scene!" Her sand tray (Figure 9.6) had

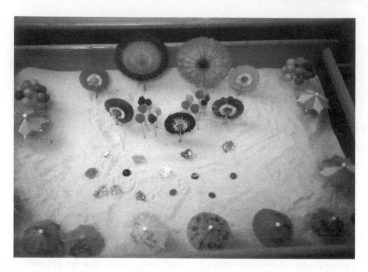

FIGURE 9.6. Birthday party celebration. *Description of the tray:* Cocktail umbrellas line the bottom of this dry tray, while two umbrellas are placed evenly on the right and left sides of the tray. An oval of fans and small cocktail fake fruits on sticks are placed in the back center of the tray. Stones and crystals make three lines in the center of the tray.

the beauty and numinous sense that characterize a constellation-of-the-self tray (a midpoint tray in which the person acknowledges the beauty of his or her "inner self").

With this celebratory tray, Stella claims her sense of selfhood. She is both celebrant and observer (e.g., "quite the little birthday scene"). She brings in another culture, a Mexican motif, with her selection of bright colors and demonstrates an emotional availability in a way that she had not done previously. There are seven fans in an oval shape, dominating the back center of the tray, signifying her seventh birthday year. Stella uses my first name during the creation of this tray, without the "Dr." in front of it, bringing me into the space in what I experienced as an intimate way, as a special friend. I felt honored by her display of feeling. This tray is an exquisite representation of the beauty and depth of her inner resources. With the additional introduction in the session of making the dreamcatcher with one of my shells, she activates a new healing energy. I told her she could choose a shell from my jar of collected seashells in the playroom, and we wove it into the sticks of the dreamcatcher, which she proudly took home to hang over her bed.

Resolutions Surface

Another pivotal scene occurred 4 months into therapy, when I came into the waiting room to find a red-faced, unusually inarticulate Stella on the brink of what looked like hysteria, trying to get back a new stuffed animal Dalmatian puppy that her sister had taken from her. Her sister just wanted to play with the puppy, Stella's mother said pleadingly, couldn't Stella just let her sister keep it during the time Stella was with me in session? Her sister began a full-scale tantrum. I bent down to Stella's sister and firmly told her that she needed to be quiet and to give Stella's puppy back to her. To everyone's surprise but mine, Stella was handed her puppy, and we went to our session.

At a previous session approximately a month before, I had worked with Stella's mom individually to identify some of the most distressing parts of their mother–daughter relationship. It became obvious that Stella's mother would benefit from individual psychotherapy herself, and I recommended this to Mom, suggesting that when she was ready, I would refer her to a colleague. After coming into the playroom following the waiting room scene, Stella proudly showed off her new pups and their different markings. She added softly, "Mommy says when I'm done, *she* wants to come to play therapy." I reassured Stella that she would stop therapy only when she was ready, and that I would help her mom find someone else to talk and play with. Stella then built and rebuilt a fence made of loose bricks on the play therapy table. She constructed another sand tray, using three bricks. Stella made a bridge carefully and placed a starfish in the tray last. She then quietly left the room.

Was Stella showing herself and me how difficult it was to set and keep boundaries at home, particularly with her mother, in her play on the table? I know that the scene in the waiting room was very difficult for everyone. I realized that her mother could not protect Stella in the way she needed at that point in time. I needed to strongly reassure Stella that I knew how to respect and contain boundaries. The bridge upon which the Dalmatian stands is flimsy and covered with paper. But it is a bridge whose path leads over the water to the hut. This time, the white ornamental fencing used in a previous tray secures and underscores the path over the pond. The stone wall enclosure is empty; the cage with the tiger pups occupied this space in an earlier tray. I wondered what would this space contain at some future point in time? The sea star appears set in a small hollow in the left front of the tray, possibly representing the deepest part of herself.

Stella came into the following session very focused, happy, and bubbly. She wasn't critical or controlling at all, which was a very big change from other interactions we'd had. Her quietness was connected to her focus, not to the usual feeling of withholding. Stella created Figure 9.7, which she named "Sinking sand." She put the Dalmatian female in and stood her up in the middle of the circle.

During this session, Stella was able to express ambivalent feelings safely and more comfortably with me. This was a huge step for her, and for our relationship, which she trusted to hold shadow material at a more conscious level. The quicksand in the shape of a nest rings the lone Dalmatian female. It can be seen as expressing her sadness and feelings of abandonment again in a very intense way. But it can also be seen as an expression of her vulnerability in a very beautiful yet scary place. It is as if she pauses to reflect nonverbally about her fear of her mother not being there for her, as well as her mother's fears of loss as well. It is, after all, an adult female, not a pup, in this scene. Is she afraid that she is not strongly anchored in herself? The dog looks directly at the place I sat. Is she looking to me for grounding and reassurance? I believe so.

At this session, after talking about Stella's summer vacation plans, I told Stella about a long vacation trip I would be taking in August and

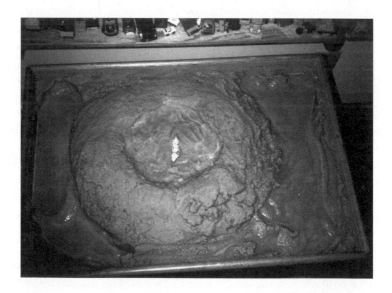

FIGURE 9.7. Sinking sand. *Description of the tray:* An adult Dalmatian is placed in the center space of this extremely wet (muddy) tray, ringed by a donut-sized ring of wet sand, surrounded by smoothed mud.

reassured her of my return. Stella then quietly said, "I'm going to miss you when you're gone." I hugged her gently, and she returned the hug. This period begins what I believe is the start of the third quadrant of her sandplay journey integration work.

Transitions Occur

Stella began to alternate between creating wet and dry trays fairly consistently from this point forward. In the dry trays she places a bridge over the pond, signifying a union of opposites in her journey. It is as if she is able to draw on a deep core of feeling energy. The bridge is strongly constructed; no paper lines the path, only sturdy clay tiles. She is definitely on "firmer footing" here than in the previous tray. The sea star, decorated with greenery, anchors her self-image to the tray. Young (1997) notes that the Chinese symbol for patience contains both "knife" and "edge" over the "heart" symbol: "When the heart lives on the cutting edge," he says, "it calls for care and endurance. This is patience" (p. 21). My wish for Stella during this time was that she learn to hold onto this meaning of patience.

"This is a rather rich place, indeed!" as Stella so wonderfully exclaimed while creating another sand tray. Stella first asks "where should the dog live?" I believe she is asking in which realm: the watery, feeling realm, or the cooler, intellectually drier landscape of pine tree forest. For now, Stella places a bone, treasures, and food within the stone enclosure in the dry tray.

Stella's efforts on the next sandtray (Figure 9.8) depict the true *hieros gamos* (i.e., the marriage of opposites) using the two puppies, male and female. The tray is beautifully balanced with its scattered shell and sea star aspects (feminine) and its three sentinel-like fir trees (masculine). The three trees anchor the tray and are reminders of what is most enduring about life. The altar contains a tiny white open shell on top, possibly symbolic of her acceptance of the feminine in herself, and a way to demonstrate her centering. She places it closest to where she stands while creating this tray. The puppies have everything they need to keep them nurtured and sheltered in the stone enclosure. They feel complete, and the container of the tray appears secure.

At our next session, we held a party that included her favorite food before I left for 3 months at what appeared to be a very sensitive juncture in our work together. Stella brought me a poem, "The Rose" (see p. 199), which she herself composed. In the last several sessions, Stella's cotransference with me had deepened to include both negative and pos-

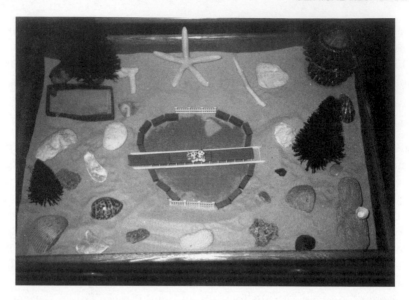

FIGURE 9.8. Dalmatian puppy happiness. *Description of the tray:* A pair of Dalmatian puppies face the center front of this dry tray on a "bridge" made of clay tiles over a long white fire engine ladder. The ladder is placed over a pond made with the bottom of the tray, which has ceramic bricks around it. The same three pine trees from trays in Figures 9.2 and 9.3 ring this tray as well. At the back left of the tray, a stone enclosure encases an area containing drink, food, and a blanket. Sea shells and a stone "altar" with a cowrie shell placed in an open position on top rings the pond. A straw hut is placed in the back right corner; a sea star (starfish) is placed standing up in the sand in the back center of the tray.

itive mother aspects. The rose is the symbol of Mary, and my name. The beautiful rose poem speaks to our strong bond and to Stella's growing connection to the spiritual as well. I believe that her last act in that session, in which she buried a fish miniature, speaks to her understanding that I would return to her.

After my return in early September, Stella's mom related that her daughter was having difficulty finishing her schoolwork in this new school year (which had started in mid-August). Stella was making some very negative comments again (e.g., "I wish I were dead"). This time, Mom didn't get overly upset; instead she just listened to her daughter. Mom told Stella, sympathetically and matter-of-factly, that she herself had felt yucky inside like that before.

Coming into the play therapy room, Stella commented, "It seems like nothing will stay where it belongs these days." For her next trays she began to use the two adult Dalmatians (Pongo and Perdita) I'd found on my trip. Using the lookout tower elevates her perspective now; her energy is moving out from the unconscious. She has always been more comfortable in the intellectual sphere, and this realm is where she places Pongo and Perdita, who look off in the distance. Underneath the tower, in a dark but secured place, she places fruits and vegetables perhaps signifying that a mother–daughter bond is growing and strengthening. Mother and daughter are not just coming to an accommodation; they are truly communicating. Stella is learning that her mother can nurture her and that they can be positively connected. Stella again left her hand-print in the front right section of the tray, claiming the place as her own, with me as witness.

For the first time, dining implements appear in the stone enclosure. Eating is shown as closer to real life, not in the abstract as in previous trays. Food is harvested in the basket, ready for sustenance. The sea star continues to stand as an anchor in the back of the tray, with a large white shell opposite as emphasis.

Stella continued to question herself during this phase of her work. She was aware that she was still missing something. Although most of her sand trays during this period are filled with resources, with treasures and sustenance abundantly available, she is still anxious and uncertain. All of these positive aspects of her learning and growth also activate her negative beliefs about being truly able to get what she needs, as well as her deep grief from 3 years ago when her sister was born. Stella was back in the deepest place in her psyche. The alternation within each session of emotional flooding and more typical adjustment seems to reflect her ambivalence as well as her increasing desire to modulate her affect and intellect, effectively bridging their split.

Stella created a messy "emotional" pool for what she called Pongo and Perdita's "anniversary," using seven large decorated marbles to delineate the boundaries. The pond in this tray is less ornamental than previous ponds and deeply set into mounded sides. Somehow, perfection has gone by the wayside. She named this sand tray "Quicksand" (Figure 9.9), putting Pongo and Perdita in the middle of the pond and suddenly yelling, "Quicksand warning—it's everywhere! Oops, the balls are getting stuck!"

Quick temper, quicksand, impatience: Stella has been wary of learning tolerance—particularly with regard to her mother and herself. Here in the flooded tray, she places beautiful treasures, seven ornamental balls. Metaphorically, Pongo and Perdita are working out the tensions between the opposites of aggression and vulnerability. This tray and the

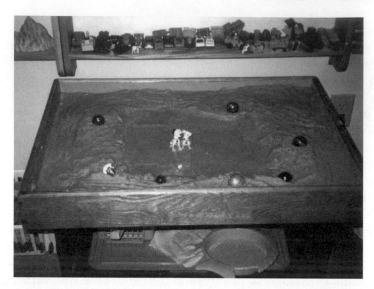

FIGURE 9.9. Quicksand. *Description of the tray:* Two adult Dalmatians are placed in the center space of this extremely wet (muddy) tray, which looks like a watery pool in a larger muddy area. Seven large and patterned marble balls ring the "pool."

next reflect separate realms again. She demonstrates that she is working hard to be present emotionally and to balance her ambivalence.

Closure

Ascent imagery now characterizes Stella's journey in the creation of her next tray, in the fourth and last part of her cycle. Stella continues to work on integrating what she has learned in the next few trays and on "bringing it home," back to daily life. Stella is clearly in quadrant 4, returning to the collective realm of society.

In this tray she moves the Dalmatians to the left side of the tray, with a garden below them. The order and peace of this tray are pervasive. Ritual lighting and anniversary partying, wine, fruit, and presents all combine in a simple way here.

The emotional depths are present in her next, very wet tray. They are contained in a relativized and centered way, anchored again by the sea star self-symbol. Soon it will be harvest time. I understood from this tray that Stella was consolidating her learning and preparing to approach termination with me.

Stella created her last tray (Figure 9.10) by first putting colorful plants all over, stating, "It's so quiet here, you can hear the clock ticking. It's Pongo and Perdita's anniversary!" She scattered the rest of the treasures around the tray. I noted that this would be her last session for a while, and that I would be there for her if she ever needed me. She built this tray with love and thoughtfulness and care in every movement. "This one in front is a statue of a Dalmatian, up here," she noted. She put in another shell by the Dalmatian statue, and then filled up the grapes with water from the blue container. After naming the tray, her last sand tray act was to gently place the blanket in the lookout tower. "Isn't it surprising that the Dalmatians can both fit in there?" she asked.

With much care, Stella demonstrated how to hold the space inside of herself so bravely and well. This tray was breathtaking in its beauty. The two Dalmatians stand facing the hidden treasure, buried under the

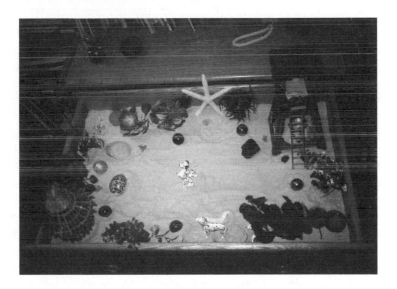

FIGURE 9.10. Dalmatian plantation. *Description of the tray:* Two adult Dalmatians placed in the center face the left side of this dry tray. A lookout tower at the back on the right with a blanket in it has a ladder placed in the front. Hollow plastic grapes and other plastic "food" line the area underneath the tower. Colorful plants, patterned marbles, and seashells are scattered along the sides of the tray. The straw hut is placed in the left front of the tray. A Dalmatian statue stands on the stone "altar" in the center front of the tray. Buried in the left center of the tray near the two adult Dalmatians are crystal treasures under a cowrie shell (from the tray in Figure 9.8). A small ceramic pond was placed on the right front of the tray as well.

cowrie shell from an earlier tray. The guardian Dalmatian (possibly representative of her incorporation of the healer archetype) stands proudly on the altar, facing the same direction as the two dogs. Around the tray is the "Plantation": by definition, a self-sustaining environment of singular loveliness and nurturance—sustained, however, through hard work. All is presided over by the sea star. There is harmony, color, lush growth, places to eat in style, sleep in comfort, and drink in peace.

SUMMARY OF CLINICAL IMPRESSIONS

The transformative journey Stella made through sandplay enabled her to remember what is most important about life: that we live it with love and compassion for others and ourselves. About 2 months into therapy, Stella had her first "best friend" sleepover since moving to the area. Within 4 months of beginning therapy (and within 2 months of receiving AG consultation), Stella began showing evidence of enjoying school, having a better relationship with peers and her teacher, and doing her homework as soon as she got home from school. All of these suggest some symptom relief. By the end of our work together, she was more comfortable with her feelings: She expressed herself dramatically, as always, but she was more open, and generally happy. Her mother wrote to tell me of Stella's continued success and delight in school and in herself, her growing circle of friends, and her familial relationships. Her mother emphasized that the family felt "that we have gotten our bubbly daughter back." I believe that Stella accomplished the goal of recovering her sense of self-worth, that treasure within. This sense of self-worth had been threatened by Stella's acute fears (some her own, some she picked up in her mother's family dynamics) of abandonment and the loss of her mother's love. Stella perceived the birth of her sibling as traumatic, as some children do; it was the goal of therapy to allow Stella to explore, identify, and process the depth of her anxiety regarding her mother. In doing so, Stella's mother was forced to confront her personal history and acknowledge that the lack of resolution in her narrative might have contributed to Stella's hypersensitivity to a perceived maternal loss.

Stella wrote the following poem for me. Love, treasure found, and heart's desire—all are present. Thank you, Stella, for the honor of working with you and presenting your work to people who will learn from your courage, as I have.

The Rose

The Rose's red is so pure,
Nothing as beautiful in the world, I'm sure.
The joyful doves fly all around
Near the soft and gentle ground.
But one dove seemed to think
That the color of the rose meant love.

ACKNOWLEDGMENTS

This chapter is reprinted from Heiko, R. L. (2008). Finding the treasure within: The sandplay journey of Stella. *Journal of Sandplay Therapy, 17*(1). Copyright © 2008 by the Sandplay Therapists of America. Adapted with permission.

REFERENCES

Campbell, J. (1949). *The hero with a thousand faces.* Princeton, NJ: Princeton University Press.

Cirlot, J. F. (1995). *A dictionary of symbols.* New York: Barnes & Noble

Clift, J. D., & Clift, W. B. (1988). *The hero journey in dreams.* New York: The Crossroad Publishing Company.

Dickerson, K. (1993). *The forgotten filly.* New York: Harper Paperbacks.

Estes, C. P. (1996). *Women who run with the wolves.* New York: Ballantine Books.

Jackson, B. (2008). Mapping the cycle of sandplay process. In H. S. Friedman & R. R. Mitchell, (Eds.), *Supervision of sandplay therapy.* New York: Routledge.

Johnson, D. M. (1999). Fairy tale symbolism applied to sandplay. *Journal of Sandplay Therapy, 8*(2), 65–86.

Jung, C. G. (1968). *Man and his symbols.* (J. L. Henderson, J. Jacobi, & A. Jaffe Eds.). New York: Dell.

Reece, S. (1995). The mound as healing image in sandplay. *Journal of Sandplay Therapy, 4*(2), 15–31.

Skutina, V. (1991). *Nobody has time for me: A modern fairy tale.* Chicago: Wellington.

Townsley-Murray, M. (1995). Bones. *Journal of Sandplay Therapy, 5*(1), 96–107.

Walker, B. G. (1988). *The women's dictionary of symbols and sacred objects.* San Francisco: HarperSanFrancisco.

Woloy, E. M. (1990). *The symbol of the dog in the human psyche: A study of the human–dog bond.* New York: Chiron.

Young, E. (1997). *Voices of the heart.* New York: Scholastic.

CHAPTER 10

"Stitches Are Stronger Than Glue"

A Child Directs the Healing of Her Shattered Heart

DAVID A. CRENSHAW

The drive for self-repair, healing, and growth are evident even in babies born prematurely. Rachel Naomi Remen, MD, a premature infant herself, described in her book *Kitchen Table Wisdom: Stories That Heal* that as a young pediatrician she worked in a premature intensive-care nursery using far more advanced technology than was available at the time of her birth. But she questioned whether it was the high-tech medical equipment that kept these early arrivals alive or something innate, some unnamed strength in those tiny human beings that enable them to survive. She stated, "There is a tenacity toward life which is present at the intracellular level without which even the most sophisticated of medical interventions would not succeed" (Remen, 1996, p. 8). The

---

This chapter is dedicated to Garry Landreth who once said, "You can't buy in a store what you can take away in your heart forever." What Garry Landreth has taught me and so many others about the art of healing is something that I will cherish in my heart forever.

drive to live, to grow, and to heal is a vital force in every child, as the inspiring premature infants remind us as they fight to live with each labored breath.

Charles Dickens had a dream as a child to seek a quality education, but his quest was derailed by the family debts that incarcerated his father for a short time in a debtor's prison and required him to go to work in a shoe polish factory. The experiences of his family in the Marshalsea debtors' prison and his own experiences working under the harsh conditions at the shoe polish factory fueled his passion to bring to the attention of the privileged classes the devaluation and deprived conditions endured by working-class people and those living in abject poverty. He became a champion of social change and children's rights, using the unhappy conditions of his childhood as the creative springboard for literary characters that continue to capture the imaginations of countless readers—as evidenced by the fact that none of Dickens's books has ever gone out of print (Swift, 2007). Dickens's drive for self-repair and growth, evident in childhood, found creative expression in writing that made visible the nameless and forgotten poor.

Rainer Maria Rilke, regarded as one of the greatest poets of the 20th century, began life as a "replacement child" (Cain & Cain, 1964). The term *replacement child* was coined to describe how parents, devastated by the death of a baby, may be tempted to conceive and raise a baby to "replace" the child who died. Rilke was a replacement child for his grieving parents, especially his mother, who had lost a baby girl just a week after her birth the year before Rilke was born. He was given the feminine name of Maria and was, for the first 5 years of life, made to wear dresses (Freedman, 1996). His childhood was marked by illness and unhappiness, yet he became one of the best known of all German-speaking poets. His loneliness in childhood and his insistence on abundant solitude in adult life were the wellspring of his creativity and genius. It is not unusual for a child who is withdrawn, lonely, and isolated in childhood to develop a rich inner world and to become quite gifted in an artistic or creative way. In addition to his poetry and published writings, Rilke wrote over 11,000 letters in his own exquisite penmanship (Baer, 2005). The child's capacity for self-repair echoes poetically through the life and work of Rilke. Although, Camila, the 9-year-old girl described below, has not become famous yet, she has been just as heroic as the examples cited above, in her determination to overcome the obstacles she has faced in a life so far marked by multiple heartbreaking losses.

CASE REFERRAL INFORMATION

Camila was referred to me by her parents for the first of four short-term treatment episodes when she was 5 years old. All the relatively brief treatments, ranging from 7 to 12 sessions, were precipitated by losses that Camila experienced as devastating. An only child, Camila is strongly attached to both of her parents: her mother is Hispanic and her father is European American. The initial referral was the result of the parents' separation and Camila's severe reaction to it. Gil (1991) stated emphatically that we should never assume trauma; only the child can tell us what an experience meant or represented to him or her. Some children appear to handle the separation and divorce of parents without breaking their developmental stride. Other children, such as Camila, are deeply affected, due in no small part to the degree to which they are attached to both parents. When Camila came in to the first session with both of her parents, her sadness was readily visible.

FORMULATION OF THE PROBLEM

Camila's parents both had extensive experience working in the field of child mental health, so their alarm at the intensity of Camila's grief and rage reactions added to the sense of urgency in the initial intervention. Camila was having difficulty sleeping, and she was not accepting the major changes in her life. The ground on which she stood was suddenly shaky, and she was shocked. It was the hope of both the parents and the therapist that the intensity of her grief and anger at the parents' separation could be eased by a combination of verbalization, play, and creative expressive techniques. However, the formidable problem encountered in the first round of sessions was that the loss was so unbearably painful to this child that she couldn't approach it in even the safe haven of play or artistic expression.

INVITATION TO PLAY THERAPY

The specific example of self-directed repair through play that I describe with this child came in the third treatment sequence, but it is important to know where we started. After the usual efforts to invite Camila to engage in play or drawings had failed, due to the extreme vulnerability she was feeling and her inability to focus on anything that might bring up the unbearable pain, I tried to "set the stage." In retrospect, I view that as a mistake. I was responding to the sense of alarm in the parents and the wish to do something quickly to ease Camila's pain. I am now convinced that the child-centered approach to play therapy, as eloquently articulated by Garry Landreth (2002), was the only correct way to give ample room for Camila's unusual capacity for self-healing. The evidence that I was off-track came convincingly from Camila herself. In "setting the stage" I asked her to pick a puppet for her to use and one for me. She chose a little brown rabbit for herself, expressing poignantly her sense of vulnerability. She couldn't have been more "stinging" in her feedback to me than when she picked the bumblebee puppet for me. She was telling me that my attempts to encourage and cajole her to expose her pain, even in indirect ways through drawings and puppet play, were "stinging" to her, insensitive, and disrespectful to her emotional state. She drove this point home even more dramatically when I started circling as the bumblebee overhead and saying in the "voice" of the bumblebee, "Oh, look, there is a little bunny down there, and that bunny looks sad. I wonder what's wrong. Maybe there is some way I can help." Camila said, "Do you have any duct tape?" When I handed her the duct tape from the cabinet, she taped shut the mouth of the bumblebee so that it then could make only muffled speech sounds. Camila found the attempts of the bumblebee to make these sounds hilarious.

Over the next few sessions she was able to draw pictures depicting her sadness, usually with tears streaming down her face, and her parents reported fewer episodes of uncontrolled sobbing or rage reactions. In a session with her father she was able to verbalize her fears that when he goes away, she was afraid he wouldn't come back. In symbolic play she also played out an angry female throwing the males out of the house. Her anger was expressed again in scenes where she played a nurse who took delight in giving repeated shots to the puppets brought to the nurse (by the therapist). She was not deterred by the therapist's reflections of how scared the different animal puppets felt and their protests about their harsh treatment. Gradually she verbalized more directly her painful feelings, although there were sessions when she absolutely refused to talk about her anger and sadness.

In another session of child-directed symbolic play, a cruel guy stole everybody's gold. He pretended to be a cool guy, but he was really a cruel robber. The robber went down a chimney at a little girl's house, a girl named Camila. She had a brother in the play drama named Anthony, who was 7 years old. Her brother was really nice to her. The robber took all the gold and stuffed animals of both Camila and her brother. When they woke up, the children noticed that their toys were missing, and they cried. Then their mother and father showed up, and they all fought the robber, including Camila—even though she had a sword in her heart. They were able to use all the powers of their hearts to kill the mean robber. Then they all went to have dinner, and they were happy together forever after. Even though Camila was only 5 years old and 4 months when she created this scene, her use of metaphor and symbolism was remarkable. The cruel robber (separation and divorce) invaded their house to take what was valuable (gold) and what made her feel comfortable (stuffed animals). This was a sudden and shocking event like the separation and divorce. The extent of her pain and anger is strikingly portrayed by her fighting with all her might, along with the rest of the family, with a sword piercing her heart. Of course, her wish for reunion of the family was also expressed in the play drama.

The playful interaction between us and her remarkable sense of humor even in the midst of her overwhelming pain were not only gifts that she would call on again and again as she incurred further losses; they kept the therapy from crashing and burning at this initial stage of our work together. I never again made that mistake with Camila in all the subsequent episodes of treatment. She has directed her own healing ever since.

CASE ILLUSTRATION OF SELF-DIRECTED TRAUMA PLAY

The second episode of treatment occurred 2 years later, after both parents had established committed relationships with new partners. Camila, who in addition to her many other strengths (e.g., creativity, sense of humor, warmth, intelligence), approaches everything she does in a wholehearted way, including making new attachments. After some initial hesitation she became attached to both of the new partners in her parents' lives because she naturally didn't want to get hurt again. Her mother called for an appointment because she was worried about Camila. An appointment was made, and again, as a show of support both of her parents came to the session, as they usually did, and in keeping with Camila's wishes participated in the sessions. Once again Camila was faced with a loss that shattered her heart. She had gotten quite close to her mother's live-in partner, and they had recently bought a house together and moved into it. Quite suddenly the mother's partner, who had a prior history of substance abuse, relapsed and left without saying goodbye to Camila. She was grief-stricken but was also quite worried about her mother, who was also in shock and in the throes of acute grief.

The Beginning: Setting the Stage

Camila did not hesitate, at age 7, to engage in play or artwork when she was unable to convey her feelings in words. Her mother said that Camila was happy to come back to therapy. Camila directed the play scenes often assigning parts to her parents, although her father was not always involved in this particular group of sessions since the loss she was feeling was primarily shared with her mother. At times she asked me to videotape the play scenes so that she could see the replays on the TV monitor in my office. In particular, she enjoyed watching the replays of the scenes in which she and her mother, and sometimes her father, in characters of the puppets, would give a good telling off to the man who had left her without saying goodbye. In some of the play scenes her confusion and ambivalence about this man, fictitiously named Larry, were demonstrated by yelling at him, calling 911, and asking the police to arrest him, whereas in other scenes in which she would confront Larry, she would tell him that she still loved him. These conflicting feelings were also expressed in her artwork and when she would write notes to Larry. On one card from the Heartfelt Feelings Coloring Card Strategy (HFCCS; Crenshaw, 2008a), she wrote, "Larry, I do not know what to say. Write me a card but tell the truth on the card. You are the best. I love you!" Then she drew hearts all around the card. This, of course, was not a card she actually sent; it was used in therapy as a safe way to work through her feelings. She both feared and longed to encounter him at the mall or on the streets of her town. She brought in pictures of happier times that depicted the obvious affection that she and Larry shared for one another. Eventually, Camila was standing on firmer ground, was sleeping better, and the intense sobbing incidents and rage reactions had stopped.

My practice model is similar to a family practitioner's. When Camila, her parents, and I agreed that we had gone as far as Camila could go at this particular point in time, we put sessions on an as-needed basis with the clear understanding that they could return at any time. I also follow the developmentally sequenced approach to child trauma outlined by Beverly James (1989). According to James, due to cognitive, emotional, and other developmental constraints, children can do only so much therapeutic work at any one stage of their young lives. So a 5-year-old, for example, grieving the death of a parent would only be able to tolerate and do helpful emotional work to a limited extent. The same child, however, at age 9 might be able to do further work because he or she now has new cognitive tools and emotional resources to undertake demanding and taxing grief work. In adolescence the same child might return to do still more therapeutic work because he or she is able to understand the loss in a new way, and perhaps assign a different meaning to the loss, because he or she now possesses additional cognitive and emotional resources to work toward accommodating such a devastating loss.

The Middle: The Work Deepens and Moves

The third sequence of treatment was initiated by Camila herself. She became anxious and worried when her mother developed a committed relationship with a man who had three children, a girl 2 years older than Camila and two older brothers, ages 14 and 17. As the mother's relationship became more serious, the stakes for Camila increased because she too was becoming attached to the mother's new partner, Rick, as well as to his children, especially Gina, his daughter. Camila had longed for siblings, and now there was a potential for a slightly older sister and two older brothers. But with the stakes higher, the question that terrified Camila was, "What if something goes wrong?" She knew full well the answer, based on previous losses, only this time she would lose an entire family to whom she was becoming increasingly attached.

The threat of future loss dramatically resurfaced the prior losses and, in particular the more recent loss of Larry. Even though Camila had done considerable emotional work in the prior treatment sequence to accommodate to the abandonment by Larry, this loss was particularly troubling to her because it had multiple features of traumatic grief. It certainly was sudden and unexpected. Neither her mother nor Camila had any forewarning. Although her parents' separation was unexpected, that loss was different. Not only did her parents support and help her through this painful period in her life but they both continued to be a consistent, loving presence helping her not only with the original loss occasioned by their separation but each of the subsequent losses. Camila suffered the loss of the intact family with all the attendant dreams, hopes, and plans that were a part of the original family—a harrowing loss—but she didn't lose her mother or father. They both remain a vital part of her life and she counts on that always being the case. When Larry left, it was not only sudden, it was final. She didn't see him again, and she had no opportunity to say goodbye. The inability to say goodbye became a significant focus of the reparative work that Camila orchestrated out of her abundant inner resources and strong desire to heal.

A key feature of Larry's troubling abandonment of Camila and her mother was the sense of betrayal. Camila had slowly allowed herself to become vulnerable to an extreme degree. She loved Larry, and the two had shared many fun times. The degree of affection between them was revealed clearly in the photos that Camila shared with me; pictures taken during their happy times together. The trust and faith placed in Larry not only by Camila but by her mother was evidenced when her mother and Larry bought a house together. Larry's relapse into his drug habit caused not only the relationship to forcefully hit the wall but the house that they had just bought and moved into had to be put on the market immediately because it was no longer possible for her mother to afford the house on her own.

Clinical experience repeatedly reveals that betrayal provokes rage of uncommon proportion. Betrayal cruelly ruptures the bond of trust to the point that some who suffer betrayal never completely trust again. This was the deep hurt that surfaced intrusively when Camila found the ties to Rick and his family becoming stronger in both her mother's and her own heart.

Camila, who was 9 years old at the initiation of the third round of treatment, was unusually verbal, reflecting her superior level of intelligence, insight, and psychological mindedness. Nevertheless, about 15 minutes into the first family session Camila stopped talking abruptly, turned to me, and said, "I can't tell you, can I show you?" I said, "Sure, how would you like to show me?" She immediately went to the drawing table and started drawing a picture of herself with a disproportionately large heart (Figure 10.1).

The large heart quite aptly captures Camila's strength but also her liability. She has a big heart. She is capable of great love and attachment, and she is vulnerable to great heartbreak when those relationships end. In Camila's heart, in the upper right-hand quadrant, was a jagged wound, a wound that didn't encompass the entire heart but a significant injury that would be hard to heal due to its deep and ragged nature (betrayal?). Quite strikingly in the picture, in her left hand she is holding a large can of glue. I asked Camila about the reason for the can of glue. She said without a pause, "My parents [who were in the room] think that this glue will be strong enough to hold my heart together and keep it from breaking into pieces again." But she quickly added, "But my parents are wrong. The glue is not strong enough. If something else happens to break my heart, the glue will not be strong enough." I

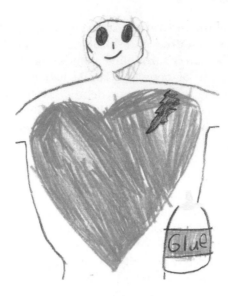

FIGURE 10.1. Camila's drawing of her big heart with a jagged wound.

said, "Well, what would be strong enough to hold your heart together?" She replied immediately, "Stitches. My heart needs stitches! Stitches are stronger than glue."

Resolutions Surface

Camila had identified clearly and decisively what was needed to make her heart stronger. She knew well that she was once again risking considerable vulnerability to her heart as her attachments to Rick's family grew stronger. It was abundantly clear that Camila was one of those remarkable youngsters that Eliana Gil (1991, 1995, 2006) identified as possessing an inner compass that directs them toward their own healing. As her therapist I simply needed to get out of her way.

Through her artwork Camila had produced a rich metaphor that would guide the therapy from that point forward: "My heart needs stitches." I would simply ask her at the beginning of each session, "What do you need to do today about the stitches needed in your heart?" Camila would take it from there. She would decide whether to draw, use the family house or school playhouse, the puppets, the play animals, the rescue vehicles, just talk, or any combination thereof. In some of the play scenes she would recruit her mother or father or both, and sometimes me, to play parts; in others she simply requested that we quietly witness the play drama. Gil (1994) described a model for family play therapy in which the family play is done under the instructions of the therapist, although the family would huddle together to decide how to carry out the therapist's directives. Gil, for example, might ask family members to come up with a story that they could play out with the puppets. While the family was working on the plan for their play drama, Gil might leave the room, to give the family time and space to plan, and return when the family was ready to do the play action. In contrast, the family play in Camila's case was strictly under her direction. She would assign parts and instruct the family and/or therapist as to how to carry out each part. She was the playwright and the director as well as the principal actor in the drama that evolved.

Another interesting feature of Camila's play dramas, going back to even the first treatment sequence, was her intermittent requests for me to videotape the play action. Frequently we would watch the video playback together. In some scenes she would express intense anger toward Larry by either telling him off or whacking him with a stick. In other scenes she would have the puppet representing herself call 911, and the police would arrive and arrest him. In still other play scenes she would have Larry appear in court before the judge (a part she played). The judge would give him a good telling off and then throw him in jail. These were the scenes she particularly delighted in seeing on video replay. Her wonderful sense of humor would lead to gales of laughter in the room, and the playfulness and fun helped to counteract some of the pain and anxiety associated with the serious and difficult content of the play that she was attempting to master and assimilate. She was working hard to create, through the symbolism of her play, a cohesive narrative, an essential component of child trauma work (Cohen, Mannarino, & Deblinger, 2006; Gil, 2006).

After each session Camila would decide how many stitches she was able to put in the heart. The range was from 4 to a high of 30 stitches in one session. Typically, Camila would assign a low number of stitches to a session when she needed to focus on a current problem, such as her relationship with peers in school. She reserved the higher number of stitches for sessions when she focused on the deeper and ongoing emotional pain, such as the betrayal by Larry and her conflicting feelings of rage and love for Larry. Watching some of the scenes on video replay was so validating for her (e.g., seeing herself in action, telling Larry off) that she decided it added an extra 10 stitches. Camila's estimate of the number of stitches that would be needed in the beginning of this remarkable self-directed reparative work was 200.

Transitions Occur

As we approached, however, the number of stitches (200) needed to repair her heart, the sessions resulted in fewer and fewer stitches. Clearly this child, who in her short life had experienced devastating losses, was reluctant to break off the therapeutic relationship—still another loss for her. For children with an abundance of loss, transitions are hard. It reminds them of the breakdowns and disruptions that led to the heart-breaking experiences that they are seeking to master.

Finally, the session came when there was only one more stitch needed. She stated at the beginning of the session that this would be our last session, at least for now. At the end of the session, however, she said, "I was mistaken—there were two stitches needed, and we were able to only do one, so we will need one more session." Once again, Camila knew what she needed in order to properly manage this transition. She was flexible enough to be able to adjust her plan and timetable and the strength to make her needs clear to the rest of us.

Closure

At the next session, the last stitch was placed in her heart and we didn't make any further appointments. Camila and her parents were well aware of my remaining available to them if the need for further treatment arose. Her creative development of the metaphor "my heart needs stitches" because the glue was simply not strong enough, guided our work over a period of 4 months of intensive therapy.

SUMMARY OF CLINICAL IMPRESSIONS AND FOLLOW-UP

Camila did come in for follow-up sessions when a specific need arose during the following 6 months. For example, she came in when she was quite shaken by an angry blowup between Rick and his older son. She was not accustomed to seeing such open displays of anger within the family. In the session, Camila once again knew exactly what she needed to do. She used the family playhouse to play out the angry exchange, and then she had fire trucks and rescue vehicles arrive quickly to evacuate the family members and take them to a place of safety. The impact of the scene she witnessed while visiting in the home of her new potential blended family was heightened by the fact that Camila has conflicts about her own anger. Although she has been able to express anger in the realm of symbolic play—initially toward her parents for separating in the first sequence of treatment, then toward Larry in the second and third sequences of treatment—she found it hard to acknowledge directly her angry feelings, and when she did she was clearly uneasy and experienced guilt. Often the anger was quickly put aside. So a key therapeutic objective on follow-up visits became validating her anger and encouraging her to embrace these feelings as legitimate and empowering as long as they were expressed constructively. The experience of observing the overt anger between Rick and his older son was used to normalize the experience of anger in families and discuss constructive choices for expressing it. I stressed that the open expression of anger between family members doesn't necessarily mean that the family is unraveling or that the family is in crisis. It was suggested that Camila try to figure out if the anger openly expressed between Rick and his son helped "to clear the air" and make things better between them, make things worse, or whether their relationship remained the same. She later reported that she thought things were better between Rick and his older son and agreed that sometimes openly expressing anger between family members can have a positive effect.

Fourth Episode of Treatment

As I write this chapter, I am currently seeing Camila for the fourth sequence of treatment. She will be 10 in 3 months. The fourth round of treatment was initiated by still another devastating loss. Her father's live-in partner, with whom she had been close for the past 4 years, decided to leave the relationship. At my suggestion, her father and his partner Connie sat down together to tell Camila about 2 weeks before Connie moved out.

When the day came for Connie to move out, Camila took it very hard. When I saw her with her parents, she looked as visibly sad as when I first met her after her parents had separated. She didn't seem like the Camila I had known since then. The spark, the zest, and the spirit that were her trademarks were missing. Again, she knew what she needed to do. She wasn't in the mood to talk much, but she went to the drawing table and drew a heart (Figure 10.2).

You can see from her drawing that the heart has a wound that extends its entire length, splitting the heart down the middle. Most of

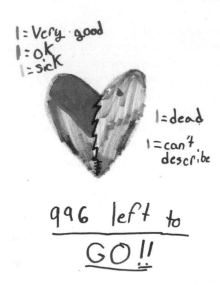

FIGURE 10.2. Camila's drawing of her heart with "sick" and "dead" parts.

her heart was either very good, as illustrated by the proportions colored pink for very good or orange for okay in a smaller but still significant section of the drawing. A small section of the heart, in the upper right quadrant and the lower right quadrant, is colored yellow and labeled "sick." A smaller portion in a ball shape, located in the upper right quadrant, was colored green by Camila, who labeled it "dead." In the lower quadrants of the heart on both the left and right periphery are small rectangular-shaped areas that she colored blue and labeled, "I can't describe." The wound that split her heart down the middle was described by Camila as requiring 1,000 stitches, and she thought we would be able to put 4 of those stitches in during that session, leaving a total of 996 stitches needed. In Figure 10.3, Camila further elaborated the meaning of the blue and green portions of her heart.

In the graph the blue section of the heart is depicted on the left-hand side of the drawing by Camila showing up in my office in a state of desperation, revealed by her saying "I don't know what to do" and by her T-shirt's message "I need help." The sense of helplessness she felt was underscored by the mouse at her foot that said "I can't help you, I am a mouse."

The green portion of Camila's graph (depicted on the right-hand side of the drawing) represents the dead portion of her heart with a very prominent tombstone emitting the words "Cry," "Weep," and "Oh no my

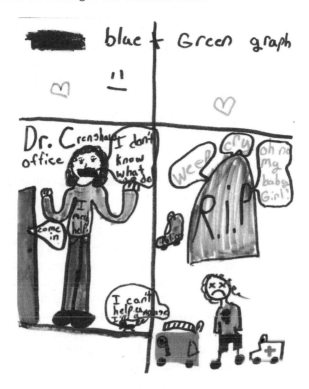

FIGURE 10.3. Camila's drawing of her blue and green graph.

baby girl." A police car, a fire engine, and an ambulance are included in the picture with a dejected looking Camila, concordant with the mood she evidenced on that day she appeared in my office. She has X's for eyes, and a frown that is uncharacteristic of her but authentically expressive of her state at that moment in time. I said to Camila, "You feel very, very sad, a part of your heart feels sick, a part feels dead, and another part you can't find words to describe. You must be wondering who you can trust not to hurt you." I continued, "But I am amazed that most of your heart is very good or okay in spite of all this heartbreak. Also, your parents are still here. They have not gone away." Camila said, "And I've got you, Dr. Crenshaw." I don't make a habit of crying in sessions, but my eyes got moist not only because of what Camila said but how she said it, with so much feeling and conviction behind it. It reinforced in my mind an e-mail exchange I had with Garry Landreth (March 9, 11, and 12, 2009), in which we both strongly agreed that in therapy, "doing is the easy part, being is the hard part." What meant so much to Camila at that moment in time when the earth under her feet was very shaky was that both her parents and her therapist were simply able to be fully present. Simply "being" with this child as she experienced her life falling apart counted for more than any "doing" in all the time we had been together over the last 5 years.

This is an ironic admission, given that I wrote two books about "doing" (Crenshaw, 2006, 2008a) before editing two books about "being" (Crenshaw, 2008b, 2009). The books about "doing" are likely to attract more readers than the books about "being" because we are creatures driven to master our world, including the challenges we face in therapy. It takes considerable ripening and maturity as a therapist to fully appreciate both the importance and the difficulty of fully "being" with those whom we seek to help.

Given Camila's despondent emotional state, I was quite concerned that a part of her heart was labeled *sick* and another small part *dead*. But she then explained that the rest of her heart was okay. In exploring this area further with Camila, it became clear that although her use of the terms *sick* and *dead* were alarming, when I asked her to compare the condition of her heart when Larry left to the situation now, she emphatically stated that it was far worse when Larry left. She made it clear that even though she was quite sad, hurt, and angry about this latest sudden departure from her life, most of her heart was healthy. We also talked about how the previous losses had perhaps made her heart stronger so that only a small portion of her heart (less than 10%) was "sick" or "dead" as a result of this latest loss.

There were several other key elements of this latest loss that were troubling for Camila. The timing was most unfortunate. Although Camila had seen signs that the relationship between her father and his live-in partner was not going well, when the ending came it was a shock for her. In addition, the ending of that relationship coincided with her mother and Camila's move into a recently renovated house with Rick and his three children. This big change, on its own, would have generated anxiety for Camila, but in addition it brought up the painful memories of Larry's sudden departure right after they had moved into their new house together. Still another factor weighing heavily on Camila's mind was that she was extremely angry with Connie. She didn't like being angry with Connie. She is a loving and forgiving child, and it was alien for her to be angry with someone, especially someone such as Connie with whom she had been so close. Part of her anger was related to her protectiveness of her father, who was extremely sad and upset that the relationship had ended. Another part of Camila's anger was related to her view that Connie had been selfish in removing the amount of furniture she took from the house upon leaving. Camila was angry that the house was quite bare and depressing for her father and for her when visiting her dad.

By the next session Camila appeared more like her typical spirited self. In the week between sessions Connie had called Camila's mother and expressed concern for Camila. Connie also told Camila's mother that she wanted to continue to stay in communication with Camila if Camila wanted to do so. Camila immediately sent a lengthy e-mail to Connie, and although the contents were not discussed, it clearly lightened the load significantly for Camila. She reported that she no longer felt that any part of her heart was "dead" or "sick" but simply that part of her love for Connie was "sickly" and "dead." Instead of 996 stitches that she thought would be required, she was sure that it would be much fewer. Camila discussed her worries for her father because he was so lonely and sad after Connie had left. She also expressed worries for her mother because something could go wrong in the relationship with Rick and the joining together of the two families.

It was clear that this 9-year-old girl was shouldering a lot of worries. I suggested to her that, since her heart had gotten stronger as a result of surviving the heartbreaks that she has been through, maybe her parents were also stronger than she was giving them credit for, because they had also survived a lot of heartbreak. I suggested to her that maybe, just maybe, it would be okay for her to simply be a 9-year-old girl and not be weighed down like a much older person with all these heavy burdens.

Camila knew, as always, exactly what to do. She started clowning around, making faces, laughing and enjoying just being playful. I suggested that her parents could help remind her that she was only 9 and that they were perfectly capable of handling their own sadness, loneliness, and heartbreak. Her parents readily agreed that they would like to remind Camila, as often as needed, that she is just a young girl.

SUMMARY OF CLINICAL IMPRESSIONS

Camila's emphasis on the heart as a symbol of both the woundedness and the center of healing is fascinating and compelling. Besides her own experience of approaching relationships and life wholeheartedly and her sense of vulnerability that accompanied trusting and loving others is a personal example of the heart as a symbol. On a collective level, the heart shape has occupied a special place in the history of many cultures and religions. In ancient Egyptian writings, the heart was considered the emotional center of the person, the life blood, passion, but also the conscience, as captured by the expression of a "heavy heart" (Biedermann, 1992). In the Bible the heart symbolizes the inner person. In the book of *I Samuel* (16:7) the passage reads, "The Lord seeth not as man seeth; for man looketh on the outward appearance, but the Lord looketh on the heart." In Hinduism the heart is considered to be the counterpart in the human of the Absolute (Brahman). In Islam the heart is viewed as the center of spirituality and contemplation (Biedermann, 1992). Since the late Middle Ages in the Western world the heart has occupied a central place in poetry and art as a symbol of romantic love, with arrows to the heart indicating the most painful of suffering. In Christian teachings the arrow penetrating the heart often symbolizes the sacrifice and suffering of Christ for all humanity (Biedermann, 1992). In the *Book of Proverbs* (15:13) it reads, "A merry heart maketh a cheerful countenance: but by sorrow of the heart the spirit is broken."

David Whyte (2009), a contemporary poet, pointed out in a lecture at the Psychotherapy Networker Symposium that the derivation of the word *courage* is from a French Norman word, *corage,* that means heart. Whyte noted that the courageous life is the heartfelt life. It takes courage to live a life in keeping with the path determined by our heart. It requires us to risk being hurt in the world in order to follow where our heart might lead us. This is the inspiring example set by Camila. She lives with courage a heartfelt life.

For the last two decades child development researchers have argued that resilience to aversive childhood events and toxic environments results from a complicated interaction of individual variables (e.g., disposition, consisting of proneness to positive mood, personality) and sociocultural (e.g., available familial and community support systems), risk, and protective factors (Garmezy, 1991; Rutter, 1999; Werner, 1995). The availability of strong social and familial support systems has been found to promote resilience in the face of extreme stress (Brewin, Andrews, & Valentine, 2000; Davidson, Hughes, Blazer, & George, 1991). The strong and consistent support of Camila's parents, as well as caring and supportive teachers, contributed to her ability to recover from her multiple losses. In addition, Camila manifests a number of individual variables that also are consistent with resiliency in children: her positive mood, intelligence, determination, flexibility, internal locus of control, and sense of humor were all important contributing factors.

Clinical issues that remain integral to the work with Camila include the delicate balance that I, as the therapist, must carefully maintain between honoring her considerable strengths without minimizing her suffering (Crenshaw, 2009). I was not convinced that, in the last session reported above, Camila had recovered so quickly and dramatically as a result of her communication with Connie. Although I think it relieved her mind greatly that the relationship with Connie wasn't going to repeat the complete abandonment she experienced when Larry left, I worried that her "flight into health" reaction may have been a form of minimizing her own suffering in order to make the adults in her life (including her therapist) feel less worried. This concern was pursued in the next session, and the parents were encouraged to consistently support her age-appropriate functioning and to convince her that they are capable of handling their own emotional burdens.

It is interesting that Camila forged such a strong bond with me, given that our relationship got off to a rocky start. My misstep could have led to a rupture in the relationship at that early point. Credit goes to Camila, once again, for her ability to be so forgiving, and for her good sense of humor that allowed her to overlook my flawed initial approach. It also speaks to the healing power of play. Although at that early period of the therapy even working within the metaphor of the play was too threatening for her, nevertheless the playfulness and ensuing laughter tended to reduce Camila's anxiety and threat level to the point that she was able to reveal more of her overwhelming pain even as we progressed through the remaining portion of that first sequence of treatment. Camila was able to leave therapy with positive memories that made her quite willing to come back for the second sequence, when needed. The therapeutic alliance was strongly established by the third sequence, as indicated by Camila, herself, who initiated the request to resume treatment.

More therapeutic work is needed to enable Camila to be fully comfortable with the anger that she legitimately feels in relation to all the losses, disappointments, and changes she has endured as a result of ruptured relationships. It will be a challenge for Camila to adjust to the major changes approaching, as she becomes part of a larger blended family with older stepsiblings. Working out each of those relationships, as well as with Rick, will involve negotiations within a more complex social field than she has thus far experienced. Hanging over those adjustments will be a pervasive anxiety expressed by Camila in our last family meeting: "Will something go wrong again?" and the implied question "Where would I be then?"

REFERENCES

Baer, U. (Ed. & Trans.). (2005). *The poet's guide to life: The wisdom of Rilke.* New York: Modern Library.

Biedermann, H. (1992). *Dictionary of symbolism: Cultural icons, and the meaning behind them* (J. Hubert, Trans.). New York: Meridian.

Brewin, C. R., Andrews, B., & Valentine, J. D. (2000). Meta-analysis of risk factors for posttraumatic stress disorder in trauma-exposed adults. *Journal of Consulting and Clinical Psychology, 68,* 748–766.

Cain, A., & Cain, B. (1964) On replacing a child. *Journal of the American Academy of Child Psychiatry, 3,* 443–456.

Cohen, J. A., Mannarino, A. P., & Deblinger, E. (2006). *Treating trauma and traumatic grief in children and adolescents.* New York: Guilford Press.

Crenshaw, D. A. (2006). *Evocative strategies in child and adolescent psychotherapy.* Lanham, MD: Jason Aronson.

Crenshaw, D. A. (2008a). *Therapeutic engagement of children and adolescents: Play, symbol, drawing and storytelling strategies.* Lanham, MD: Jason Aronson.

Crenshaw, D. A. (Ed.). (2008b). *Child and adolescent psychotherapy: Wounded spirits and healing paths.* Lanham, MD: Jason Aronson.

Crenshaw, D. A. (Ed.). (2009). *Reverence in healing: Honoring strengths without trivializing suffering.* Lanham, MD: Jason Aronson.

Davidson, J. R., Hughes, D., Blazer, D. G., & George, L. K. (1991). Post-traumatic stress disorder in the community: An epidemiological study. *Psychological Medicine, 21,* 713–721.

Freedman, R. (1996). *Life of a poet: Rainer Maria Rilke.* New York: Farrar, Straus & Giroux.

Garmezy, N. (1991). Resilience and vulnerability to adverse developmental outcomes associated with poverty. *American Behavioral Scientist, 34,* 416–430.

Gil, E. (1991). *The healing power of play.* New York: Guilford Press.

Gil, E. (1994). *Play in family therapy.* New York: Guilford Press.

Gil, E. (1995, May). *Healing in play therapy the abused and traumatized child.* Presentation cosponsored by the Astor Home for Children and Dutchess Community College, Poughkeepsie, New York.

Gil, E. (2006). *Helping abused and traumatized children: Integrating directive and nondirective approaches.* New York: Guilford Press.

James, B. (1989). *Treating traumatized children: New insights and creative interventions.* Lexington, MA: Lexington Books.

Landreth, G. (2002). *Play therapy: The art of relationship* (2nd ed.). New York: Routledge.

Remen, R. N. (1996). *Kitchen table wisdom: Stories that heal.* New York: Riverhead Books.

Rutter, M. (1999). Resilience concepts and findings: Implications for family therapy. *Journal of Family Therapy, 21,* 119–144.

Swift, S. (2007, April 28). What the Dickens? *The Guardian,* p. 12. Retrieved July 5, 2009, from *www.guardian.co.uk/books/2007/apr/18/classics.travelnews/ print.*

Werner, E. E. (1995). Resilience in development. *Current Directions in Psychological Science, 4,* 81–85.

Whyte, D. (2009, March). *The language of discovery.* Keynote address at the 2009 Psychotherapy Networker Symposium. Washington, DC.

CHAPTER 11

Manny's Story

A Soul Ascending

ERIC J. GREEN

Wherefore my counsel is that we hold fast ever to the heavenly way
and follow after justice and virtue always, considering that the soul is
immortal and able to endure every sort of good and every sort of evil.
                                                    —PLATO, *The Republic*

CASE REFERRAL INFORMATION

Manny, an 11-year-old European American male, was referred for play
therapy treatment by his middle school counselor within a county
located in the Southern portion of the United States. Manny was the
victim of chronic interpersonal trauma. Manny's Aunt Sheila met with
me to provide the data for the clinical interview and intake. The courts
revoked Manny's biological mother's parental rights and awarded Sheila
custody of Manny when he was 7 years old. Manny's biological father was
deceased. Sheila was awarded custody because Manny was neglected,
physically and verbally abused, and sexually assaulted by his biological
mother and her boyfriend. Manny's mother did not provide him with
adequate sustenance from the time he was 4 to 7 years old. The child
was malnourished, diagnosed with idiopathic growth failure, and was
physically and emotionally delayed in his development. He was exceedingly thin, diminutive in stature compared to his peers, and pale. His

mother, who suffered from depression, was dating a male close to her age. They routinely smoked crack cocaine in the home. They would go on drug binges, sometimes lasting several days, without eating or providing Manny with nourishment.

In addition to the neglect Manny endured, his mother and her boyfriend regularly incorporated Manny into their sexual activities while high on illicit substances. Manny remembers his mother's boyfriend saying that Manny was their "sex toy." Manny was sexually molested repeatedly over a period of 1½ years. Furthermore, Manny was exposed to domestic violence, as the mother's boyfriend would sometimes physically assault her after coming down from a drug high. The mother and her boyfriend would also harshly discipline Manny, frequently imposing corporal punishment along with branding Manny an "ungrateful bastard" when he would be disinclined to partake in the horrendous sexual assaults.

Sheila eventually began to suspect that something was terribly wrong when Manny, age 6, disclosed to her one day that he was engaging in oral sex with his mother's boyfriend. Sheila also discovered bruises on Manny's back where the boyfriend had beaten him with a wrought-iron candlestick holder the preceding night. Sheila immediately contacted Child Protective Services, who removed Manny from the home within a couple of days. Manny was placed in Sheila's temporary custody while the investigation and legal proceedings ensued. Eventually, the courts awarded Sheila full custody of Manny, and the mother was awarded a 1-hour monthly supervised visit. Because of a lack of evidence to corroborate the sexual abuse and Manny's inability to disclose the details of the abuse to investigators, neither the mother nor her boyfriend served jail time. The courts removed Manny from his mother's custody due to "severe medical neglect."

Manny was despondent and unresponsive for the first 8 months of living with his aunt. He was placed in an elementary school, but his transition was riddled with chaos. Manny would often become dysregulated by minor changes in his routine. He was apprehensive, suspicious, and anxious around others. Sheila reported that Manny was highly sensitive to sudden loud sounds, alarms, touch, and smells, many of which would cause him to panic. Manny was referred to the school's psychologist for a battery of psychological tests: He was diagnosed with posttraumatic stress disorder (PTSD); attention-deficit/hyperactivity disorder (ADHD), predominantly inattentive type; and a learning disorder. Because Manny was diagnosed with an emotional disability and suffered from acute, debilitating symptoms related to ADHD, the psychologist recommended that he be taken to a child psychiatrist and to a pediatric neurologist.

After myriad psychological and neurological diagnostic tests (e.g., Child Behavior Checklist, Wechsler Intelligence Scale for Children, fourth edition), Manny was found to exhibit elevated levels of anxiety and hypervigilance to his surroundings. These two traits are symptoms affiliated with PTSD in children, as traumatized children often perceive their world as unpredictable and people as threatening (Green, 2008). Accordingly, traumatized children typically exhibit hypervigilance, excessive self-monitoring of themselves and others, and require a need for consistent routines. Also, Manny (1) was unable to sustain attention, (2) had impaired short-term memory, (3) was ineffective at problem solving, and (4) was disorganized. Children diagnosed with PTSD commonly have weak executive functioning skills, a deficit that manifests in the inability to generate solutions to problems and may exacerbate anxiety. Moreover, his executive functioning was diminished primarily as a result of the early interpersonal trauma he experienced. Executive functioning is a cognitive domain that encompasses skills related to self-regulation (e.g., problem solving, planning skills, organization, and impulse control). The psychiatrist noted that because of his interpersonal trauma history, Manny focused much of his mental energy inward, which made him less available to apply his efforts to external tasks requiring sustained cognitive processing.

Manny's psychopharmacological regimen consisted of 20 mg of Focalin daily and 0.5 mg of Risperdal at bedtime. The Focalin was administered to attenuate his ADHD; the Risperdal, an antipsychotic, is sometimes prescribed in small doses to young children to treat significant anxiety. Sheila commented how one of the side effects of Focalin was that Manny appeared as though he was in a foggy, dreamlike state, especially in the mornings. Manny was also taking hormones to accelerate his physiological growth patterns, which were stunted.

At school, Manny's teachers reported that he (1) was forgetful, (2) did not remain seated, (3) did not follow rules, (4) was shy and timid, (5) made careless errors, (6) was messy and disorganized, (7) was mean and aggressive with his peers, and (8) talked out inappropriately. Manny appeared to give up easily when he was assigned a challenging task or one that he judged may require sustained effort. He had one friend at school, a boy who was 3 years younger and diagnosed with Asperger disorder. He and the boy would play with toy cars and trucks at recess and converse about topics befitting children much younger, such as watching the cartoon *SpongeBob SquarePants*. Manny was reading at a second-grade level, and his progress reports contained some failing grades, but mostly C's and D's. At home, Manny had difficulties falling asleep at night without his aunt staying in the room. Sheila noted that he had poor sleeping habits, nightmares, would sleepwalk, and sometimes wet the bed. Additionally, Manny could not sit still for more than 20 minutes in the evenings to complete homework, thereby complicating his evening routine.

Aunt Sheila had custody of Manny for approximately 5 years before he began play therapy. He did see a social worker for a year long period with unsuccessful results. Manny's presenting problems upon the referral were (1) "shutting down" at school, (2) dysfunctional social relationships with peers, and (3) difficulties falling asleep at night.

FORMULATION OF THE PROBLEM

First, I'd like to explore the meaning of childhood trauma from a Jungian perspective, as this will help the reader understand how I conceptualized the case. When interpersonal trauma, such as chronic sexual assault of a child, has rendered psychic integration untreatable, children may dissociate (Green, 2009; Jung, 1959). In dissociation, the child's psyche tricks itself into cutting off the harmful, unbearable external elements of trauma and suppresses them in the unconscious, so that the trauma becomes removed (or suppressed) from consciousness. For children who have experienced the trauma of the destruction of their delicate egos (the center of consciousness, the "I" as we know ourselves), as happened to Manny during the first few years of his life, the psychological sequelae of the trauma become poisonous to their interior psychological state (Green, 2009). Specifically, Jung (1963) stated that these trauma-induced complexes—strong images surrounded by gripping emotions—are represented in children's dreams, fantasies, play, and artwork by diabolical images (e.g., monsters, villains, dark figures, violence, death). For example, Manny often described a recurring dream of being chased by a dark red monster in a tunnel from which he could not escape. He recalled being terrified by this monster who wanted to "rip him apart." Sometimes the dream was so intense that Manny would wake up screaming. He often drew pictures of red monsters, violent activities, and prickly objects that he said were dead.

When an unbearable level of anxiety engulfs a child's vulnerable ego, as in the case of Manny who was chronically neglected by his primary caretakers, psychological degeneration occurs throughout the child's personality (Jung, 1964). To repair this annihilation, according to Kalsched (1996), an archetypal self-care system assists the child—an archaic mechanism that creates a defensive splitting to protect the child's personality by suppressing in to the unconscious (Green, 2009). The child's psychic defense against intolerable pain sends an archetypal *daimon,* or an image from the self-care system, to help the child dissociate from the immense anguish.

When a child is sexually assaulted by the very person who is the primary caretaker and is supposed to provide safety, the child's "transitional space" may become tenuous (Winnicott, 1971). The transitional space is the realm between the inner and outer world where the child learns how to use the *spiritus phantasticus,* or creative spirit, to play within symbols. Traumatic anxiety disassembles the transitional space and thwarts the child's creative efforts in symbolic play, thereby inducing a dreamlike state that is deceptively soothing (Green, 2009). For example, Manny often dissociated without realizing it. He would vicariously live through cartoon characters' lives so that he would not have to face his own psychic hell. He was fearful of befriending age-appropriate peers because he said they did not understand him and taunted him for being different. Manny often saw the world as unsafe and unstable, based upon isolated, negative interactions with peers.

Jung (1959) believed that representational communication, such as symbolic play, which may be momentarily disconnected during acute trauma, directs a child toward healing and fulfillment by linking the unconscious psyche to the ego (Allan, 1988). Children who are victims of interpersonal trauma suffer a *disconnection* from their ego's stability in managing the external world (Green, 2009). Specifically, children often exhibit a deprived connection with their unconscious because of the erosion of the transitional space between their outer and inner worlds due to the destabilization of their "good-enough" parental introjects (Winnicott, 1971) (e.g., images and the feelings associated with those images of the good mother or good father archetypes that provide safety). Since birth, Manny was exposed to ambivalent parenting, which culminated in rape and violence. His internal schemas of safety and stability, typically formed when children are cared for and nurtured as infants, were eradicated. He had no psychic referral point of a nurturing, caring, safe love. His cognitive representations of parental introjects were likely intensely frightening and insecure, thereby creating a void in his personality.

For the child's ego to resolve the devastating effects of interpersonal trauma, a significant assimilation must occur (Green, 2009). Assimilation, according to Kalsched (1996), occurs when children's bodily exci-tations are given mental representation by transitional archetypal fig-ures so that they eventually can reach verbal or symbolic expression and be shared with a trusting, kind individual. Helping the child recover the tenuous transitional space, so that his or her creative abilities are restored requires enrichment of the link between the unconscious and conscious (Allan, 1988; Green, 2009; Jung, 1963) and this results in an intensification of the child's ego.

Through analysis and therapeutic support, the Jungian-based ther-apist accentuates the strengths of the child and the family and builds upon those assets in a strengths-based approach to psychic healing. Manny and his family have several strengths that are important to exam-ine when generating the case conceptualization. Manny is of moderate intelligence and is capable of regulating some of his impulses (e.g., when he completes homework segments for 20 minutes at a time at home in the evenings). Manny is also extremely resilient; he survived malevolent parenting practices over an extended period of time without succumb-ing. Other strengths include Sheila's maternal desire to care for Manny and her good parenting skills. She permits Manny to make his own deci-sions, and she praises him appropriately for his successes.

Manny's case can be delineated further by examining the familial variables and how Manny's severed attachment may contribute to his pre-senting problems. The interpersonal trauma may have created breaks in the ego—self axis (i.e., the relationship between the exterior and inte-rior life) and thereby disrupted typical ego maturation (Edinger, 1992). The traumatic and sexualized mother—son attachment may have led to highly reactive states associated with internalized shame and dejection. These feelings may have manifested behaviorally through Manny's rage at home and school.

The sexual assault combined with the lack of nutrition, proper emo-tional care, and Manny's interpretation of these events culminated in the activation of the image schema of *splitting* (dissociation), the opposite of *containment*. This splitting is most likely due to cognitive misattributions of Manny's egocentric state of development (e.g., Manny often blamed himself for his mother's physical beatings and sexual/emotional abuse). Good-enough parent images in children provide an experience of safety and containment, wherein their world is perceived as stable and secure. In contrast, caretakers who sexually assault their children may activate the archetype (or image schema) of splitting/dissociation. Throughout childhood, Manny internalized the experiences of his caretaker rela-tionships and stored them as generalized patterns in implicit memory in the form of *internal working models* (Bowlby, 1979; Knox, 2003). These split archetypes, not innately hardwired structures but fluid, emergent, spatial patterns, are the underpinnings of the metaphorical meanings in Manny's life.

Through the analytical process of play therapy, images of containment activate and create the conditions in which inhibited image schemas can resume. I believed that through play therapy, Manny would produce unconscious imagery that would guide the analytic exploration. The facilitation of unconscious symbols, the emotionally and physically safe, trusting, nonjudgmental therapeutic relationship, along with the *temenos* (or sacred space within the playroom) would coordinate to activate the archetype of containment.

Throughout the first 6 weeks of play therapy, I observed Manny at his school twice, consulted with his teachers, had numerous discussions with his aunt, and conducted an extended developmental assessment. Based upon the subjective/projective assessments in the playroom, in addition to the psychometric tests I conducted, I substantiated the previous findings that Manny was grappling with posttraumatic stress, significant impairment from ADHD, poor self-esteem, and low levels of social functioning. His problems partially stemmed from the unresolved early trauma he had experienced, as well as physiological and neurological impairments that further exacerbated his distress and weakened his academic and social functioning.

INVITATION TO PLAY THERAPY

It took Sheila some coaxing to get Manny to show up for his first appointment with me. I was a bit anxious, or maybe excited, about meeting this child. Upon arriving, Manny scanned me carefully with his eyes, seemingly to ascertain what type of threat I might pose. He was well dressed and his hair was combed. I stated, "Manny, this is our special play time and in here you can play with all of the toys in most of the ways you'd like. If there's something that may hurt you or me, I'll let you know." He seemed curious about the items in the playroom and began engaging in exploratory play. After a few minutes of being silent, he quietly, almost inaudibly, uttered to me the types of toy cars he brought with him to our first visit. The door remained slightly ajar so that he could see that his aunt was right outside in the waiting room. He was quiet and incredibly apprehensive. I showed him the toy cars, and he asked me to play with the cars with him. He labeled each car. Next, he spent most of the session playing in the sand tray. He smoothed the sand with his hand over and over again and placed additional sand in the sand tray from an alternate container. He placed only the toy cars he brought with him in the sand tray. He did not speak during this time. He also traced several circles in the sand with his fingers. Then, without hesitation, he looked at me and said, "Thank you," and walked out into the waiting room. It had only been 15 minutes since we started, and we had 30 minutes remaining. I smiled at him and told him I would see him next week. I sensed that this was the right thing to do. I would typically have said, "I can see that you're ready to leave, but we still have 30 minutes of play time left. Let me show you the board games I have—maybe we can find one you like." I knew instinctively this was not the appropriate response for this child. Then he walked out and his aunt followed him, smiling.

My interpretation of his first invitation into the playroom and the initiating process was that Manny was curious about life and wanted to escape the haze of melancholy and pain. He seemed robotic-like, with no human emotion visible. He was not capable of speaking more than one word or two at a time. He had flat affect and seemed detached from his environment. For the first time, I could tell just by looking at this child, perhaps because of his stunted growth and disconnected affect, that he was suffering with deep, inconsolable psychological pain. I could see years of sorrow in his eyes. He appeared like an old, troubled soul, ravaged by a lifetime of disappointment and heartbreak; yet he was only 11. But there was something within him that was deeply moving, a sense of resiliency coupled with shame, that made me wonder.

I hypothesized that Manny would benefit from long-term psychotherapy; group counseling with same-sex, age-appropriate peers; filial therapy with Aunt Sheila; advocacy at his school environment; and coordination of psychotropic and behavioral services between his doctors, school system, and home life. After our first few appointments, I spent several days creating a comprehensive treatment plan, replete with cognitive-behavioral, evidence-based techniques. What happened next, during the course of therapy with Manny, has forever changed the way I conduct psychotherapy with children. Manny was unresponsive to techniques. He was unresponsive to me as a therapist who combined nondirective and directive play modalities. He was unwilling to participate in anything that remotely appeared as therapeutic. He was highly distrustful and disinterested, and rightfully so. Most of the adults in his life had let him down . . . terribly. All of my analytical training, use of evidence-based techniques, and belief in the play therapy process as a linear event that evolved from a trusting relationship were radically "thrown out the window." This child showed me how children heal themselves, in the purest sense of the term. He organically devised his own "treatment plan." He led the process, not me, and I will never approach play therapy the same way again.

CASE ILLUSTRATION OF SELF-DIRECTED TRAUMA PLAY

The Beginning: Setting the Stage

Throughout the first 3 months or so of therapy, Manny and I slowly developed a trusting relationship by routinely spending time together during our weekly session, occasionally discussing his worries related to school, and frequently discussing cars and comics (especially *Sponge-Bob*). Sheila would often provide me with information related to Manny's failing grades or a teacher complaint about his poor socialization. Taking a child-centered angle, I would allow Manny to lead the few verbal discussions we had, and I would not ask specific questions about information I obtained from Sheila for fear of alienating him. Infrequently, Manny would describe problems he was experiencing with peers (e.g., being teased and excluded). I would facilitate these conversations using reflective questions and providing empathic understanding, such as, "I'm wondering what it would be like if you could confront your friends at school about being mean to you, and the teasing would stop. What would that look like?" Because Manny was uncomfortable sharing difficult school experiences, and because he did not have the developmental capacity to do so effectively, I used an arsenal of directive art techniques to provide Manny with a nonthreatening mechanism of play through which he could voluntarily disclose his worries. I never brought up the abuse or asked him questions about it, and he did not speak of it or allude to it during our sessions. He was not ready to reveal his trauma narrative. I also attempted to engage him in Jungian sandplay on multiple occasions. I used this approach with him because he was tactile and enjoyed playing with his cars and exploring the playroom with his hands, whereas some traumatized children explore with only their eyes. Again, he would participate in creating worlds in the sand, but he would eventually go back to having a typical, casual conversation with me about cars or the toys he had brought into the playroom during that session. His sand worlds (elaborate scenes created in a sandbox with sand miniatures) were often related to illusory things, such as storylines from comics he viewed on TV. My conclusion was that he wanted to therapeutically bond with me, but not on my clinical terms.

As the months progressed, and Manny and I started to build a modicum of trust and confort with each other, I began to feel as if something about our sessions was lacking. Manny seemed disinclined to participate in activities or even to be in the playroom for an hour at a time. When he did participate in directed activities, he did so tentatively. Also, he would often look at the clock or his watch while we were in the play-room, checking the time frequently. He had a fixation with his watch: He never took it off. He told me once that knowing the current time was important. During our filial sessions, Sheila would describe Manny's eagerness to attend sessions with me and how he would ask during the week if it was time yet to see Dr. Green. So, while I was concerned that Manny was not interested in play therapy or something about our thera-peutic chemistry was preventing us from progressing, he articulated to his aunt and to me in subtle ways that he enjoyed something about our time together.

At times, Manny seemed anxious and discontented in the playroom during our weekly sessions. I'm not referring to symptoms related to his ADHD diagnosis that made him unable to sit still for periods of time; instead, it was as if he was trying to communicate to me that this artificial setting was insufficient for his healing. In his own way, he tried to communicate this message to me by sometimes bringing the play or therapeutic activity back to a discussion of his toy cars and trucks. Manny had an extensive knowledge of toy cars and trucks, because he collected them. He would often bring toy model vehicles to our weekly sessions and share their detailed history. Again, I would permit him to lead the content of our conversations.

One day Manny asked if we could go outside and play during our session. I told him we needed to speak to his aunt about the request, and we would make a decision as a team. His aunt was agreeable to Manny's request to go outdoors. Manny thrived while being physically active and in nature. Alongside my office was a pond with a mini-waterfall, geese, lush trees, plants and flowers, and large rocks to climb. This natural-istic setting afforded us an opportunity to be in Manny's element. He set the stage: He asked if we could spend half of our sessions playing outside and the other half in the playroom. So began our next phase of his play therapy: moving out of the artificial setting of the playroom and diversifying our time with physical activity outside, especially at the pond.

The Middle: The Work Deepens and Moves

Manny's verbal interactions with me increased when we started playing outside during the play therapy sessions. I noticed that he checked his watch less frequently. Manny still brought toys from home to show me and play with, including remote-controlled boats that we placed in the pond. There was a palpable difference in the quality of our time spent together once we moved the play outdoors and into nature. Specifically, Manny began to show a caring, sensitive side to himself that he did not reveal within the clinical playroom. He invited Sheila to play with us sometimes because he thought she might be bored, and he wanted her to "have fun too." Instead of just showing me toys and trucks and talking to me about them, now he would have me tell him what I remembered about the toys. Moreover, our play became more interactive and dynamic. When he brought his boats to play with in the pond, he would demonstrate his trust by asking me to steer the boats with the remote. In fact, he would sometimes bring me my own boat with which to play at the pond. This act of sharing was significant for Manny for a couple of reasons. First, Manny valued his toys highly, especially his remote-controlled cars and boats. He did not permit anyone to play with them, typically. However, he was okay showing others his toys and describing them. So the play began to deepen as Manny eventually began to view me as a trusted adult who could play with the miniature boats without destroying them. His aunt commented that I was the first person, besides herself, that Manny had allowed to play with the boats. Second, I noticed that Manny began to appear less constricted when expressing his thoughts and emotions. He slowly began to change from a withdrawn, shy, timid child to a young boy with some energy, passion for the outdoors, and a sense of humor.

The first time I ever heard Manny laugh was month 4 into play therapy. We were building a complex model car out of the box, with glue and all. I inadvertently glued the wheels upside down, not particularly paying attention to the smallest of details required to successfully build a replica model car. As I was gluing the tires onto the car's body upside down, I noticed that Manny had disengaged and was watching me intently, with his hand over his mouth. He was holding the laughter in, waiting for me to finish my upside down wheels! He quickly grabbed the car and stated in an animated voice, "Dr. Green, are you going to drive upside down, too?" With that, I realized the mistake I had made and began to laugh. And once I started to laugh, Manny began to laugh. And we both laughed until Manny was teary-eyed with laughter. This was a profound deepening in our playtime together; I had not seen Manny smile much over the past several months, much less laugh. His aunt could hear Manny's roaring laughter from outside, in the waiting room. After the session ended, she asked Manny, "What was so funny?"

He replied, "Oh, nothing. Just that Dr. Green is supposed to be smart but doesn't know how tires go on a car." Then we both started laughing again. It was a magical moment: This mistake I made, however minor, led Manny to a respite in his somber reality. I saw, for the first time, the child within him, peeking from the proverbial clouded veil, and looking for comfort through laughter.

The most significant event in the deepening of our therapeutic work occurred outside one day with Manny and another child I was counseling. After almost 6 months of individual play therapy, Manny mentioned that he was ready to have another child participate in group play therapy with us. Manny had met Jack, one of my other patients, on multiple occasions, as their sessions were back to back. Jack and Manny were the same age, and both liked sports. We had conducted a couple of group play sessions outside, mainly doing "feeling throws" with a miniature football, collecting rocks by the pond and "giving the rocks a life story," and playing with Manny's remote-controlled boat. Manny would not permit Jack to play with the boat, but he did talk to him about it extensively and showed him how far/fast it could travel in the pond. After our third group play therapy session outside, Manny conceded to Jack's repeated requests to take control of the boat in the pond. With reluctance, Manny permitted Jack to take the remote control, place the boat in the pond, and play with it, but "only for 10 minutes." I told Manny that I could see him working on his trust with others, and he smiled. Unfortunately, Jack steered the boat into a floating log while going at a fast speed, and the boat capsized in the middle of the pond. Manny had an adverse reaction to this event. Because there was no life-size boat with which to retrieve Manny's toy boat, we had no way to get the toy boat back. Jack profusely apologized to Manny, but Manny was filled with anger. He told Jack that he would have to buy him a new boat, and that these boats cost "several hundred dollars or thousands." This conflict between the boys was a prime opportunity for me to observe Manny's deficient self-regulation and social skills. Additionally, he displayed a tremendous amount of rage, culminating in crying and running away from the pond.

I got the entire group together—Sheila, Manny, and Jack and his mom—minutes after the event occurred. Jack's mother told Manny that they would give his Aunt Sheila the money to buy a new toy boat. They were apologetic, and Jack obviously felt concerned over Manny's temper. Manny was screaming, "I don't want their money, Aunt Sheila. I want that boy to swim in that pond and get me my boat back, now!" Manny was clearly frustrated and demonstrating his rage by making unreasonable demands, speaking sternly and loudly, pacing back and forth, then finally running off, crying.

Aunt Sheila began to follow Manny to console him, but I stopped her. As the drama was unfolding in real time, outside in the middle of the day, I realized that safety and containment were of paramount importance for both Manny and Jack. Manny must be permitted to express his rage and not keep it bottled up. This was the first time I had seen any significant emotional display from Manny. However, when a child is drowning, it's not the best time to teach him or her how to swim. I walked over to him and reflected back to him how angry he was at Jack for wrecking his boat, and how I wondered if he was disappointed with me for arranging the group play therapy in the first place. Again, this was the definitive turning point in therapy. After the simple reflective statements, Manny began to calm down. Because he was not yelled at or punished for displaying his rage, he paradoxically calmed himself. I commented on how different it must be to be able to get this angry and not be in trouble for it. I was trying to give his rage a voice and carry it for him, if only for a short period of time. After a couple of seconds, Manny hugged me. Then he ran over to Jack and apologized to him and his mother for yelling. He asked Jack if they could split the cost of the boat, since they both were playing with it. Jack and his mother and Aunt Sheila all agreed to this compromise. After Jack and his mother left, I walked Manny and his aunt to their car to say goodbye. It was an intensely emotional play session, and I ended it early as Manny seemed depleted. It was not until this incident that I realized Manny was, in fact, leading the healing, not me. Manny would heal himself on his own terms when he was ready.

From this experience, I realized that therapy isn't therapeutic because it's therapy. Therapy can be therapeutic just by two people being there for each other, without fancy interpretations or elegant interventions. Specifically, Manny had not ever hugged me (nor had I seen him hug his aunt) during our entire time of therapy up until the sinking of the ship. Manny and I affectionately referred to this turning point in play therapy, this painful and deepening piece of our therapeutic work, as our "Titanic day." It was not until "Titanic day," when the ship was stranded and all hope seemed to be lost for Manny, literally and figuratively, that he allowed himself to sit with the pain, reach out to someone he trusted, and employ the social skills he had learned during our previous work in play therapy to come up with a resolution. Later, during filial therapy, Sheila remembered this day quite well and commented that it wasn't until Manny allowed himself to be vulnerable and feel safe at the same time, thereby allowing him to reach out for help, that he began to know in his heart that he didn't have to carry the pain and hurt any longer.

Resolutions Surface

After our "Titanic day," Manny began formulating his trauma narrative on his own terms and at his own pace. It was during his retelling of the trauma symbolically that resolutions began to surface. The first session after the boating incident, after which Manny felt safe to express deep-felt emotions without being judged, he asked me if his aunt had told me what happened to him as a child with his mother. I responded that she did, in fact, share with me the things that his mother did to him. I asked him if he wanted to share anything about that time in his life with me or if he had any questions. He said that he didn't remember most of what happened because he was too young, but he did remember feeling scared and sad a lot of the time. When I tried to facilitate his retelling or symbolically reconstructing the trauma narrative, he told me that he knew what I was doing. Amazingly, this child thanked me for trying to get him to "get the bad stuff off his chest." However, he also, again, confirmed that he was in control of his own healing. When I asked him to create his world in the sand tray, he told me that he didn't need to retell his story to get past it. He commented that he already told it several times to his aunt, the police, lawyers, and a judge, and that doing so hadn't helped him to feel any better about it. What he said that he needed to heal from the trauma was for me just to be there with him. "Dr. Green, I know what you're trying to do, and I appreciate it. You're trying to help me get all the bad stuff off my chest. If you really want to help me, maybe you'll just be my friend and listen to me. Maybe if I'm sad sometimes because someone is mean to me at school. Or maybe you'll play with me sometimes, like you do now, when I feel like no one else likes to play with me. I'm wondering if that will maybe help me the most?" I explained to Manny that he was in control of his own healing trajectory at this point, and that I was still in his life to provide therapeutic support whenever he needed. Again, Manny knew that what he needed most was not to produce a trauma narrative in sandplay, or through a series of artworks, or through a verbal reconstruction with me helping him correct misattributions and cognitive distortions. He needed me to simply be there with him during this time of healing. Once I accepted this difficult truth and let go of the image I conjured to be an "effective" therapist, the resolutions paradoxically began to appear.

There was a significant resolution that surfaced during the middle to end point of therapy: forgiveness. First, Manny changed from attending a public to a Catholic school due to his aunt's belief that he was not getting the individualized attention he needed in public school. This change occurred while Manny was in therapy with me. After a few weeks of attending his new school, Manny told me that he was required to have one period of class time a day titled "Religion." The first lesson in the course was about souls and heaven. Manny said that he wasn't sure if he believed in God, but that maybe people did have souls. He began to explain a rather sophisticated understanding of spirituality. When I asked him to tell me more, he commented that he thought people clung to the concept of God to feel better about the bad things that happened to them or to feel forgiveness for the bad things they did to other people.

One afternoon during our play therapy session, we were at the pond. Manny was fascinated with a family of geese that lived at the pond. We saw the family frequently, which consisted of two adult geese and three small baby geese. I would often ask Manny what was going on with the family that day, and part of our time together would involve his telling me a story about the goose family. He would often use current struggles from his life but transferred unto the geese. This was similar to using puppets with young children to help them disclose painful pieces of information that may be too difficult to do unless done through a symbolic outlet. On this specific day, Manny, who had never talked about anything metaphysical or spiritual with me when describing the geese and assigning these "stories" to them, told me and his aunt that they were all looking for their souls. I inquired, "Manny, what are souls and what happened to them?" Manny said that a soul is a part of everyone and is invisible. He said that if you are good, your soul goes to heaven, and if you're bad, your soul goes to hell. Furthermore, he said, the goose family had gotten into a big argument that day, and they couldn't find their souls. I asked him to explain the fight. He said that the mother goose and father goose had mistreated their three children by not feeding them since the week before. They did this because they were mad at the children for quacking too loudly and sometimes attracting an alligator who could maybe eat them. Once the children learned that they were being starved for quacking too loudly, they became angry and retaliated against their parents. They purposefully began quacking louder and louder so an alligator would come and eat their parents. Because everyone had been mean to each other, Manny said, the goose family had lost their souls.

Two weeks later we were at the pond again, and Manny was watching the goose family intently. I asked him if they had found their souls yet, and he replied that the children had, because they were too young to know any better and didn't really want the alligator to eat their parents. So they were forgiven, and their souls returned. But the parents' souls were gone because they were purposively mean. I asked Manny, "Do you think the baby geese will ever forgive their parents for not getting them food for a week?" Manny responded, "Maybe so, because everyone deserves a chance to be forgiven." About a month later, when we were at the pond again, I asked Manny to tell me his final story of the geese, as I knew that termination would be happening soon. Manny said that all the geese had found their souls, and they were happy . . . except the mother goose. He said that the mother's soul had risen to heaven because she was the sorriest for what she had done to her babies. And then he unexpectedly broke with the metaphor and asked me, "Dr. Green, do you think my mom has her soul after what she did to me?" After a brief hesitation, I replied, "Manny, what your mom did to you was a terrible thing. And I know that it caused you to be sad for a long time. I think what you're asking me is if it's okay to forgive her. And my answer is yes . . . whenever you're ready." Manny replied, "Okay." To me, this represented Manny beginning to come to terms with forgiving his mother for inflicting harrowing psychological and physical pain upon him as a toddler, while still maintaining his dignity.

Transitions Occur

Most of the transitions that occurred in Manny during the course of therapy were positive. He transitioned to a Catholic school where he received individualized care and attention. His grades dramatically improved within the first grading period. Over the course of the year in therapy, he also transitioned from being an emotionally immature, developmentally delayed boy to a child who faced his fears, found the strength to trust in others again, and started developing rapidly. One of his primary transitions was in his physical appearance. His pale white skin and disheveled hair, along with flat affect, all changed. He became a child full of color and life from playing outside and being in the sun. He started grooming himself in the mornings, and his affect was dynamic and engaging.

Another significant transition occurred in his ability to feel and express emotions. I remember his aunt telling me once, with a humorous, playful tone, "Dr. Green—what have you done to this child? He's now so in touch with his emotions that we can't get him to shut up about them!" As he continued on his own path in healing, his psyche knew that he must connect to his emotions and express them in appropriate ways. While he still felt rage and anger at times, he would walk away from the situation or the person and not lash out at them like he had done previously. He would count to 10 or participate in an alternate type of diffusing activity before reengaging. I can best describe this transition as the child going from unhappy and cold (without the capacity to express any of his emotions) to feeling like a real human being again, replete with warmth, anger, and depth.

Manny transitioned out of his solitude and began playing with age-appropriate peers. He would invite friends over for play dates on weekends, and conversely, he felt okay going to his friends' homes and playing with them as well. This behavior was in stark contrast to that of the child who came into my office at the beginning of therapy. He had no friends except an autistic child with whom he fought frequently, and he was afraid to leave his aunt's house except to go to school. Manny also experienced a qualitative shift in his views of himself and the world around him. His aunt told me that for the first time in many years, she saw that he felt secure in his abilities. I believe it was a combination of his internal representations changing from negative to positive, as he let himself feel emotions again, and the fact that he was able to hear positive feedback about himself. Also, the change in school environment was helpful in improving his grades, which may have further improved his self-esteem.

Two other practical transition pieces that I must share are small things, but nonetheless items I will not soon forget. Sometimes Manny and his aunt would call me between sessions (when they began to be held every 2 weeks instead of every week due to termination approaching) to update me on Manny's progress or a situation occurring in the household that they wanted to share. Manny's aunt said that in the years he had lived with her, he had refused to speak on the phone. When he would talk to relatives, he would make beeping noises similar to that of a toy robot. This was the first time Sheila had seen her nephew feel comfortable with telephone conversations. Second, as we (child psychotherapists) are sometimes viewed as extensions of the family, I accepted an invitation to join Manny, Sheila, and her husband for Manny's celebratory birthday dinner. Manny spoke to the waitress, ordered his own food, played with my iPhone, laughed, and was socially interactive. After the meal ended, Sheila got teary-eyed and thanked me for joining them. She said that this was the first time in a long time that she had seen her nephew smiling and happy. It was around this time that I began planning for termination. I knew that Manny would continue to benefit from psychotherapy, as I provided referrals, but that his time in individual play therapy with me had gone as far as it could go. Manny had self-developed the tools to be more successful at school, at home, and with his newfound friends.

Closure

Closure was a difficult event for myself, Manny, and Sheila. Though I had given everyone the 4-week warning, then 3-week, then 2-, it still was one of the most challenging "goodbye celebrations" I've experienced. I had bonded with this child and his family over a year's period and had witnessed his profound psychological development. I wanted to have an encouraging goodbye, where we both would be allowed to leave on our own terms, so to speak. As I sit here typing this and recalling the closure in my mind, I am getting teary-eyed. For all of the "success" stories I had been a part of with children and their families previously, this child and his story really made a significant impact on me as a clinician, but more importantly, as a human being. I had prepared, as I typically do, a presentation to review with the child wherein we discuss the play therapy experience with me, like a timeline. I had his artwork to review, pictures of his sandplay, and a couple of significant moments that I wanted to share during the course of the therapy (e.g., "Titanic day").

When Manny and his aunt arrived for the last session, I was already heavy-hearted. Just as Manny had determined the course of therapy, he now knew what he needed to do to end it. It was not being in the playroom for 50 minutes, reviewing my presentation, allowing him to say his goodbye, then having a "goodbye celebration" with his Aunt and me. I realized later that my plan was a product of my need for closure combined with methods I had obtained from previous trainings or a textbook, and not his. Our closure was simple. He came in, told me goodbye, cried, gave me a hug, and asked me to keep in touch. I told him that I would be checking in with his aunt from time to time about his progress and hoped that we would have an opportunity to talk about what was going on in his life. Before he left, he gave me a small duck made of wood. He said that he wanted me to remember him by it. Our closure was analogous to his play therapy: It was relationship-based and on Manny's terms. It was not overly clinical or something to be learned from a training manual.

SUMMARY OF CLINICAL IMPRESSIONS AND FOLLOW-UP

Many of us in the mental health field comment that we aren't the ones that do the healing, we're just there to witness children heal themselves. I had said this myself many times before my work with Manny, but I didn't quite buy it. I just said it because it sounded like the humble and most appropriate thing to say. Somewhere deep inside I knew that we had a small part to do with children's healing, though. What I have deduced from working with Manny is that my part as a clinician is mainly to step aside and just "be" there with the child, providing social comfort and support through play. But it has taken me many years of education, clinical experience, and children telling me this over and over in their own way to finally "hear" it from Manny. Why was this child's story and time with me different? I don't know, and I'm okay with admitting that I can't understand everything that occurs within play therapy. My clinical impression of this case was that a wounded child came to a wounded healer, and through recognizing and accepting our own limitations and strengths, we, like the alchemists before us, transmuted the charred rocks, or *prima materia,* into precious elements. Once Manny was provided with a safe, therapeutic relationship, he began working on himself and rebuilding trust in others. He also began practicing forgiveness, which helped him feel better about himself and the world around him.

Since termination, I have spoken to Manny and Sheila a couple of times. Sheila reports that Manny continues to grow and mature every month, including receiving an award at the end of the school year for being "Most Improved Student." He and Sheila expressed pride in this accomplishment. I told Manny that I was writing this book chapter, and his response was that one day he wanted to go on the Oprah Winfrey Show and tell people his story. I asked how he would tell his story, and he said, "I would talk about my strength and let them know it's okay to feel bad about yourself if someone hurts you, but maybe someone will be there to help you too. I would also tell them about the geese at the pond." Manny not only self-healed some of the wounds inflicted from the sexual abuse he experienced as a toddler, but he also came to a place spiritually where he felt compelled to share his story to help other abused children cope with their own difficult feelings. Manny is one of the most courageous children I know. One day, when he's an adult and reads this chapter, hopefully he will recognize and appreciate the central role he played in his own recovery and what a profound impact his legacy has had on me.

REFERENCES

Allan, J. (1988). *Inscapes of the child's world: Jungian counseling in schools and clinics.* Dallas, TX: Spring.

Bowlby, J. (1979). *The making and breaking of affectional bonds.* London: Tavistock.

Edinger, E. (1991). *Ego and archetype.* Boston: Shambala.

Green, E. J. (2008). Re-envisioning a Jungian analytical play therapy approach with child sexual assault survivors. *International Journal of Play Therapy, 17*(2), 102–121.

Green, E. J. (2009). Jungian analytical play therapy. In K. J. O'Connor & L. D. Braverman (Eds.), *Play therapy theory and practice: Comparing theories and techniques* (2nd ed.) (pp. 83–122). Hoboken, NJ: Wiley.

Kalsched, D. (1996). *The inner world of trauma: Archetypal defenses of the personal spirit.* New York: Routledge.

Knox, J. (2003). *Archetype, attachment, analysis: Jungian psychology and the emergent mind.* New York: Brunner-Rutledge.

Jung, C. G. (1959). *The Collected works of C. G. Jung. Vol. 9: The archetypes and the collective unconscious.* New York: Pantheon.

Jung, C. G. (1963). *Memories, dreams, reflections.* New York: Pantheon.

Jung, C. G. (1964). *Man and his symbols.* Garden City, NY: Doubleday.

Winnicott, D. W. (1971). *Playing and reality.* London: Routledge.

CHAPTER 12

"I Am an Artist"

A Sexually Traumatized Girl's Self-Portraits in Paint and Clay

BARBARA SOBOL

NaTasha, at this writing, is approaching her 14th birthday. She is a bright, energetic, and athletic African American girl who does well in school, loves art, and loves dance in all its forms. She is also argumentative, demanding, and moody. From her first session with me, in a long and necessarily intermittent course of therapy over the past 10 years, she has taken the lead on many occasions. In this chapter, I focus on six sessions, late in therapy, that exemplify her powerful spontaneous responses to my open invitation to do art. They also show the value of the therapist's nonintrusive stance and of his or her intuitive knowing about when, and how, to respond to the child's lead.

CASE REFERRAL INFORMATION

NaTasha B., just shy of her fourth birthday, was referred to the DC Rape Crisis Center (DCRCC) in the earliest weeks of its new children's program. It was a program that I had helped to design and that funded up to 18 months of individual and/or family therapy for children who had experienced sexual abuse. NaTasha had just completed 6 weeks of evaluation, psychoeducation, and basic abuse counseling at the local Child Avocacy Center, which did not at the time offer continuing long-term therapy. The recommendation for follow-up therapy noted the involvement of social services and the need for counseling to be established in order for the family to maintain care and custody of their daughter. NaTasha had been sexually molested by her 15-year-old (paternal) half-brother during a period when her parents were separated. Each parent blamed the other for having created the situation that allowed this to happen—each saw the other as neglectful in allowing the troubled 15-year-old to babysit his sister. (He was subsequently charged, entered a therapeutic program for young offenders, and moved out of his father's home to live with his biological mother.)

BACKGROUND AND FAMILY HISTORY

NaTasha's parents are Eddie B. and Sandra T., a couple who were in their 40s at the time I met them. They had recently separated (just prior to the abuse), after having lived together for several years, raising their only biological child, NaTasha, Eddie's adolescent son, and Sandra's two elementary school-age children. Their turbulent relationship had always been punctuated with heated arguments, separations, and reunifications. Both parents are intelligent and articulate, and by their own acknowledgment, emotionally volatile. Physically, they were polar opposites: Eddie was thin, wiry, and filled with nervous energy. Sandra was sedentary and often seemed preoccupied. Both parents had significant health issues that affected their ability to work, so the family often lived on the edge of poverty. Mr. B. owned the house they shared and, within that household, he characterized himself as the breadwinner, head of the family, and rule maker. Despite chronic pain, he worked long hours as a self-employed car mechanic. At home, he appeared to require that Sandra accept a traditional "housewife" role: cooking, keeping the house clean, minding the children. Neither he nor Sandra talked about how much sexual intimacy there was between them. Both parents, however, expressed a strong commitment to their daughter. Eddie, while often defensive, was remorseful and ashamed at having exposed NaTasha to abuse. Sandra, who was able to acknowledge unresolved issues of familial sexual abuse in her own childhood that had left her depressed for much of her adult life, was the driving force behind NaTasha's therapy.

Because neither parent had been able to complete college, they shared a sense of the dream deferred—the hope that this child, the last for both of them—would be the one who might fulfill her own promise.

Whatever tenderness or commitment Eddie and Sandra may have had with each other at some earlier time had eroded by the time they brought NaTasha to my office. Within the first months of therapy, they attempted a reunification for NaTasha's sake, followed by another dramatic separation. It became apparent that although the household could become physically safe, it was not emotionally safe and NaTasha lived in an environment of great tension and emotional chaos. When living in the home, Sandra was often irresponsible with money. When very angry or fearful, Eddie would suspect Sandra of using drugs or engaging in prostitution, accusations she vehemently denied. There were incidents of threatened violence and calls to the police, and, while there was no overt physical violence between the two, there had been at least one physical altercation between Eddie and Sandra's older brother, requiring police intervention. NaTasha had been a witness.

FORMULATION OF THE PROBLEM

The treatment of NaTasha, begun in the wake of sexual abuse, attempted to combine two models of therapy: trauma-focused cognitive-behavioral therapy (CBT) and attachment-focused therapy, both using art therapy as the primary means of expression and communication. The goals of CBT and those of attachment-based therapy are compatible in work with traumatized children, but often the "feel" of the art sessions is different from that of CBT sessions that are primarily verbal.

The value of CBT work—and CBT as it is addressed in art therapy—has been documented abundantly and discussed by many authors, both in general (Rosal, 2001) and specifically in relationship to trauma-focused work (e.g., Prifalo, 2009; Tinnin & Gantt, 2000). In using art therapy to further CBT goals, the therapist may present art directives, seeking to use the content of the artwork to challenge and restructure old beliefs and to give a child tools for self-reflection and self-repair.

Attachment theory, from its inception, has contained strong cognitive elements, including John Bowlby's (see Wallin, 2007, pp. 27–28) description of "internal working models" of self and other. Based on children's felt security or felt insecurity in early development, such models or maps comprise deeply held belief systems that shape personality and influence thought and behavior. In recent years, neurobiological research has had a profound influence on attachment theory, creating a strong emphasis on the subjective aspects of relationship. Current writers focus on the nonverbal communication of affect and on affective attunement, or the achievement of a subjective sense of emotional resonance with another person. According to Schore and Schore (2008, p. 10), attachment theory has shifted to a theory of affect and affect regulation. Siegel (2003, pp. 38–40) notes the importance in childrearing of several "ingredients": *reflective dialogue* (in which a parent shows a sensitivity and responsiveness to the subjective life of the child), *repair of ruptures in attunement* between child and caregiver as they occur, *emotional communication* (the sharing of positive emotions, the soothing of negative emotions), the creation of a *coherent narrative* of a child's life, and *contingent communication,* which Siegel describes as an ongoing transactional process between parent and child that involves: "(a) perception of the child's signals, (b) making sense of the signals in terms of what they mean for the child, and (c) a timely and effective response." From this process, the child may "then experience the sensation of 'feeling felt' by the parent." In early childhhood the signals, both sent and received, are primarily nonverbal, transmitted through, for example, eye contact, gesture, and tone of voice.

In beginning to work with NaTasha and her family, I thought that the trauma work would eventually require significant use of CBT in order to replace her incoherent life narrative, her distorted beliefs, and her confusion. However, my early experience with the family led me to formulate some issues more prominently in attachment terms, given the disrupted and unrepaired affective attunement between NaTasha and her mother.

Since I considered spontaneous art expression to be a form of Siegal's nonverbal contingent communication, I planned to encourage NaTasha to draw, paint, and sculpt freely in an atmosphere of acceptance and interest. My goals for therapy also included establishing and maintaining affective attunement. This meant that I would take the time to become aware of and responsive to NaTasha's immediate mood and shifts in mood, mainly through my receptivity to her expressive art and play. Moreover, in keeping with Siegel's note (2003, p. 42) that the "most robust predictor of disorganized attachment is a parent's unresolved state of mind," I planned to counter the disorganization by helping NaTasha create a coherent narrative of her life within the family. To this end, I hoped to engage one or both parents in the work of clarifying the story of the family through one or more family art sessions as the individual work progressed. Because the specific trauma of sexual

abuse was embedded within the larger story of the difficult relationships of this household, I saw these sessions as essential in establishing a
sense of emotional security before NaTasha would be able to resolve her
feelings about the abuse.

INVITATION TO PLAY AND ART THERAPY

The original therapeutic framework of the DC Rape Crisis children's
program was a three-stage trauma model using art therapy (see Sobol,
1998). The stages involved the development of trust, the trauma work
proper, and self-repair, including creating new relationships. One of
the four initial or intake sessions in the program presented an invitation to free play and/or art in the play therapy room similar to the first
session(s) of the assessment protocol articulated and later authored by
Gil and Green (2004). This format was balanced by more structured art
assessments in subsequent sessions.

In the free-play session, NaTasha chose to play in the dollhouse,
where she created a loving couple, with the wife-doll cooking for the
husband, calling him "honey," and then joining him to take in a little
stray girl whose own mother, in the story, had abandoned her. When
NaTasha tired of this story, she turned to the life-size African American
infant doll. She dressed the baby in pull-ups and a dress and engaged
in nurturing play, but at the end of the session she would not relinquish
the baby, refusing to put the doll in her crib, as suggested. She informed
me that she was taking the baby doll home with her, because "This . . .
baby . . . loves . . . ME!" She said she would tell her dad that her mother
had bought the doll for her but then decided instead that she would
tell her mother (who was in the waiting room) that I had said she could
keep the doll. At my invitation Sandra then joined us, at first trying to
gently persuade the pouting, crying, defiant NaTasha to let go her grasp
of the doll. Sandra soon became impatient. NaTasha sensed the change
in mother's tone of voice and released her grip. After the family left the
clinic, I found NaTasha's jacket and followed them out into the street to
return it. It was evening and the urban street corner was busy. NaTasha
was no longer crying, and she greeted me cheerfully. She had stopped to
admonish a homeless woman who was unrolling blankets in a doorway:
"You can't make a bedroom in the street! You have to go home now and
go to sleep in your own bed." The spontaneous dollhouse play and doll
play as well as the street corner scene quickly brought part of NaTasha's
internal world to light. In her fantasy world, domestic life was loving and

generous, and she had the power to prevent someone she loved (and who loved her) from ever being taken from her and by the force of her will, adults would listen and behave as she needed them to do. While all children must undergo realistic disillusionment, NaTasha's interior schema for life was brittle and was particularly thwarted by her real-life experience.

An early portrait made with tempera paints at age 5 (Figure 12.1) captures some of NaTasha's magical thinking bravado. A child's face (hers) dominates a landscape of silvery mountain peaks. The central mountain sits directly over her head and serves visually as a hat (its shape suggests a magician's or a witch's pointed hat), reinforcing the sense of omnipotence that the nearly bodiless child belies.

NaTasha, in fact, had the daunting real-life task of navigating the confusing emotional terrain between her two parents. Eddie was harsh and rough-edged but devoted, steady, and predictable; Sandra, who was more emotionally attuned in the moment and more openly expressive and loving, was unfortunately unpredictable and preoccupied. Her departures and absences grew longer and longer as time went by, and

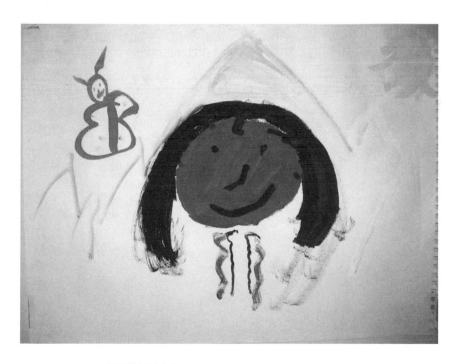

FIGURE 12.1. NaTasha's self-portrait at age 5.

there was less and less chance for repair of their disrupted relationship. NaTasha alternated in her presentation and identification between these two poles. When she came to sessions with Sandra, NaTasha withheld her anger and sought to please her mom. If she lost her mother's attention in the moment, she would become clingy or coy. When she came to session accompanied by Eddie, she struggled to find a way to communicate with him. Her coyness or other attempts to be appealing (in the way a younger child might be) elicited impatience from Eddie. Failing to "get her own way" (Eddie's words), NaTasha turned angry and defiant toward her father, withdrawing only when he threatened consequences.

When she was in the presence of *both* parents, NaTasha could become disorganized and agitated. In order to better understand how she was able to regulate her emotionl life in the midst of this chaotic stimulation, I asked the family (several months into the therapy and during a period of reunification) to do a family art evaluation (FAE), a procedure that elucidates family dynamics through art (Gil & Sobol, 2000). Her drawings shown here (Figures 12.2, 12.3, and 12.4) are three sequential attempts to respond to a single directive "Draw a portrait of your family." The unmistakable affective arousal that can be seen in the haste, carelessness, and disorganization of her images illustrates the effects of the extreme affective polarity in the home. NaTasha's efforts

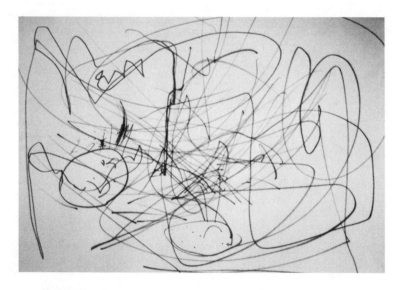

FIGURE 12.2. NaTasha's family drawing, first attempt, age 4.

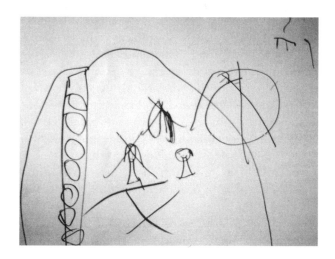

FIGURE 12.3. NaTasha's family drawing, second attempt, age 4.

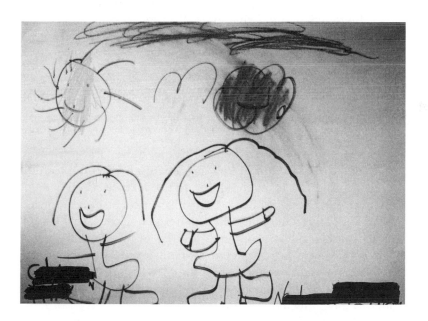

FIGURE 12.4. NaTasha's family drawing, final attempt, age 4.

to regulate her out-of-control feelings included connecting to her older half-sister (Sandra's daughter, then 9-year-old Nichelle) and copying images from Nichelle's more organized drawings. The polarity of the two parents was amply demonstrated in the parents' artwork, made during the same session. Eddie made a meticulously rendered replica of the pyramid image on the dollar bill, an image of an idealized family home (the children are playing in the yard, Sandra is calling them all in for lunch), and one of a man and woman talking (the profile of the woman has no mouth). Sandra's drawings, on the other hand, seemed to bubble up from an internal preoccupation with longing and loss. Particularly striking and unusual was her drawing of an abstract "family tree" done in vivid magenta and black, with herself as the trunk and many significant family members as stubby branches, including adults, children, and miscarried babies whom she was still mourning. While neither parent was willing to attend regular sessions as a couple or as individuals, when caught off-guard—as they were in the family art session—both could acknowledge some longing for help with their own significant losses. Almost a year later, in the last therapy session with NaTasha before she drifted out of contact with her daughter, Sandra made a nearly identical image of the family tree drawing, only this time in clay. The clay piece was emotionally invested but poorly constructed, and sadly, it broke into pieces while in the kiln.

CASE ILLUSTRATION OF SELF-DIRECTED TRAUMATIC PLAY AND ART

Before NaTasha's eighth birthday, Sandra had moved out permanently and had subsequently relinquished custody of all her minor children (two to her brother, NaTasha to Eddie). In the years between her eighth and eleventh birthdays, Eddie was sensitive to NaTasha's sadness and anger and would try to arrange visits with her siblings or with her mother. Eventually, he became discouraged, and he grew emotionally warier than ever. He alternated between lavishing expensive material gifts on NaTasha and angrily withdrawing the gifts as punishment for poor grades or disrespectful behavior. NaTasha, too, had begun to withdraw emotionally. She affected a controlled and stereotypical drawing style (Figure 12.5), which, although spontaneous (i.e., generated by NaTasha and not in response to any directive from me), effectively masked, or rather caricatured, her genuine feelings. Cartoons can serve a number of defensive needs for many children (see Kramer, 1993, p. 49). This

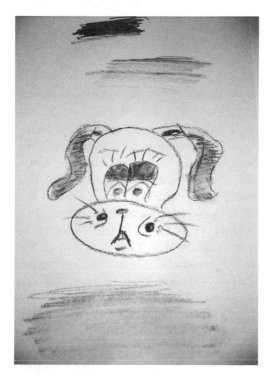

FIGURE 12.5. NaTasha's "signature" cartoon rabbit, age 9.

particular drawing, which she repeated, could also be understood as a communication. Behind the bunny's exaggerated features is an unhappy expression, perhaps asking or hoping for someone to pay attention and to provide the contingent communication stressed by Siegel. The bid for attention, however, is disguised, embedded in convention and exaggerated silliness—almost guaranteeing that it will not be heard. In a subsequent session, also filled with cartoon drawings, NaTasha scribbled on a scrap of paper, "My father will not listen to me or believe me about what happens in school."

NaTasha's retreat into cartoon art suggested to me that she was no longer able or willing to risk exposing genuine feelings directly. Just as earlier, when Natasha's artwork had fallen into disorganization, in the presence of both parents, it seemed likely that in the environment of her father's avoidance of emotional expression, she responded by unconsciously sending her own emotional expression underground. Perhaps the most useful response to such art is to, paradoxically, "take it seriously" as opposed to discounting it as the "joke" it appears to be. Also paradoxically, NaTasha's highly controlled and defensive bunny with its frozen facial expression may have been the clearest "cry for help" she was able to produce during a time when she was instinctively shutting down as much affect as possible. While "funny," the rabbit was indeed communicating. I said to NaTasha, "I wish I could talk rabbit talk, so that I could understand what this rabbit might be saying."

Recalling the odd mountain peak/hat in then 5-year-old NaTasha's self-portrait, as well as the out-of-control and affect-laden drawings from the FAE session, I could discern a pattern in her use of art. Perhaps NaTasha' s *internal working model* was of a child who felt out of control, fantasized herself as omnipotent, and then retreated to a "safer" defensive position. The therapy itself had already tracked the responses in a world that was not providing much in the way of attunement or repair, etc., so that she could less and less risk being vulnerable, disappointed, and hurt. I felt that in NaTasha's case, my most important contribution would be to provide emotional safety to a possibly despairing child. In retrospect, I would refine my statement to her to emphasize my wish to understand her subjective world: "I wish I knew more about how this rabbit *feels inside,* so I could understand what its eyes want to say."

Invitation to Art

The changes in drawing style reflected not only the natural changes of age and cognitive development; they also reflected the inconsistency in NaTasha's life and the need for connection. Her therapy, for one, was not consistent; there were months of regular sessions, but also long periods taken off for school vacations and for her father's illness. Eddie held a certain amount of skepticism for the long-term therapy process, despite my arguments with him, he would include therapy in his reward-and-punishment system for his daughter. When I stopped consulting to the DCRCC, I made a decision both to keep this as a pro bono case and to be extremely flexible. I tried to keep my communication with NaTasha clear and consistent, even where the scheduling was not. It was important to not replicate a disappearing mother with a disappearing therapist and attachment figure. It was also important to reestablish my receptive stance, or in attachment terms, to reestablish the attunement between us, especially if several weeks or even months went by between sessions.

Over time, it became clear that NaTasha's parents, despite their intentions, might remain emotionally locked down (Eddie) or too distraught and incoherent (Sandra) to provide an environment in which NaTasha could safely express and process her thoughts and feelings. I understood that I would need to construct an ongoing safe place in the therapy room where the attachment work might be done. I would come to rely on NaTasha's expanding world—particularly her school counselor and her father's close friend Linda—to also provide listening and guidance and to raise an alert when NaTasha's behavior or moods signaled a level of distress that could not be talked through or solved within her close environment. My office and the primarily nondirective approach, at least during this period, became the safe haven[1] for genuine expression. Eventually, she emerged from her cartoon period and began to paint.

As an art therapist (and a counselor), I have set up my office to be as inviting as I can make it to both children and adults. There are shelves of art books on painting, drawing, photography, sculpture; some instructional books; and a substantial array of supplies that includes fine art supplies, ample collage material, cloth and sewing supplies, wood scraps and elementary woodworking tools. It was easy for NaTasha to make a transition from using tempera paints to experimenting with both acrylic and watercolor as she grew older and more skilled. I also have a CD player with an assortment of instrumental and vocal music that I have collected over time. If a client wishes, we will have music playing during a session. My sessions run longer than talk therapy sessions, allowing time for a client to drift through the supplies and find what he or she would like to do. The therapeutic frame consists of the beginning or talk time, followed by the invitation to do art or imaginative play, which in turn is followed by at least 10 minutes to close down the session and create a verbal bridge to anticipate the next session. In NaTasha's case, we called the beginning part "checking in" (e.g., "Let's talk for a while about how things are and what's going on," or "Here is what I know from what your teacher or your dad has said . . . "). As I have noted earlier, when the work is clearly cognitive, I may use a specific directive and then process it with the child. When the child takes the lead spontaneously (or accepts my invitation to take the lead), there is only a brief

---

[1]By the time NaTasha was 5, I had changed the setting in which she and I did therapy. I began working in my private practice office, maintaining this case under my consultant contract with the DCRCC. While the room in my private office was larger than our original room, I either kept or duplicated most of the play therapy materials so that I had an identical dollhouse, most of the same puppets, an expanded set of sand tray figures, and especially the identical baby dolls and doll bed she had come to love and identified with our work together.

check-in. I do not give a specific directive; instead, I allow ample time for the child's hypnotic drift among the art supplies.

The Beginning: Setting the Stage

Between the ages of 10 and 12, NaTasha drifted in and out of therapy, not by her own choice. She continued to live with her father, moving once to an apartment in what he hoped would be a safe urban neighborhood. She was attending a public charter school, where she did fairly well but was seen by her teachers as a gifted child who undermined her own talents by her anger and sometimes "superior" attitude (report card, age 11). At certain times such as birthdays and holidays she would seem depressed. But she had begun to write music and poetry and was active in her after-school cheerleader group, one of the few activities permitted by her father.

Eddie was almost relentlessly protective of NaTasha. He drove her to and from school and kept her with him while he worked on cars in their parking lot until dinnertime. She was not allowed out alone in the neighborhood, and there seemed to be only one trusted babysitter: Linda, Eddie's long-time friend. Linda often took NaTasha out to get her hair braided or go with her to the shopping mall or to see a film, activities that Eddie felt properly belonged in the domain of women and girls. And although the family had drifted away from therapy, a call for an appointment would come during times of crisis—most often after NaTasha had spent some time with her mother, when her longing and sense of loss had been reactivated. When this happened, NaTasha's grades or school behavior would usually reflect her stirred feelings. Of course, the problem would come to the attention of the school guidance counselor, who in turn would bring it to Eddie's attention and mine as well. Depending on how Eddie assessed the school situation, he would either fiercely defend his child's rights (if he felt she was being unfairly treated) or be harshly punitive (if he suspected she was being disrespectful or lazy). He did not use physical punishment, but rather withheld or took back gifts, cancelled planned celebrations, and cancelled therapy. When I talked with Eddie, he was able to understand how his daughter's unresolved sadness and anger could lead to her "bad" behavior, but he could not see how his own rigidity might contribute to it as well. He continued to take great pride in providing a good school and material goods for NaTasha. Although he continued to engage with me, he avoided my admonitions about the effects of his harsh behavioral regulation system.

He also avoided my invitations to work on issues of emotional communication. Not able to see the value of emotional expression for himself, he was unable to see the point of it for his daughter.

After about a year's absence from therapy, NaTasha, now 12, returned to several months of regular sessions. At our first meeting, I saw that she had lost her little girl look and had the powerful appearance of an emerging adolescent. She was appropriately and fashionably dressed, and she was proud of her meticulously braided hair. She was still outspoken. She wanted me to know that she was drawing and painting in school, and that she and Linda were "working on" her dad to allow her to join an after-school dance club. She had little professed interest in boys, more interest in designing clothes, dancing, and writing songs. She showed me some songs she had written. In fact, it had been a deeply sad song about her mother that had come to the attention of her school counselor and then me.

We spent a little time doing our ritual recollections and reminiscences that chronicled and organized a cohesive narrative about our therapy together: "*Remember when you would not give me the doll?; Remember when you and your dad made the clay mash together?; Remember when your mom came in and made a sculpture with you, but it broke?*" The remembering created a strong thread of continuity in the discontinuous treatment.

The Middle: The Work Deepens and Moves

The Dance (Three Sessions)

NaTasha wanted to show me the cheers she was learning in her after-school cheerleading class and the modern dance and ballet movements she was learning in physical education. After a few cheers, she asked for music and we selected both a celestial-sounding meditation CD of harp music and a Brahms piano concerto that shifted in and out of darkness and tenderness. We pushed furniture back and I sat to one side, acting as her audience. As she began to spin and whirl to the harp music, she seemed to go into a trance. Soon she picked up my larger-than-life rag doll, dressed to look like a young adolescent. (The doll had elastic bands on her cloth "shoes," so that a child could slip his or her own feet under the bands and propel the doll around the floor as a dance partner.) NaTasha filled the entire therapy hour with silent movement and told me that she wanted to do this again in the next session, when she would want to use the second (Brahms) recording.

The following week, she again danced for an hour, lost in the shifting emotions evoked by the music. She danced the gamut of feelings. Her gestures—she used her whole body—were by turns aggressive and angry, even murderous, tender and sweetly maternal, joyful, introspective, and profoundly sad. Once when she was dancing, she had a look of great fear. She had wrapped the doll's arms around her neck in a gesture of strangulation. She fell to the floor and was "dead" for more than a minute before suddenly leaping back to life and resuming her dance. This went on for a third week. Then it stopped and she said nothing more about it. As I remember, the comment I made, after an awed silence, was "Wow! It seems that you've danced out every emotion that any human being has ever felt." I also asked "How are you feeling after that?" primarily to reestablish my connection to NaTasha through as many senses as possible. I did not, however, offer my interpretation that she had created both a recapitulation of her parents' relationship and, simultaneously, the externalized expression of her own deepest feelings. To provide an interpretation at the conclusion of her dancing would have been an attempt to direct or process the emotional information at a moment when my intuition was guiding me to simply receive and accept it. The quiet moments after the dance were intended to extend the momentum of the dance, allowing the mood to deepen so that NaTasha might feel "felt" by the therapist as well as know that her full range of feeling had been accepted and appreciated. The dance, which had exemplified an affective self-regulating process and had received approval rather than criticsm or shaming, would be internalized and become part of NaTasha's process of learning how to self-regulate when there was no therapy room dance floor. Our nonverbal contingent communication would need to be followed by reflective verbal exchanges, cognitive tools, and a great deal of practice in their use.

The Painting (One Session)

The week immediately following the last of her three dances, NaTasha came in the door and said, "I want to paint." This was not an unfamiliar request. She had loved experimenting with acrylic paint and with watercolor long before she had been taught techniques with these media in school. More than once, she had declared with great certainty, "I am an artist." We sat in relative silence across from one another at the small art table as she mixed acrylic paints. There was little conversation other than quiet discussion about mixing colors. Also, I did not take any notes that could disturb her process in any way.

Figure 12.6 is a landscape with two pine or spruce trees, one large and one smaller, at the right and left edges of the paper, somewhat isolated from each other on either side of a divide (a river or cleft in the otherwise smooth landscape). A sky, painted with a mixture of blue and white, appears cloudy and perhaps windy. Because the color is subdued (the greens are quite dark, the sky more blue-gray than blue), the subjective moment of the scene seems to be at a time toward evening. But there is a small sun high in the sky, in the upper right-hand corner of the page. The sun is just above the smaller tree. NaTasha seemed quietly pleased with her work and said that when it dried, she would want to take it home.

As in the aftermath of the dance, I let my own subjective response emerge and develop. But I chose again to say very little out loud. I experienced NaTasha's painting as a symbolic externalization of her internalized family: two trees and a sun, separated from one another but held within the larger framework of ground and sky. I was also aware that the

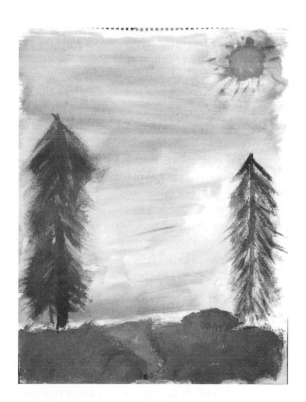

FIGURE 12.6. NaTasha's landscape "portrait," age 12.

painting reflected her continued love of painting landscapes, going all the way back to the time she was 5 and had painted herself among the mountains. Subjectively, I understood this new painting as a portrait of the implicit self, expressed as a landscape.

Art therapist Edith Kramer (2001) has written extensively on the subject of sublimation in children's art. The term refers to a complex defensive process in which both primary and secondary process thinking are involved, and, "as secondary process thinking takes over, symbolic representations lose their protean, driven quality and become stable. Imagination replaces fantasy" (p. 39). Kramer states that "art retells the story of transformation. . . . and only what emerges within an ambience of supportive but nonintrusive contact can feel real to the person who brings it forth" (p. 39). Kramer supports a range of responses to a child who is making art, from direct help with the artistic process, to noninterference, to active verbal interpretation. The principles of attachment are compatible with this psychoanalytic understanding of the art process. However, the emphasis in attachment theory is on the relationship between the child and the therapist, because it gives the child the necessary sense of being loved and understood, in Siegel's words, "felt" through attunement, repair, and contingent communication. The linking of the drawing to the earlier landscapes may also have provided a subtle element of coherent narrative making. With just a few graphic elements, the painting had evoked unspoken emotion, and our silent gazing at it had created an experience of attunement.

It should be noted that asking clients to create an imagined landscape that "might represent your current emotional state" (Cohen, Barnes, & Rankin, 1995, p. 41) can be an art directive that may be given in the hope of eliciting some discussion afterwards. That I chose to say little or nothing and did not interpret meaning simply reflects my sense of the moment, as described earlier, that it was a lucid "portrait" resonating with implicit knowledge of self and could remain safely in the domain of wordlessness.

Resolutions Surface: The Clay Sculpture
(Two Sessions, a Month Apart)

The following week, NaTasha came in and declared her intention to do another painting. While getting out the supplies, she saw a clay sculpture made by an adult client. It had been set out to dry on a shelf in the storeroom. She was taken by the piece: two hands slightly smaller than life-size were pressed together to create an open cup. Within the "cup" were at least a dozen small marble-size clay balls, each meant to be the head of a baby. One "baby" was outside the perimeter of the area that held all the others. I imagine NaTasha caught the poignancy of that lost baby and sensed that there was a story and a meaning to this work. When she asked what the sculpture was about, I asked her what she thought it might be about. She described the piece, then again asked, "What is it supposed to be about?" I answered that the person who made the sculpture said that sometimes she feels that she is made up of many different parts of herself with many different feelings inside. "Oh," she said, "well, I want to make one of these sculptures about myself."

NaTasha proceeded to work with clay for the next 45 minutes, with great focus and investment. She could not replicate the hands of the adult client's sculpture or copy my hands held in a similar pose, and she grew frustrated before she found a solution. The two hands she was trying to make looked better to her when she fused them into a single form. As she worked, the "hands" began to take on the shape of a chair. By fusing the individual fingers she had attempted to shape, she soon had made a throne-like chair with a high back, capable of holding within its arms and on its seat a number of marble-like heads (Figures 12.7 and 12.8). These, she said, would be her own "many different feelings inside."

Transitions Occur

As she worked, the concept continued to evolve into something more and more her own: She asked me to make a tiny hand "like the one the lady made," and I did. She dug out a niche in the seat in which to place the hand, then she rolled a clay marble, incised facial features on it, placed it in the little hand, and then placed the hand and head into the niche on the seat. She next made several more clay ball faces, each with a distinct hastily carved expression: She called these "excited," "in your face," "angry," "goofy," and "happy." One unnamed face had a blank look; another seemed to show fear. These were placed at intervals within the throne cavity and along the top of the throne back. When I asked her to notice which feeling was missing, she answered quickly and without defensiveness, "Oh, it's sadness. That's a feeling I never let people see!" But she then turned to the back of the throne and incised

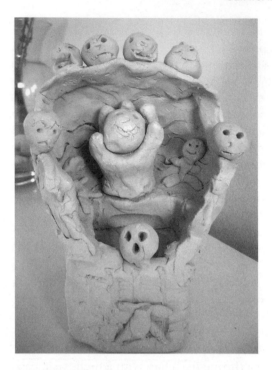

FIGURE 12.7. NaTasha's clay throne, age 12.

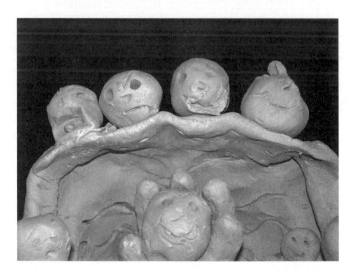

FIGURE 12.8. NaTasha's clay throne, closeup, age 12.

a little sad face in the wet clay, as if to acknowledge the feeling that she did not easily expose.

Because I knew she would not be back for several weeks, I told her that I would let the throne dry and then have it fired. About a month later, she did a hasty glazing with bright opaque clay glazes in several colors: a vivid "Caribbean blue," a sunny yellow, a bright yellow-green, and a midnight blue, almost black. The hasty and uninvested glazing seemed to me to be an afterthought. The power of the piece was in the imagery; the color, in this instance, was decorative. Perhaps the time between sessions allowed NaTasha to reorganize somehat internally and to begin the process of dismissing, trivializing, or distancing herself from an important image.

Closure and Summary of My Art Treatment with NaTasha

In retrospect, the process seems simple. During the intense sessions of dance, NaTasha poured out deeply felt emotions, so much so that she was both exhausted and unburdened. In the wake of these experiences, she was able to make an eloquent painting that expressed a deep and lucid implicit sense of self. Following this, there seemed to be no need to paint again for a while. Instead she produced a complex sculpture that externalized the structure of her internal world. As she worked on the clay piece, she talked, asked questions, and was seeking answers, suggesting that this piece marked a new level of trust—and perhaps a more strongly felt internal need to resolve some troubling parts of her earlier childhood that continued to affect her life. The clay piece provides an extraordinary amount of information about NaTasha that she and I were able to use in our subsequent work on past trauma, unresolved loss and grief, and rage.

If NaTasha's painting is the implicit accepting self, then the clay piece is the complex map of her rich interior world. It contains part selves, affects, or ego states, both revealed and hidden, harmonious and in conflict. It suggests an underlying narcissism in the child who can create a throne but cannot copy the gently cupped clay hands. Its metaphor of the small hand embedded in the center of the throne suggests the assignment of a central but removable place for me. The piece suggests the sense of underlying trauma and loss in the unconscious replication of the "lost baby" in a figure without a head that adorns the front of the throne. And the more I look at this remarkable piece, the more it suggests the unexplored identification between NaTasha and her mother.

Perhaps the "lost baby" is Sandra. Or perhaps the organization of the whole piece is an echo of Sandra's early drawing and sculpture of her "family tree" with their many parts related to a central holding element. Sandra's trees may also have been "portraits" of her internal life: a truncated branched tree, imbued with loss and disorganized to a point that leaves her unable to give her daughter the tools with which to organize her own internal world.

The visual similarity between Sandra's early works and NaTasha's spontaneous adaptation of another person's work raises an important point about spontaneous artwork. It seems possible that Sandra's powerful image may have remained almost intact in NaTasha's mind for several years and was evoked by my adult client's sculpture. This possibility suggests what we intuitively know to be true: Images stored in the right brain are evocative of powerful feeling states, memories, and other less-defined aspects of our interior life. They can be reignited, combined, and recombined in the creative process.

The painting and the clay work that emerged out of NaTasha's choices made in a creative "drift" are communications from the right brain and suggest how important it is to have a trusted person—a parent, a therapist—present to receive, accept, and respond.

In NaTasha's case, I have been privileged to have a gift of time, so that I have been able to see her through a period of mistrust and emotional "stuckness" (the era of the stereotypical drawings) to a point where she became ready to work more consciously on her traumatic and chaotic earlier childhood. The process has been helped enormously by NaTasha's father's willingness to return her to therapy at her request. Despite his innate skepticism and distrust of the power of emotions, his support of therapy has continued and remains pivotal in our being able to continue this work.

I view NaTasha's artwork as a continuously unfolding "story" of her internal responses to as yet unresolved trauma and loss. I can trace her cautious move toward openness and her relinquishment of the more rigid defenses, and I sense a new willingness in her to engage in reflective verbal exploration of her experiences and beliefs. While I anticipate more focused cognitive tasks involving identifying and challenging her beliefs, I consider that the attachment-focused spontaneous art making will remain the foundation of her therapy. Her most recent landscape, an evocative, richly colored painting (Fig. 12.9), suggests that she has the emotional strength for this upcoming phase of the work.

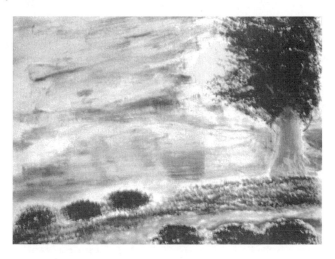

FIGURE 12.9. NaTasha's landscape painting, age 13.

REFERENCES

Cohen, B., Barnes, M. M., & Rankin, A. B. (1995). *Managing traumatic stress through art: Drawing from the center.* Baltimore: Sidran Press.

Gil, E., & Green, N. (2004). *Extended play-based developmental assessments. Clinicians guide.* Unpublished protocol.

Gil, E., & Sobol, B. (2000). Engaging families in therapeutic play. In C. E. Baily (Ed.), *Children in therapy: Using the family as a resource* (pp. 353–357). New York: Norton.

Kramer, E. (1993). *Art as therapy with children.* Chicago: Magnolia Street Publishers.

Kramer, E. (2001). Sublimation and art therapy. In J. A. Rubin (Ed.), *Approaches to art therapy: Theory and technique* (2nd ed.). Philadelphia: Brunner- Routledge.

Pifalo, T. (2007). Jogging the cogs: Trauma-focused art therapy and cognitive behavioral therapy with sexually abused children. *Art Therapy: Journal of the American Art Therapy Association, 24,*(4), 170–176.

Rosal, M. (2001). Cognitive-behavioral art therapy. In J. A. Rubin (Ed.), *Approaches to art therapy: Theory and technique* (2nd ed.). Philadelphia: Brunner-Routledge.

Schore, J. R., & Schore, A. N. (2008). Modern attachment theory: The central role of affect regulation in development and treatment. *Clinical Social Work Journal, 36,* 9–20.

Siegel, D. J. (2003). An interpersonal neurobiology of psychotherapy: The developing mind and the resolution of trauma. In M. F. Solomon & D. J. Siegel (Eds.), *Healing trauma: Attachment, mind, body, and brain.* New York: Norton.

Sobol, B. (1998). Art therapy with children who dissociate. In J. Silberg (Ed.), *The dissociative child: Diagnosis, treatment, and management* (pp. 193–210). New York: Guilford Press.

Tinnin, L. W., & Gantt, L. (2000). *The Trauma Recovery Institute treatment manual.* Morgantown, WV: Gargoyle Press.

Wallin, D. J. (2007). *Attachment in psychotherapy.* New York: Guilford Press.

CHAPTER 13

The Gift of Time

Helping to Heal through Long-Term Treatment Involving Complex Trauma and Cultural Issues

ATHENA A. DREWES

I worked with Tancisha for 3 years in a residential treatment setting. She was placed in this setting to deal with complex trauma from physical abuse, possible sexual abuse, attachment disorder, multiple separations, grief, and acculturation issues. She was seen in individual child-led therapy, once weekly for 50-minute sessions. Taneisha was nonverbal during most of her sessions due to expressive language difficulties and her preference to be selectively mute.

Her story is one of courage and perseverance in the face of serious emotional difficulty. Through her play she was able to "rebirth" herself, healing the wounds of her past. Her play was able to nurture and transform her feelings and behaviors, and raise her functioning to age level, opening the door for a positive and successful future. She taught me a lot about resilience and the therapeutic power of play (Schaefer & Drewes, 2010).

CASE REFERRAL INFORMATION

Taneisha was an attractive, overweight child with ebony skin and expressive dark brown eyes that appeared to pierce whomever she was looking at. She had a beautiful, engaging, and ready smile. She often appeared disheveled and rumpled, although she dressed in clean and appropriately fitting clothes. She was happy to receive one-on-one attention, and often would run up to strangers and staff to greet them and try to hug them. Her hugs and greetings had a superficial quality to them, rather than appearing to come from a genuine feeling of joy or warmth at seeing that person. Her expressive language skills lagged behind her receptive language ability. As English was a second language, she spoke using simple sentences, and had a strong accent that made it difficult at times for me and others to understand her. Taneisha often preferred to be selectively mute, not wishing to have to repeat what she said in order to be understood. She would linger in the background observing adults and peers until she was invited into an activity. Whenever I asked about her feelings, she was able to say that sometimes she felt sad, although her affect on the surface was cheerful and playful. Often beneath the surface was an undertone of anxiety and hostility, however.

Taneisha was almost 7 years old when she was admitted to the residential treatment facility, having just been discharged from a 3-month stay at a local psychiatric hospital. Prior to hospitalization, she was reported to have exhibited regressive and aggressive behaviors, including smearing feces all over the house, as well as herself, having increasingly aggressive outbursts toward adults and children that included hitting and punching, and increasing impulsivity including stealing and riding her bicycle into a busy highway. A possible precipitant to the escalation of her behaviors was a visit from her older sister.

Strengths

Over the course of treatment, I witnessed Taneisha's tremendous courage, extraordinary growth, and development of a number of important strengths. She was athletically coordinated, loved to participate in sports such as basketball, swimming, and track, and also showed an aptitude for horseback riding. She came to display a wide range of interests, including reading, music, popular culture, and expressive arts activities. And she particularly enjoyed and actively participated in an African dance program. I was struck by how well Taneisha responded to structure, and when willing, was able to follow directions. She could be genuinely affectionate at times and engaging and friendly. She was able to make good use of therapeutic modalities.

Taneisha's Developmental History

Taneisha was the product of a full-term uncomplicated pregnancy and was reportedly healthy during the neonatal period. At 6 months of age she had a high fever with a respiratory infection and was hospitalized for 1 week. It is not likely that her mother remained with her. At around 1½ years of age she was again hospitalized for a respiratory infection. The length of stay is unknown, as well as whether her mother was available.

Developmental milestones were reportedly attained at normal time frames. She also had a history of recurrent vaginal infections. Taneisha's first few years of care were inconsistent. Due to her mother's drug and alcohol abuse and prostitution, Taneisha was occasionally cared for by her maternal grandmother, who also had alcohol abuse issues. Although sexual abuse was not documented, there were suspicions voiced by the psychiatric hospital staff.

Around age 24 months, Taneisha experienced a near drowning. It was at this point that Kayleen, her mother, felt she could not manage her daughter's care. She consequently decided to send Taneisha to live with her adult older sister, who was living in the Caribbean. Taneisha remained there for the next 4 years. Her sister, being extremely fair-skinned, was favored by the mother. Tancisha's skin was very dark, darker than her mother's. Kayleen was very proud of her eldest daughter and especially her light skin, often referring to her as "Snow White." Her culture valued skin tone. Upper-class citizens in her home culture are descended from European settlers and have lighter skin than lower-class citizens, who are darker-skinned and descended from African slaves or Haitians. Social class determines access to power and position in her country, and there is little social mobility (Gil & Drewes, 2005). Kayleen had great hopes for "Snow White" and her children. On the other hand, Kayleen saw Taneisha as even below herself in status due to her dark skin.

In spite of the strong family allegiance and the extended family social network, Kayleen reported that Taneisha was physically and verbally abused by her older sister during her stay. Overwhelmed with trying to raise her own children, "Snow White" found Taneisha's highly active behaviors difficult to manage. Although Kayleen knew about the severe discipline, she did not intervene; she did not consider it atypical parenting, given how she herself was raised. While in the Caribbean,

Taneisha's contact with her mother was mainly by telephone, and once-yearly visits.

Because of her behaviors, Taneisha's sister decided not to enroll her in school, even though primary education was free and compulsory from ages 5 through 14. In her culture, networking is an important part of getting into a higher-class status and allows for extending a base of contacts (Drewes, 2008a). "Snow White" did not want to jeopardize her good standing and contacts in the school setting by Taneisha's negative behaviors, and she was not willing to trade in her favors to maintain Taneisha in school. As a result, Taneisha received limited education from her sister. She spoke mainly Spanish and had few academic skills.

When Taneisha was 6 years old, her mother, having dramatically changed her life, and hearing of her older daughter's intolerance of Taneisha's behaviors and not sending her to school, decided to bring Taneisha back to the United States to live with her. Her mother arrived in the Caribbean, unannounced, and took Taneisha back with her without any advance planning or an adequate farewell to her sister and cousins.

Once back in her mother's care, along with her mother's new boyfriend, Taneisha had difficulty adjusting. She would not respond to her mother's limits, was defiant, and extremely active to the point of being dangerous. She demanded constant adult attention and would become destructive if she did not receive it. Within a year of being with her mother, Taneisha required psychiatric hospitalization. While she was at the psychiatric hospital, Taneisha wet her bed, smeared feces, and was resistant to direction from medical staff. Due to her behavioral problems she was put on medication for attention-deficit/hyperactivity disorder (ADHD) and depression. Taneisha also engaged in self-injurious behaviors. She often picked her nose until it bled, and picked at her toenails until they became infected.

After 6 months in residential treatment, her self-destructive behaviors still increased after visits from her mother, and her self-injurious behaviors continued to the point that she required surgery to have the toenails on her big toes removed. Her picking at the lining of her nose and inside of her mouth became so severe that she was close to requiring reconstructive nose surgery. She was also eating from the garbage, and her level of motivation decreased. Her attention span and affect tolerance declined, and she seemed intent on punishing herself. She would chew on inedible objects, such as staples or items found in the garbage, and she would intentionally urinate on herself, on the floor, or on furniture.

Family Issues

At the time of admission, Taneisha's mother verbally stated that she wished to have her daughter live with her and to rebuild a relationship. Our first meeting focused on obtaining history.

Mother's History

Taneisha's mother, Kayleen, was born and raised by her grandmother, on a Caribbean island, and closely identifies to this day with its culture. She had a history of drug and alcohol abuse, which was supported from age 11 through prostitution. Taneisha's father is unknown, and likely her conception was the result of her mother's prostitution. It is possible that Taneisha was exposed to drugs and alcohol in utero.

Kayleen reported that her life in the Caribbean was fraught with poverty and physical abuse. Her mother and grandmother beat her as a child, and she often had little to eat, living with her four siblings. At age 10 she began to experiment with drugs and turned to prostitution to support her habit at age 11. She was pregnant with her first daughter by age 12, at which point her mother threw her out of the house. She was taken in by her maternal grandmother, who allowed her to remain in her care after the birth of her daughter. She talked lovingly of her first daughter, whom she doted on as though she were a "porcelain doll." She and her daughter remained in her grandmother's care, in spite of her grandmother's punitive verbal and at times physical abuse of Kayleen. Kayleen continued to abuse alcohol, at times drinking heavily, as did her grandmother. Periodically Kayleen turned to prostitution when money was low or her daughter needed things. When her daughter was 17 years old, Kayleen was able to immigrate to the United States, leaving her daughter behind. At age 29, Kayleen found work initially cleaning houses. But after a few years she soon found herself returning to prostitution to help support herself. This setting led her back into using drugs and alcohol. At one point she was arrested and deported to the Caribbean, but was somehow able to return to the United States after 6 months. She again returned to prostitution, drugs and alcohol, and at age 32, was pregnant with Taneisha. She stated that she had limited schooling, learning only how to read, write, and speak English, and do basic math before dropping out.

She wished she could be a better mother to Taneisha, but she has had no stable role models from her own life to guide her. Her country's poverty and high unemployment gave her little opportunity to learn skills for employment and no social mobility because of her class and skin color. She loved to sing and dance to merengue music, which made her attractive to the men she solicited as a prostitute. She felt lucky to have met her current boyfriend, who was not abusive to her. He was the motivating force in getting Taneisha to come live with them—he was hoping for a family.

However, upon returning to her mother's care, Taneisha was defiant, aggressive, controlling, and demanding of attention. She would become destructive when she did not receive attention and began to hurt herself. Her mother felt uncertain that Taneisha would ever be able to come live with her, as she has begun to create problems within the relationship with her boyfriend.

Psychological Testing

Psychological testing showed low-average intelligence, which was felt to be a minimal estimate of Taneisha's abilities because she was uncooperative, displaying off-task behaviors and periodically openly refusing to continue. Projectives noted that she did not appear to recognize common social clues and had difficulty interpreting her world accurately. She was more vulnerable to confused thinking than other children her age. Her hospital diagnosis of ADHD was equivocal according to the residential treatment psychiatrist, who felt that her interpersonal problems, depressive symptomatology, and range of symptoms (night terrors, "acts jumpy") seemed to be consistent with a diagnosis of posttraumatic stress disorder (PTSD) and attachment disorder issues. It was felt that her acting-out behaviors had more to do with events that triggered strong affective responses than with distorted perceptions of her world.

Taneisha's drawings suggested a need for nurturance and attachment but a fear of reaching out to others. She seemed to feel insecure, lonely, and abandoned. Her drawings were somewhat regressed, suggesting a history of trauma and a tendency to express anger in passive–aggressive ways. She also expressed feelings of self-degradation and sorrow.

Academics

Taneisha had significant learning and expressive language difficulties, and had been placed in a special education kindergarten and first grade in the residential treatment school. She received speech and language services. In school she simply refused to do her work or became passive–aggressive and smeared her feces.

Taneisha would go through periods in which she was removed from class on a daily basis and required frequent therapeutic holds. Her self-destructive, self-abusive, defiant, and destructive behaviors often fluctuated. She would intentionally urinate on herself, and had periods of inappropriate sexual behavior and stealing. She would sabotage positive experiences and rewards, ripping up her certificates or acting out so that she could not go on special trips.

She had low self-esteem, stating, "I hate me." She was shunned by her peers due to her offensive behaviors. She had difficulty settling for sleep. She would jump on her bed, play, or do anything to distract herself from sleeping. She did enjoy individualized attention, and it seemed important for her to control the interactions to the best of her ability. When limits were placed on her negative behaviors, she would continue her behaviors and smile, as if her behavior and caregiver directions were part of a game or joke. When staff would ask her why she thought she was in the residential setting, she readily stated "My mother doesn't want me." She denied any history of having been hit, hurt, or touched in a way she did not like.

FORMULATION OF THE PROBLEM

Taneisha is a child with a chronic complex trauma history, including possible intrauterine exposure to drugs and/or alcohol and a chaotic early life due to maternal substance abuse and prostitution. A significant attachment disorder is evident from several disruptions with her primary attachment due to two hospitalizations in infancy, being sent to her older sister's care at age 2, and then being abruptly removed from her sister's care at age 6. There is also the possibility of anoxia from the near drowning. Her longstanding history of behavior problems, depression, and high activity appear to be the result of many stressors and the chronic trauma of physical and possible sexual abuse, as well as loss of her primary caretaker and multiple moves. Acculturation issues further compounded her complex trauma, with difficulties adjusting to a predominantly English-speaking culture, disorientation to a new culture and living environment, and mourning the loss of a country with which she had begun to identify culturally and emotionally (Drewes, 2008a).

She displayed further vulnerabilities in the form of learning difficulties, in large part due to English being her second language and with expressive language deficits prominent.

As a result of her significant attachment disorder, Taneisha appeared to feel a tremendous need to control others to ensure that her needs were met (Drewes, 2001). She used both passive–aggressive and aggressive means to do so. Her regressive and self-injurious behaviors appeared to serve several purposes. For example, they appeared to be an expression of her self-loathing as well as her anger toward others, and they also may play the part of putting her in control of the rejection she experiences and expects from others. She may fear that if she does well, she will have to return to live with her mother, which she was ambivalent about, and so was maintaining her control over the likelihood of discharge via her regressive and self-injurious behaviors. It is also possible that she is a regressed child who is utilizing self-stimulation and provocation of all those around her to create a diversion from her own overwhelming affects. Further, her self-injurious behaviors may be a way for Taneisha to physically feel she is alive, having lost feelings of pain from the dissociative processes that typically accompany chronic trauma and abuse.

Taneisha also appeared to feel grief and anger toward her mother for her inability to care for her and nurture her appropriately. She felt a tremendous need to control others to ensure that her needs were met and craved individualized attention but lacked basic trust (Drewes, 2001). She could not tolerate the loss of control she experienced in genuine interpersonal engagement. Milieu therapy was essential as a way to offer a safe and secure environment for Taneisha to begin to master age-appropriate developmental tasks and to become more able to function without constant one-on-one attention from adults.

Treatment goals for Taneisha included (1) decreasing behavioral dysregulation (including impulsivity, aggression, and sexual acting out), (2) increasing coping skills and frustration tolerance, (3) addressing loss regarding mother and country, and (4) increasing academic functioning.

CASE ILLUSTRATION OF SELF-DIRECTED TRAUMA PLAY

Taneisha was seen in once weekly individual nondirective play therapy over the course of 3 years.

Initial Session

Taneisha ran up to me, hugging me around my waist, eagerly following me into the play therapy room. Once inside she stopped and looking slowly around, visually taking in all the toys, looking in cabinets and at items without saying a word (Drewes, 2001). She saw a map of the world lying on the cabinet, and quickly ran over to it, scanning it for her Caribbean Island. She soon found it, and clapped her hands together with glee, saying "*Mi casa, mi casa*"! Then she slowly turned and, with head down and a sad expression, took one of the dolls from the crib. She specifically chose a white doll over all the others and began to hold it to her chest, rocking it slowly and softly singing to it, in what sounded like a Spanish lullaby.

Suddenly, she put down the doll and turned to me, yelling, "*Estupido*," and in broken English ordered me about. She yelled at me that I was bad, stupid, and a "blackie." She gestured for me to kneel down and said in Spanish that I was kneeling on "rice" as punishment for being such a bad girl. I was ordered about, and no matter what I was told to do, I could not do it right. I complied with her directions, following her lead despite the discomfort of kneeling. When the discomfort became too great, I told Taneisha I had to stand up (using my therapist voice). She would then have me stand in a corner instead.

She then took out the doctor kit, intrigued by the stethoscope, and wanted to see if she could hear my heart and her own with it. She nurtured the white baby doll, then hit it hard and said it was bad. She briefly held up the African doll, studied it, and then threw it aside.

The toy kitchen set interested her. She explored the Hispanic food items that were in the stove and began to prepare a taco dinner for me, with rice and hot sauce. What started out as appearing to be a nurturing act soon turned sadistic, with Taneisha pouring "hot sauce" over the food and adding potions to it. She silently then forced me to eat it, while she laughed as she said "*Caliente*" at it being so hot it burned my tongue.

Next Taneisha spied the sand tray and went over to it. She put her hands in the sand and said she missed the beach and water of her home. She looked around at the miniatures that were available and slowly and silently began to take out a few babies and people, stones and horses, and buried them all under the sand.

When it was time to leave the session, Taneisha had a hard time leaving the room. She wanted to be the one to determine our ending and how we were to leave. She ordered me around and told me she was the "boss of me" and that we would now leave. Following her lead, I allowed her control of the ending.

Sessions 2–5

Taneisha returned each week and began her time with the sand tray. She would put her hands in the sand tray, and then she would put my hands in the tray and cover them over. She would then pull on my arms, indicating that I should uncover them, and then would push my hands back in, covering them up again and again. She would also bury babies, people, and snakes in the sand. She often spilled colored stones across the surface. Her affect was serious, but there was also calmness at times as she was silently involved in the self-soothing task of feeling the sand and burying items.

During these sessions Taneisha would make concoctions out of the sand, mixing water with it and stirring it up. She said I was "*dos años*" (2 years old), and she would then "force" me to eat what she made, saying that the food was good for me, and then laughing after I "ate" it, saying it was feces. In spite of repeatedly being tricked, my role was to comply, being made to feel her past experiences of betrayal of trust.

She would take the white doll and gently hold it and rock it, staring at its face and stroking its arm. She said she missed her "mama." It was unclear to which person she was referring: her biological mother or her older sister who helped raise her. Then she quickly got angry, threw the doll, began cursing at it in Spanish, kicked the doll, and laughed.

Next she went over to the large oversized stuffed lion, hit it, giving it a "bloody nose," and said that it was me. She stood on it and told me to make sounds of pain and groans. She ordered me about, through her gestures and motions. No matter how much I tried to comply, my efforts were in vain, and she repeatedly made me kneel down on "rice" as punishment for being bad and stupid. I would comment "No matter what I do, I am punished. I try and try but it is never good enough."

In session 5 she added a puppet show, first with animals and then using the people dolls. The animals would begin to be friendly and then were mean to each other until the wolf came and ate them all up. The people puppets wanted to know how old I was, and she told me to say I was "32" (old enough to be her mother).

Repeatedly over these few sessions, themes of control were played out with power struggles over making me do things that could "hurt" me, and deciding when it was time for the session to end and how. It appeared that my compliance was important to her and as time neared to leave the session, Taneisha would order me to be her slave or else I would get spanked and sent to my room. Just before we left the therapy room, Taneisha whispered, in broken English, that she wished she could live in the therapy room and never have to be sent to her room. These sessions were difficult for me to endure emotionally. I was careful not to allow transference reactions, monitored with help through supervision (Drewes, 2008b).

The Next 5 Months

Tancisha increased her control over me during the next 5 months of sessions. She directed my every word, gesture, and action. She was the mother and I was the daughter in most of the scenarios, but at times she would switch the roles. Often I would be ordered to say *sand* when asked what something was, as she silently held it up, even though I knew it was not sand. When I was "wrong" in naming the object (said in either English or Spanish), I was severely "beaten" and "punished." Food was concocted and fed to me that was bad, even though I was told it was good to eat, and after I "ate" it and was sick, she would then tell me she loved me. I was constantly tricked into thinking I would be given something good to eat or promised that I wouldn't be hurt, only to be repeatedly betrayed by punishment and poison. There were times when I would dread seeing Tancisha, knowing what might transpire. I would begin to comment in the play role "I don't like being tricked. I can't trust you. It's not fair." Taneisha would nod as I said this.

Taneisha often put on puppet shows for me in sessions. She would take a friendly looking puppet and then have it pinch and bite me after I petted it. She would promise it would be nice to me, and then her puppet would go try to hit me and trick me. After several sessions, the puppets (male and female) fought and cursed at each other over the woman's drinking. They repeatedly fought to the point of dying, and no matter what helpers came along, the end result was that they died too. Sometimes I would be made to recreate these puppet scenarios, with Taneisha sitting and watching the play, with the same tragic outcome. I often left the sessions feeling emotionally depleted, necessitating lots of self-care to avoid vicarious traumatization and utilizing supervision to avoid any transference or my anger interfering with the process.

Several times Taneisha added in play that there was a pretend fire alarm bell that would go off, and we would have to crouch and hide in the puppet theater. She would look around, pretend it was over, and then laugh because the "bell" would ring again and we would have to hide all over again.

Taneisha took out the doctor kit in many of the sessions, wanting to check on me and see if I was sick. Her play often was repetitious and exact, reenacting first checking my pulse, then using the blood pressure cuff, then checking my ears and putting the thermometer to my mouth. She would end with the stethoscope, having me breathe while she listened to my heart. After several months she varied the play to add that I was the mother and had to take my two babies (one white and one black baby) to the hospital after having visited Taneisha, who was the doctor. I would leave the babies in the hospital and say I would return for them, but then I never would. They would be left there crying and crying. Other times the play would switch to both of us going to the mall and buying lots of things to bring back home: food and clothes and toys for the babies.

In the sand tray Taneisha began to use a male figure and a female figure. She would take out the Disney Wicked Queen from *Snow White* and put sand all over her. She had it urinate on the male, saying he did "nasty" things on her. She took the Ninja figure and had it "cut me up" with its blade, requiring me to set limits that I was not for hurting or cutting. Taneisha wanted the lights in the room turned off, while she added two mermaids, Snow White, a wishing well, two princes, a girl figure and mother figure, along with cultural items from her country (e.g., a flag, food items, and religious figures). She set up one house at one end of the tray and added a bridge midway between it and the other house, which had all the cultural items clustered around it. She then scattered the colored stones on the surface of the sand. Taneisha would often sit silently and stare at the tray for many minutes. She would then move the figures around, leaving the house from her country and crossing over the bridge to the other house. She would often have the prince rescue the little girl and take her away from the home with the cultural items around it, but Snow White would try to get her back, and the Wicked Queen would capture her in the end, taking her to the second house. I began to see the play scenes as representing Taneisha's ambivalence over leaving her island home and starting to mourn her loss.

Each session ended with Taneisha deciding when it was time to leave and refusing to go because she was not yet finished playing. She repeatedly wanted to take an object from the room, quickly grabbing something on the way to the door. I often felt conflicted over setting limits and regaining control. I realized her need for a transitional object from me. Rather than engage in a power struggle over unmet limit setting, Taneisha gladly accepted a note, written by me, saying what toy she would play with next time. This soon became a ritual she looked forward to as we ended the sessions, often telling me just what to write and with what color marker.

Themes of loss, cultural identity, lies, deceit, lack of trust, and trickery repeated over and over throughout each session and across sessions. During this time Taneisha's attitude toward me was demanding, controlling, and yet needy for possessions and proof of my caring (Drewes, 2001).

Concurrent Family Events

During this time Taneisha had a visit from her mother for her birthday. Within the first 15 minutes of the visit, she wet herself. Her mother was extremely rejecting of her because of it and did not wish to visit with her again for several weeks. Kayleen also was not complying with Child Protective Services' requirements of obtaining a drug and alcohol evaluation, random urine tests, or her own individual therapy. It was suspected that she was drinking heavily. Kayleen also reported during the family therapy session that she had a dream about Taneisha having a knife and that she was going to kill her. In short, she was afraid of her daughter. Kayleen also said that she was entertaining the thought of signing over parental custody rights to the Department of Social Services, as she cannot manage Taneisha's behaviors when she is with her.

After day visits and phone calls with her mother, Taneisha's functioning and emotional state deteriorated. She began eating pencils and staples; inserting objects up her nose, resulting in daily nose bleeds; smearing blood-like paint on her desk or on peers; picking at her lips, fingernails, and cuticles until they bled; and wetting herself but not telling anyone resulting in a painful "diaper" rash. In school she would provoke peers until she was hit, and then she would act like a victim. She would flinch when her child care staff would try to give her affection through a hug. Taneisha would destroy her property and schoolwork, and was removed from class two or three times per day. She could not be left alone in her bedroom due to self-abusive behaviors and needed to be carefully watched during group activities or trips due to her stealing and destructive behaviors.

Session 26

Taneisha's play shifted into lots of preparations before starting her play. She would gather up the "supplies" that she needed to make an art project. She would carefully select which color paper she wanted, find the tape, look for just the right color markers, pencils, and crayons. Preparation took up most of the session time, leaving little time for Taneisha to actually make anything. When she did draw something, she would then smear clay over it at the end.

She also spent time singing into the toy tape recorder and then yelling into it. Sometimes she would sing a lullaby in Spanish or other Caribbean Island songs. She would dance and show me how to do the merengue, wrapping colorful play cloths around her head for decoration. Taneisha would also take bendable pipe cleaners and tubing and put them on my hands, wrists, and head, saying they were snakes. Then she would play out alternating between being the good and bad mother, one minute nurturing me and the next, angry, mean, and poisoning me without reason. She'd blame me, the daughter, for things I did that she, as mother, had just told me to do. She would have puppet shows with a dog or rabbit puppet needing to be protected, saying "*Ayudame, ayudame*" ("Help me, help me"). The alligator "mother" would come along and be hurtful to her puppet, hitting it after giving it a hug, or feeding it poison food, and then her alligator puppet would laugh, saying, "Only kidding." I needed to be emotionally available in the session, in spite of the quick changes of themes and return to my being the target of Taneisha's anger and punishment.

In session 27, Taneisha started our time by taking out a mother and father figure and having them play out sexual contact. She had them kissing and then having intercourse. After 5 minutes of this play, she quickly abandoned it and went to the puppet theater. She had me sit down and hold the black baby doll as I watched. She again reenacted having her puppet, the alligator, being friendly at first and gesturing to me and the baby that it wanted to pet us. As soon as we neared it, it would bite us and run away. This was reenacted four or five times, until she stopped the alligator with the policeman puppet that said "No," and then she flung the alligator puppet away. It was very difficult for Taneisha to leave this session. She wanted to take my bracelet off my wrist to take with her, which I had to set clear limits on. And she refused her usual transitional note. Instead she hid in the room and then jumped out to scare me, before finally walking out the door.

Session 28

Taneisha had the alligator puppet play out affection by tickling and hugging my rabbit puppet. She then had her puppet get shot by the policeman and die, but then it comes to life again only to get killed again. She had my rabbit puppet cry and be sad. She would alternate between having her alligator puppet seek affection and hugs from my rabbit puppet, at times tricking me, and then finally having the alligator accept the hug from the rabbit. After this scenario her play quickly shifted to wanting to pretend she was little, age 4. She sat in the wooden cart that was in the room and had me push her around and around the room. This was a turning point in our work. I could feel a shift in Taneisha's emotions, an opening up of trust and being cared for.

During this time, for a few brief moments, she would close her eyes and look like she was resting or sleeping. After this play, it was time to go and for the first time Taneisha did not ask for her note or attempt to control the ending of the session. She calmly left the session and went back to class.

Session 29

Taneisha had a hard time coming into therapy. She wanted to wander the hallway and stopped to wave hello to everyone she could find. I found it difficult to refocus her, making me feel frustrated. She would look to see if there was something on their desk or an object in the garbage she could take, requiring me to repeatedly set limits. Once in the therapy room, Taneisha began to order me about, as the daughter. She told me what to say and do, insisting I do things exactly her way. I braced myself for the onslaught of anger and punishment. No matter what my character did, it was not good enough. I was yelled at, cursed at, and punished. Nearing the end of the session, she sat on the large stuffed lion and had me sit next to her. She slowly leaned back, putting her weight against my shoulder, letting me support her weight. When the session ended, Taneisha again left the room without her note or any difficulty. Taneisha's play showed me her attempts to form a relationship. Fearing opening herself up to being cared for, defending against it, and then taking a risk to get emotionally close.

Session 30

Taneisha was extremely affectionate, seeking hugs and wanting to give me a kiss on my cheek. She would jump into my arms off of the chair, having me catch her and hold her. She repeated this play for 5 minutes, giggling each time that I caught her. She then used various animal puppets to hurt the black baby doll I held. I was supposed to protect the baby, but I would get hurt, in turn, by the animals. After several versions of this scenario, Taneisha took the policeman puppet and had it give the mother a ticket three times for drinking and speeding. The policeman sent her to jail, and in silence, gestured with her forefinger to scold her for not being a good mother. Before ending the session, Taneisha had me sit in a chair and she stood behind, playing with my hair and trying to braid it. She sang in Spanish and hummed as she tried to make rows of braids. Her ability to connect and form an attachment with me was emerging.

Session 31

Taneisha was again exceedingly controlling, gesturing and directing what I would say and play. She was angry at me for having taken a few days' vacation. She was angry over the break in attachment and feared I might not return to her. She used the sand tray briefly, having "monsters" stomp on the toy people. She added water to the sand, called it "poop," and had the toy people look disgusted and repulsed by a toy dog pooping. She would bury the poop and then dig it up, wanting me to touch the poop with her. She then built a tall block tower with wooden blocks and crashed it down on the toy people. She repeated this vignette several times, smiling and clapping when it fell on the toy people. I reflected on her actions and pleasure in her play. She really wanted to be sure the people got hurt and knew she was angry. Next she had fire drills, playing out that we had to hide. She would then trick me into believing it was over, and I could come out—only to have the bell ring again signaling that I had to hide. She then shifted her play to pretending that she was ironing her "son's" clothes with the toy iron; I was her daughter. She dictated what she wanted said and done, cleaning and cooking, and my being punished for not doing it right. Near the end of the session, she sat in the therapy chair that swivels and wanted me to spin her around in it. Leaving was difficult, with Taneisha demanding to control how the session ended. She accepted the note and, after some turmoil, left the session. I was feeling the intensity and retribution of Taneisha's anger that I wasn't there for her since I had been away.

Sessions 32–35

Taneisha's play returned to using the puppets. For example, she chose a seal, had it die and told me to be sad. She alternated between having her alligator puppet attack me and the baby, with the baby now fending it off again, saying "Help me, help me" in Spanish with the alligator puppet being nice and friendly. Then she would sit or stand on the lion and try to jump into my arms. Next she would "cook" using the sand, at times being the mean, poisoning mother, and other times being nurturing and caring toward me, the daughter. I would comment about how hard it was to know when the mother would be nice and loving, about how it would feel good to be taken care of, and about how upsetting it was when the caring turned into anger. She would try to braid my hair, humming and sharing how the times that Snow White was nice to her was when she had her hair braided. Culturally, braiding of hair was a special time, as the child had to sit at the grownups' feet for a long time while getting a chance to talk and be together (Drewes, 2008a). At the end of the sessions, she was able to leave the room after taking her note, and when I said goodbye to her at her classroom, she turned and said quickly, with her head down, "I love you" in Spanish.

Concurrent Events

During this time period, visitation and family therapy with her mother were stopped, and phone calls diminished. The Department of Social Services was working toward terminating parental rights, as Kayleen was drinking heavily and was believed to have returned to prostitution. Her grandmother hid a note written by her mother and some pictures of her mother into some gifts that she sent to Taneisha. Taneisha's behaviors deteriorated again, with increased sexualized behaviors of lifting up her shirt to boys, coming out of the shower naked into the living area in front of peers and staff, eating with her hands, and purposely defecating in her pants and smearing the feces on herself and the bathroom. Her body odor repulsed her peers, who no longer wanted to sit near or play with her. She required repeated therapeutic holds and removals from class, with increased self-abuse and destruction of her possessions.

Sessions 36–46: The Work Deepens and Moves; Significant Shifts Occur

Taneisha's play began to change significantly. While she continued to remain nonverbal during most of her sessions, she occasionally asked me personal questions through her play. She would take the toy phone, "call" me, and ask if I was married, if I had any children, if they were boys or girls, or if they were her age. She wanted to see if I was old enough to be her mother.

I would first ask her what she thought, guessing I was married (I wear a wedding band). I replied that I was married, and I did have a son, but no girls. I commented that, when children ask me those questions, that they wish they could have me as their mother. I wondered if she might be thinking that, too. Taneisha slowly nodded. She would then play out being a mean mother who ordered me around and hit me, and then she became the father who would do the same. After this punitive play, she climbed into the cart and said that she was a baby, a 2-year-old. I had to push her around, sing a lullaby to her while I "carried" her to her crib, and tuck her into "bed." She would, at times, be the angry 2-year-old and "wet" herself, throw things and bang on things in a mock tantrum, and then "hit" herself on the head with objects. (I would make sure that she was not trying to hurt herself and would have intervened if she had begun to actually harm herself.) I commented on how I wanted to keep the baby safe and didn't want her to get hurt. She would then build up a block tower and crash it down several times, before climbing on the stuffed lion and jumping off of it into my arms. She had the black baby kiss me on my cheek, and then she would take the baby bottle and pretend it was hers. Seeing her need to actually use the bottle, I bought a real baby bottle for her to use in therapy. I felt it was important that she have a bottle that she could suck on, which would only be used by her in her sessions. She was communicating to me that being able to go back to feeling and acting like a baby was an important piece of her healing.

Taneisha eagerly took the bottle. Each session she filled the bottle with water and sucked on it, drinking the water, as she leaned into me on the couch. Over the next four sessions, she went directly for the baby bottle, which I brought to each session, the moment she arrived in the therapy room. She would climb onto my lap, curl up and drink her bottle, closing her eyes and at times drifting off to sleep for most of the session. Each session this tender exchange was reenacted: Taneisha sat on my lap, in the cart, or on the swivel chair, and I gently rocked her while singing a lullaby as she sucked on her bottle. Near the end of the session she would play hide and seek, still sucking on the bottle, repeatedly having me find her and apparently relishing being a baby who got nurtured and was found (Drewes, 2001).

In Session 45 she had two houses with families living next door to each other in the sand tray. I am a mother with one child, and she is in the other family. We all eat together and live together. Periodically, before the session ended, she would play with my hair, stroking it or trying to braid it. Leaving the session was much easier for her, taking her note with her, and at times wanting me to hold her hand as I took her back to class.

In Session 46, Taneisha initially did not want the baby bottle. Instead she took the puppets and played out having the koala bear want a home and someone to care for it. "Its mother ran way. No, died." She asked if I'd find a family for her to live with and if she could live with me. I replied that it was the agency's rule that staff could not adopt children in our care, but I would work on finding a safe home for her with people who would care for her when she was ready to leave. She used the sand tray and was initially the mother cooking who then turns into a dead mother, a ghost, who comes back to get her. She makes a grave so she could be buried with the mother, because she is going to be dead, and go to hell for all the bad things she did. She feared I would leave her too if she was bad. I told Taneisha that no matter how she behaved or acted toward me I would be back for our therapy. I would be there for her. She then took the baby bottle and curled up on the swivel chair and wanted me to slowly turn her around and around, as she held a baby blanket. Near the end of the session, she opened up the bottle and drank out of it without using the nipple. Before ending the session, and leaving, I assessed how depressed she was and whether she had suicidal ideation or plans, which she denied. I said to her, "I need to be sure you won't hurt yourself. I want to keep you safe." She understood my need to keep her safe and that I cared about her. As we headed back to class she asked if I would get her a pacifier, "bunky," for her next session.

Session 47

Taneisha was happy to see both her bottle and the new pacifier. She put the pacifier in her mouth and kept it there for most of her session. As she sucked on it, she painted, smearing the paint with the brush, adding lots of colors until it was a nondescript brown color. She then put her fingers in it and started to fingerpaint on the drawing. She rinsed off her hands and moved to the sand tray, where she created a "sand story" of a baby in the bath who was in danger of things falling from the sky and making craters and destroying things. There were three houses, with a genie sleeping in one and a girl in another waiting for her Prince Charming to come. There were lots of blond-haired girls and ladies in the tray. As the end was nearing, Taneisha began to squirt the baby bottle at me and out toward the toys. She was testing limits, but she also appeared to be acting more like a 2- to 3-year-old in manner and voice.

I set limits on getting me wet, which Taneisha accepted. She left the session without difficulty.

Sessions 48–52

Taneisha wandered around the room with her pacifier and bottle. She drank water out of the bottle with the nipple top off, or she chewed on the pacifier. She went back to playing doctor but was now a caring doctor who had the babies live with another "mama." At times she built very tall and complicated block towers and then knocked them down with glee. She sought out the fingerpaint and enjoyed smearing and mixing the colors into a brown-black color. At times she tested the limits and tried to smear the paint on me or herself but readily respected the limit. Near the end of the sessions, she used the chalkboard to play school, showing me how to add numbers and learn the alphabet. Her play and demeanor appeared less babyish. She smiled and laughed as she found success in making various objects with paper and pipe cleaners. A few times she was eager to end the session so she could show her teacher what she had made. I found myself looking forward to the sessions to see the shifts and growth.

Concurrent Events

Taneisha's mother's parental rights were terminated, and she was no longer permitted to have contact with her daughter or to call. A closing session was allowed for her to say goodbye to Taneisha, together with her therapist to explain to her how her mother was not able to be the mother she wanted her to be or the mother that Taneisha needed her to be. The mother was coached to tell Taneisha that she wanted her to get a home that could keep her safe and protect her. During this span of time, Taneisha's behaviors outside of therapy showed remarkable improvement. Teachers and child care staff noted that she seemed happier and was less demanding and controlling. She started to take pride in her personal appearance and hair. After having the nails from her two big toes surgically removed from self-mutilation and infection, Taneisha lessened her self-abusive behaviors. She started to comment on feeling pain if she fell or banged herself, in stark contrast to the years of not feeling her self-abusive acts. Peers began to want to play with her, and Taneisha was included in many activities. She began to show talent in horseback riding, as well as in African dancing, winning praise from peers and staff. Her self-esteem improved, and she began to come up to child care staff and talk with them more, while seeking a hug. I felt our work together was generalizing. I could see her ability to form attachments, to express and manage feelings, and to improve her self-esteem were solidifying at a core level.

Sessions 53–63: Resolutions Surface

Taneisha began to ignore her pacifier and baby bottle, preferring to use the sand tray and other toys. She created sand tray stories about a mermaid who would approach humans but then get in trouble. The sea was filled with marbles and colored stones, along with dolphins and whales. Through the sessions, the mermaid would persevere in making contact with the humans, in spite of the disappointments from the grownups. Taneisha made increasingly elaborate trays, putting in religious figures and flags from the Caribbean, as well as water and seashells, recreating her island home. At times she buried a female figure in a coffin and put stones and crosses over the grave; at other times she buried the "Wicked Witch" or "Snow White" Disney characters in the same way. In another corner of the tray, she placed a house with a black mother holding a black baby next to it, then adding trees, stones, and toys. When a tray felt finished, she would stare at it, in silence, for long periods of time. I would comment on her long periods of looking and how much she was thinking about her scene.

Taneisha also played out, with the puppets, having me hold two babies, one black and one white. She would then throw items out of the puppet theater, hitting me and the dolls with a hat, for example, enacting her fear that I would leave her and never come back from my vacation. I commented on her wanting to trust that people she cared about and who cared about her wouldn't leave her and go away. She went back to her baby bottle for two sessions, briefly sucking on it while curled up on my lap, hugging a blanket. Some of her old play returned as she acted out affection–aggression, trickery, and promises that turn into lies and distrust. She vacillated in her play from being a 2-year-old, then an infant, then 4 years old, to finally being a teenager at age 12 or 14. She alternated between using baby talk and being pushed in the "stroller," to cooking food, to talking on the cell phone. She would suck on the pacifier while talking about having a boyfriend and having me pretend that I was her mother and keeping her safe. At times she was exceedingly clingy, seeking hugs and not wanting to let go. She would say that she was ugly, that no one likes her, and then ask if I liked her. I would comment on her shifting play and how confusing it was, with all the different feelings and needs she had.

Games of hide and seek, with mostly me having to find her, happened in each session. Like a younger child, she wanted to be found, to know I missed her and delighted in being found by me. She then began recreating sand trays with huge mounds of sand, horses on the top or climbing up the hill, and colored stones and marbles scattered around the hill. She symbolically was showing me her own success and rise to the top in mastering her past, her losses and emotional pain, and becoming triumphant. Her puppet shows now included a dog and iguana, with the dog getting bit by the iguana. But she would then nurture and hold the dog, caring for it and mending it by using the doctor kit. Her empathy and caring tenderness emerged. At times she used the magic wand to change herself or have me change her into a pretty princess who was now 10 years old, her chronological age.

At times she put the black baby in the swivel chair and slowly spun it around, and then she would become my daughter, who had her own baby for whom she was caring. I was instructed to give her money and surprise her as we were "reunited" again. She wanted me to chase her around in the room, and she asked to wear my jacket or a piece of jewelry during the sessions. I would let her use my jacket and hold onto my bracelet for just the session. She easily relinquished them at the end. Occasionally she braided my hair, other times she started to braid the black baby's hair. At times she would drink out of the bottle while she put on music and danced, sang in Spanish, and showed me African dance moves or the merengue. Often she would fill up the bottle and then leave it untouched. During this time period, it was hard, again, for Taneisha to leave the session. She tested limits as she attempted to control the timing of the end of the session and my actions. She wanted me to write her notes again at the end of the sessions, which I did, and began to insist on the ritual of getting a hug and holding hands back to class, which I also complied with.

Sessions 64–80: Transitions Occur

Taneisha would initially want her baby bottle but often decide to set it aside and play instead with the hospital set. She set up the hospital scene, intently looking at the little girl figure lying on the bed. She said it was she, having had surgery on her toenails. She began to say, in a babyish voice, that she did not want to lose her foot if it got infected and that she wished she could go back in time and be back in her mother's tummy. She then decided to play hide and seek, repeatedly wanting me to find her. When I did, she got angry with me and pushed me away, only to want me to find her again—and again. I found it confusing, trying to figure out the symbolism of her anger in being found. Taneisha began to talk more about how she wished her mother would come back for her, and take her, wishing she could be the mother she wanted. As she curled up next to me, she was able to share how sad she felt, and with tears streaming down her face, she said that somehow she was to blame for her mother not being there for her. She wasn't sure if she could love another mama, and would she be bad if she did not love her real mama any more? I told her that she was not to blame for her mother not being in her life and how her mother had her own grownup problems that prevented her from being the mother she needed and wanted. I explained that it was alright if she loved another mother and did not have the same feelings for her birth mother, that it did not make her bad; and that other children who go to a forever home feel the same. Taneisha listened carefully, soaking up my words. She then wanted to leave the session and return to her living unit.

Sessions 85–90: Closure

Taneisha's final sessions focused more and more on looking toward the future and the conclusion of her time at our residential treatment program. She would ask what type of family might she get, and she began to think of the possibility of someone being able to love her. She shared how she had earned "Top Four," highest points in the living unit, which allowed her to go on special trips with three other girls and staff. She would spend more time talking about her feelings and how she was doing in school, making drawings, or cutting up paper and making collages. She enjoyed listening to Latin music and would dance to it during the sessions. I saw much joy on her face, smiling as she danced. She occasionally worked in the sand tray and enjoyed making scenes of unicorns and horses on top of mountains, to which she would add Snow White, the Wicked Witch, and Prince Charming, along with Bambie and Simba Disney characters, in a family scenario. In another corner she would place a house with trees, a mother holding a baby, and a path leading up to the house. She happily said that this would be her home soon!

SUMMARY OF CLINICAL IMPRESSIONS AND FOLLOW-UP

Taneisha displayed severe chronic and complex trauma reactions and symptoms of PTSD, magnified by an underlying disorganized attachment disorder and acculturation issues. Through her self-directed play, Taneisha was able to work through feelings of abandonment, loss, and grief over losing her mother, older sister, and the cultural home with which she was beginning to identify. The healing aspects of play (Drewes, 2010) allowed her to utilize abreaction and catharsis in dealing with her losses and grief. She was able to slowly fill the void and emptiness of her traumatic attachment history through self-nurturing and "rebirthing" play. She began to relate and attach to me, as her therapist, and in extension to those around her. Through games of peek-a-boo (hiding from the alarm) she was able to develop a firm sense of permanency and constancy (Drewes, 2001). During our physical separations she was able to remain emotionally intact, learning that others would indeed return and that she "carried" them within her. Through her play Taneisha learned that I would continue to be there for her even after sessions filled with her angry rejecting, controlling, and punishing behavior. Slowly her view of herself, others, and the world began to shift toward a more positive template.

Taneisha's self-abusive behaviors significantly declined, and she had more positive interactions with peers and staff. Her bedtime problems resolved, and she was able to participate more appropriately in the school and living unit programs. She was socially more appropriate, was able to complete more of her work in school, and generally seemed happier. She was earning privileges and seemed more motivated by potential consequences or rewards. She was social with peers and showed more age-appropriate interests. Her affect was appropriate and congruent, and she was able to demonstrate some degree of genuine engagement and attachment.

Taneisha had shown improvement in her ability to relate in a genuine and direct manner to both peers and adults. Her self-esteem improved, although she still appeared to be vulnerable to regressions in the face of stress or any contact with her grandmother. However, she has shown a significant and lasting gain in affect tolerance, relatedness, and ability to communicate her feelings in a direct manner.

By the time Taneisha was discharged from our program, her self-abusive behavior had virtually disappeared. She was much better accepted by her peers and no longer was intentionally grossing them out or repelling them. She smiled more and appeared much happier.

She was proud of her success in horseback riding, African dance, and, as mentioned, had earned her way up the point system to the top in her living unit. She cared about her personal hygiene and appearance. In school she continued to avoid work at times, but generally, with enough motivation, she would complete her assignments. She made significant academic progress and, in general, seemed happier in school. She was awarded the school's highest honor at graduation: "Student of the Year" for her significant gains, which she was able to maintain.

Taneisha was placed in a therapeutic foster home, where she made a positive connection with her foster parents. She was successfully discharged from the residential treatment center at age 10. Currently she remains with her foster parents, who adopted her. She successfully completed high school and has been attending a community college where she is studying to become a nurse.

REFERENCES

Drewes, A. A. (2001). Developmental considerations in play and play therapy with traumatized children. In A. A. Drewes, L. Carey, & C. E. Schaefer (Eds.), *School-based play therapy* (pp. 297–314). New York. Wiley.

Drewes, A. A. (2008a). Cultural considerations of play. In K. Stagnitti & R. Cooper (Eds.), *Play as therapy* (pp. 159–173). London: Jessica Kingsley.

Drewes, A. A. (2008b). Culturally competent supervision of child and play therapists. In A. A. Drewes & J. A. Mullen (Eds.), *Supervision can be playful. Techniques for child and play therapist supervisors* (pp. 77–90). New York: Jason Aronson, Rowman & Littlefield.

Gil, E., & Drewes, A. A. (Eds.). (2005). *Cultural issues in play therapy.* New York: Guilford Press.

Schaefer, C. E., & Drewes, A. A. (2010). The therapeutic powers of play and play therapy. In A. A. Drewes & C. E. Schaefer (Eds.), *School-based play therapy* (2nd ed., pp. 3–16). New York: Wiley.

CHAPTER 14

"This Mommy Has No Milk!"

A Neglected Child's Adaptation to Loss and Hunger

ELIANA GIL

It has been nearly 30 years since I met and worked with Niki. I chronicled her case in condensed form twice (Gil, 1991, pp. 204–205; James, 2008, pp. 141–145) as a powerful illustration of what young, traumatized children could accomplish through play. I have also shared this case example in teaching play therapy as well as trauma resolution, and it serves as a great vehicle for discussion, often eliciting polarized responses. The crux of the question, as we discuss later in this chapter, is whether Niki's work could stand on its own or whether direct clinical interventions were required, desirable, or necessary in this case.

Niki made a lasting impression on me, so much so that I have revisited the case regularly, trying to deepen my understanding of Niki's evocative process of self-reparation. These periodic reevaluations have also served to strengthen my respect for the principles of humanistic theory, which suggest that human beings possess the internal resources that they need to confront both small and large challenges. It appears that sometimes these resources are not encouraged; in fact, sometimes they can be systematically dismantled, and access to them can be inadvertently blocked. But it also appears that the reparative potential is fierce and persistent, rechargeable and fortified, as long as a safe, relational context for growth exists.

My therapeutic curiosity and constant reevaluation of the reparative process, both the one that occurs naturally as well as the one that can be clinically facilitated, has led me to become more and more intrigued by pinpointing the variables or conditions that coexist in order for children to feel inspired to engage in their own reparative work. Indeed, this self-generating and often self-initiated work emerges in a pure fashion, not because of clinical suggestion and not because of fancy clinical techniques. These children are simply driven toward mastery opportunities and seem compelled to create concrete, physical, and emotional opportunities to do what they need to do to feel better and move toward health. These are the youngsters that I've previously described as "mastery-driven"—in these circumstances, clinicians "step aside," become silent witnesses, and regale in the wonder of, for lack of a better description, the natural healing process. What clinicians can provide to advance children's progress is twofold: (1) the opportunity for an emotionally connected, heart-to-heart relationship, and (2) the positive and safe environment that contains selected and appropriate symbols that children can use for expression, creation, and management of difficult, painful, and confusing traumatic experiences.

I am thrilled to be able to provide some follow-up on this case, because I was fortunate to hear from the adoptive mother over these last two decades about the life story that evolved for this child with whom I worked when she was 3 and 4 years of age. As of this writing, Niki is approximately 35 years old, teaches second grade at a local elementary school, is happily married, the mother of two birth children, and the adopted mother of a little girl whose name is Liana.

Revisiting this case seems rich in possibilities, given the amount of interest it has generated in myself and others and the deepening of insight that has continued over the decades since I saw this child with the moon-shaped eyes.

CASE REFERRAL INFORMATION

Niki was all eyes when I met her, reminiscent of the little girls drawn by the painter Margaret Keane, popular in the 1960s. Her stature was quite small, her movements even smaller. Her eyes were haunting and although her earliest work was done with her eyes turned away from me, those eyes began to change and sparkle as her work came to life.

When I got the referral about Niki, I remember sitting back and wondering how parents could be so cruel and inhumane toward their children. This was one of my earliest clinical cases as an intern, and I had not yet encountered the compelling cross-generational transmission process. I remember having read Dr. Ray Helfer's book *A Crash Course in Childhood* (no longer in print) that made the then riveting point that parents who abused and/or neglected their children were often repeating their early life experiences. Dr. Helfer went on to say that it was not reasonable to expect that parents could possibly provide to their children the nurturing that was not given to them. Thus his book emphasized that abusive parents first need a "crash course" in childhood to prepare them to make substantive shifts that would allow them to provide safe and nurturing parenting to their own children.

I was asked to keep a journal by my first supervisor, and I often revisit these innocent missives to myself: The first two questions seemed perplexing: (1) if someone was maltreated as a child, why would he or she possibly repeat those behaviors with their own children? And (2) don't all mothers have an intuitive mechanism that would trump negative experiences? These and other questions were answered over and over throughout my career: Those who abuse don't usually make conscious decisions to abuse their children. Instead, often they abuse impulsively, sometimes driven by unconscious behavioral reenactments that they cannot control at the time but that definitely signal unresolved traumas of their own. Also, I came to recognize that some mothers do not have the intuitive maternal response that we assume exists in all women who bear children. Instead, they may need to get their own needs for nurturing met first before they can learn to meet (*not* intuit) the needs of their children.

Niki was referred to me because she had been starved by her biological mother, Tamara, a 20- or 21-year-old woman who had been in and out of psychiatric hospitals and had been diagnosed with intermittent psychotic episodes, one of which bloomed with the birth of her first child, Niki. Tamara had made numerous attempts to provide her firstborn with a stable home but her efforts proved unsuccessful.

Niki was diagnosed with nonorganic failure to thrive at 32 months of age when her mother took her to a pediatrician because she could not toilet train her, and child care programs would not accept her without being fully toilet-trained. Niki had been in foster care twice briefly, and her mother had moved out of state twice, apparently in an attempt to avoid social services interventions. Tamara had hoped to break the pattern her mother had set of allowing her child to flounder in the foster care system most of her life. Tamara's best placement had lasted 3 years with her maternal grandmother, who, in a turn of fate, had been able to show Tamara the kindness and care she was not able to show her own daughter consistently. Tamara was also a graduate of the foster care system; she became pregnant with Niki shortly after becoming independent in the eyes of the law. She had wandered around visiting some of the friends she had met in foster care over the years who were now also trying to build productive lives for themselves, some more successfully than others. Space does not allow me to talk about Tamara in greater detail, but suffice to say that along with a very abused child's story is an equally distressing and compelling parental story.

In Niki's case, the separation caused by her hospitalization allowed Tamara to come to terms with the fact that she was not prepared to care for a child and that she wanted to place her for adoption. I remember being quite impressed with this mother's ability to evaluate her behavior and make the difficult decision to relinquish her parental rights. We met only once and, I was struck by how young she was chronologically and developmentally. In spite of her lack of maturity and her horrifying history of neglect and abuse, Tamara was grateful that her social worker had given her permission to consider giving up Niki for adoption. "I wish my mother had been counseled to let me go instead of putting me through all the torture she did before I was put in foster care over and over." Her willingness to allow for an uncontested termination of parental rights created positive options for an early adoption for Niki.

I visited Niki in the hospital to introduce myself; at that point Niki still looked physically gaunt and small for her age. She also looked lethargic, and my natural instinct was to sit near and whisper in hushed tones. I told her my name, that she would be coming to see me after she left the hospital, and that I had a room with lots of toys with which she could play. Niki never made eye contact with me and barely responded to anyone or her surroundings. I came back several times to simply watch her through the window; she seemed to be barely breathing. Niki went from an IV line for dehydration to small doses of liquids, then mushy food, and eventually solid food. Niki's mother had not been able or willing to notice the seriousness of her daughter's medical condition. She had begun to feel concerned about her bloating stomach only because the child was not responsive to toilet training. Amazingly, Niki was saved just in the knick of time and now was making a slow turn toward jump-starting the organs in her body and beginning to thrive. Hospital personnel told me that the true sign of a child with nonorganic failure to thrive is his or her receptivity to appropriate care and rapid and steady growth once basic needs are met. A nurse also told me another interest-ing fact: Children need touch as surely as they need food, so the fact that her mother had barely held or rocked her child was another hurdle that Niki would need to overcome.

When I visited Niki at the hospital, I also met Mrs. Tucker, Niki's future foster parent, who had decided to come visit Niki daily—she knew intuitively that this contact would be helpful for this little girl, who would soon be coming into her home. Mrs. Tucker sang to Niki and also read children's books to her. She was a naturally warm per-son, and I remember feeling happy that Niki's luck might now change. I was especially pleased to hear that Mrs. Tucker and her husband were *fost-adopt parents,* which meant that they were looking to adopt children entering the foster care system. Mrs. Tucker had also sought me out and expressed interest in Niki's therapy, so I felt optimistic for Niki's immediate future. Finally, Niki's social worker was one of the best I've ever met; not only had she worked with Tamara in a sensitive and kind way, she was also very invested in ensuring that Niki's situation would change for the better.

Niki was released from the hospital and placed in the care of Mr. and Mrs. Tucker and their 5-year-old daughter, Trisha. The Tuckers had always planned to have one biological child and adopt at least three more; however, their plans changed after adopting Niki because they didn't have the heart to adopt another child after her. They were con-cerned that she might feel displaced, since her adjustment had been challenging.

FORMULATION OF THE PROBLEM

Niki had suffered greatly at the hands of a mother with limited capaci-ties to nurture her child. It's hard to understand why anyone would or could deprive a child of food even when obvious signs of malnutrition became visible and compelling.

Although we tend to associate physical and sexual abuse and domes-tic violence with trauma, we often underestimate the impact of severe malnutrition and neglect. Niki had clearly sustained chronic trauma in which her very survival was in question. Niki's body showed the signs of severe neglect (bloated stomach and shrunken limbs), yet she also showed the tremendous resiliency that children can muster. When I vis-ited her in the hospital, I was struck by how receptive she was to human kindness and how she had adapted to her environment easily, perhaps because the attention, although anxiety-provoking, was also a relief.

I understood that Niki would likely be struggling to gain a sense of safety and security, particularly in regard to food and being fed. In my experience with other severely neglected children, I had found that they hoarded food, had anxiety about eating enough, and had to develop a basic trust (that most of us take for granted) that their most basic needs would be addressed by others. I anticipated that Niki's play would somehow reflect life and death issues, loss, and nurturing needs. Niki continued to ask for her mother and seemed sad and worried that she could not see her. These ambivalent feelings played out in the work she did in therapy.

INVITATION TO PLAY THERAPY

Niki came to therapy sessions shortly after she was released from the hospital. During this time, she had made a somewhat difficult transition into her new family. The Tuckers were patient and their foster daughter Trisha was intrigued by, and wildly enthusiastic to have, a younger sister. Niki, however, was withdrawn, passive, and seemed sad. She did not engage easily with others and often sucked her thumb and stared into space. She did not eat or sleep easily and seemed indifferent to her surroundings. Mrs. Tucker had decided to leave her full-time job in order to be a full-time mother to Niki and her older foster sister, who was now attending first grade and excited to go to "big girl school." Trisha was clearly securely attached to her parents, extremely social and outgoing, and had spent considerable time in day care, preschool, and kindergarten programs. In addition, her mother had taken her to baby gymnastics as well as dance classes very early. Trisha reportedly welcomed the idea of a sister and did not seem to mind her mother's diverted attention. Mr. Tucker had a high-powered job that required international travel, but when he was home, he was completely engaged in family life, seeking out his own bonding time with Niki. While Niki was somewhat disengaged with Mrs. Tucker, she became even more so in Mr. Tucker's presence. Trisha was the family member most likely to get a reaction out of Niki, although her smiles were fleeting.

Niki's behavior in therapy followed suit: She was slow to warm up, cautious, and separated easily from Mrs. Tucker. During our first session I showed her around the room, offering permission for her to play with whatever she liked. I touched some of the toys to model that she could do the same. I showed her the easel and paints, the feeling faces, the board games, the kitchen, the dress-up bin, the hospital, the dollhouse, the courtroom, the puppets and puppet stage, and the sand tray with miniatures on shelves. She looked around the room in a surprisingly disinterested way; nothing much seemed to catch her attention. I remember doing parallel play with her for at least 2 months, at which point she began slowly to explore her environment.[1]

I wondered what Niki would show me through her play, when and if it took form. I also wondered whether Niki would be able to use symbolic play, since she appeared to lack spontaneity, was emotionally constricted, and showed measured movements.

Mrs. Tucker had told me that Niki did best when there was a routine to follow and she knew what to expect. I had made sure, therefore, to have an opening and closing ritual that was repeated each session. I introduced her to the room each time, walking around and talking about the things that were available to her and the activities that she could undertake. At the end of the session, she was allowed to choose a butterfly sticker (which Mrs. Tucker had also told me that Niki enjoyed putting in her sticker book). Almost 2 months into the therapy process, Niki began to put her hands in the sandbox—and her sand journey began.

CASE ILLUSTRATION OF SELF-DIRECTED TRAUMATIC PLAY

The Beginning: Setting the Stage

When she first ventured into working with the sand tray, Niki's movements were quite inhibited. She sifted sand through her little fingers, sometimes looking up at me as if asking if it was okay to do what she was doing, or perhaps to communicate a sense of pleasure at this activity. I carefully picked moments to communicate verbally what I saw her do: "I see that you're letting the sand run through your fingers," or "You're patting down the sand with your hands." Sometimes I would comment on her looking at me by simply stating "and you're looking over at me while you're patting down the sand." I noticed very minute changes in Niki's

---

[1]In my first brief description of this child's play (Gil, 1991, pp. 204–205), I mistakenly stated that I worked with Niki for 7 *months* before she began her posttraumatic play. In fact, this should have said 7 *weeks*.

behavior—so small, in fact, that sometimes I would become discouraged at how slowly she was responding to nondirective play therapy. Over the years I have learned to see these early, hesitant, often constricted movements in the room as setting the context for movement ahead. Just as those who work the land prepare it by turning it over, irrigating, and eventually planting seeds and waiting for their crops, so trauma-specific play themes (or posttraumatic play) appear to need a context for emerging, and the initial work of children appears to serve a similar purpose.

Week after week Niki would enter the room and join in the development of a familiar routine. By the end of 2 months, there was an undeniable rhythm that she was both led by and led. She spent about 10 minutes looking around, touching certain objects in repetitive fashion, eventually coming to the sandbox and putting her hands in the sand, sifting and patting, sifting and patting. Her little hands seemed to have their work cut out for them, for she worked the entire rectangular sand tray from corner to corner; within 35 minutes precisely, she had touched every inch of the sand tray and had left a perfectly smooth surface. She then touched a few more things, looked at me sideways, and stood in front of the door. I would usually say, "I see that you're waiting for me to open the door. Let's go see your foster mom." She would walk slowly next to me, and Mrs. Tucker would take her hand, ask me if everything had gone well, and lead Niki to the car.

A couple of times, Niki looked back to wave goodbye. I always waited at the window in case she did. There was no rhyme or reason to when she would wave to me, so I didn't want to miss a chance of being there to receive her trust through the window once she was safe in the car with the mother she was beginning to love. Mrs. Tucker would call once during the week, and her reports were full of optimism: Niki was more responsive, had initiated a few words, pointed to the things she wanted, and had begun to smile. Mrs. Tucker also reported that Niki was beginning to develop food preferences and was no longer either apathetic or anxious during feedings. As Mrs. Tucker spoke about Niki, sharing her positive perceptions and asking questions about how to explain to Trisha why Niki was often unresponsive and unwilling to play with her, her optimism was contagious. I found myself thanking God that Niki and Mrs. Tucker had found in each other precisely what they both needed. Mrs. Tucker kept Niki close to her at all times, and what I initially had thought of as "too much holding" ended up being just enough. Mrs. Tucker reported that Niki was developing a good comfort level with her husband and sometimes sought out Trisha without prompting.

The work that Niki was preparing to do in the sand tray would soon emerge, as she was also beginning to feel her way around forming an interpersonal relationship with me. I saw her for at least 4 months during which I took a primarily nondirective stance in which she set the pace and I followed. I was peaceful, I was emotionally present, and I provided her with structure and some verbal feedback from time to time. When I first utilized reflective comments (such as the ones I shared earlier and which simply reflected back to her what she was doing), Niki sometimes ignored me completely and other times had a slight startle response. Both those responses suggested that she was used to being in her own world—neither seen nor heard. It was a world I hoped to understand as I spent more time with her.

Clearly the safety and empathic care she had found with Mrs. Tucker served me well, as Niki seemed to soften, develop more comfort, and become physically more relaxed and emotionally more expressive. She was very efficient in her verbal communication and often signaled rather than spoke. Mrs. Tucker reported that her language skills were growing substantially, but when she was with me, she rarely said much of anything, perhaps sensing that words were not as necessary between us. I did not ask questions and rarely spoke while she was in session other than to occasionally summarize what I observed. As we grew to know each other, we often experienced serenity in the room. Our sessions were void of expectation or demands. It was in this setting that Niki's sand play took form.

The Middle: The Work Deepens and Moves

The Introduction of the Mother Pig and Her Babies

This particular day Niki seemed to skip into my office. One wouldn't characterize this as a full skip but definitely something between a walk and a full run. Her hair had grown, and I remember watching it sway from side to side as I followed her to the room. In all the time she'd been interested in playing with her hands in the sand tray, she had never put objects inside it. On this day, she walked into the room, went to the shelves where the miniatures were displayed openly, and selected a large mother pig. She seemed to count the baby pigs that lay close to this mother pig and simply placed them down in a pile after touching each one. As she did this, I counted seven baby pigs (there were a few more mother pigs in my miniature collections, but they were not chosen).

Niki brought the mother pig to the sand tray, and, after smoothing the sand as usual, she used her right hand to dig out a little hole in it. Afterward, she put the mother pig in the hole and covered her with sand. She looked up at me and said, "All gone!" "Oh, it's all gone," I said, not knowing what to call this miniature now out of sight. "Mommy piggy all gone," she said, as I repeated it word for word. In this one single action, Niki had introduced both a mother figure as well as the fact that the mother figure was gone. How apropos to her experience, I thought to myself, wondering what might happen next.

Niki signaled that she wanted to put the cover on the sand tray, and I obliged. This was yet another interesting action—a way, I surmised, that she might keep this buried mother even more unavailable. It could also have been her way of ensuring the continuity of her play. Unfortunately, I was not able to secure the sand tray intact during a busy week of therapy appointments, and even though I considered putting the pig in the tray the way she had left it, I thought it best to simply allow Niki to find the tray as she always did. Hopefully, she would be able to tolerate the fact that the pig had been put back on the shelf where she had spotted it before.

When Niki came into the next session, the top was off the tray, and she went to the shelf to find the mother pig with her seven little babies. Once again she took the mother pig to the sand and buried it, asking me to place the sandbox cover on at the end of the session. She was using most of her time now preparing the sand for the uncovering of this one spot where the mother pig would be buried. She did this twice more before the next aspect of her play began.

The Search Begins

Niki buried the pig and added another component: In addition to the mother pig in the tray, two baby pigs joined her. Soon after the mother pig was buried, Niki took one pig in each hand and began calling "Mommy, mommy." Niki noticed that as she moved the baby pigs around on top of the sand, they made very small footprints. She methodically proceeded to put footprints everywhere on the surface of the sand, literally covering the sand with little markings. Once finished with this process, she took the baby pigs back to the shelf and asked to cover the tray.

Over the next 2 months, the original two baby pigs that she used were gradually joined by the other five in the miniature collection. Niki was intent on having all seven piglets walk around the sand tray, leaving footprints that covered the surface of the tray and calling out for their mommy. It was amusing to me to watch Niki with her seven baby piglets in hand, trying to ensure that each baby piglet had called out for mother at least once.

Niki's play introduced an element of danger, placing many piglets in precarious or vulnerable situations. One piglet "fell off" the sand tray while another got its head stuck in the sand. Toward the end of this stage of the play, Niki also began adding other objects such as a bridge, a tree, and a large truck. She placed one of the baby piglets under the bridge and had another fall off the tree; as the truck ran down another two, it became evident that seeking out Mother was full of perils (see Figure 14.1). During this play Niki appeared to experience affective changes. Her breathing increased, as did her movement and her sounds. She sometimes appeared to be anxious, whereas other times I would swear I heard her giggle. She was definitely engaged and invested in this play.

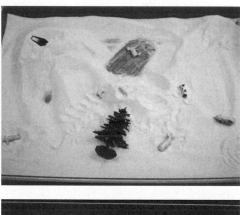

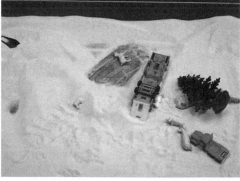

FIGURE 14.1. The perilous world without Mother.

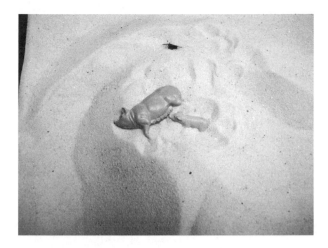

FIGURE 14.2. "This mommy has no milk."

The Search Continues

Finally the day came when one pig somehow was able to dig up the mother pig. The baby piglet in her hand appeared to help the mother pig up from under the sand to a flat surface. She laid the mother pig down on her side, exposing many nipples, as if she's ready to feed her babies. Niki brought one baby pig to the mother's nipple and, amazingly, looked up and said, "Titty has no milk." I repeated what she said, matching her tone of voice, "Titty has no milk." "No," she said, "no milk." Then I said, "The baby has no milk from Mommy," and Niki stated softly, "This mommy has no milk" (see Figure 14.2).[2]

When I asked Niki how the baby pig felt about the fact that the mommy had no milk, she responded, "The baby is sad" as her eyes watered, and she moved away from the tray. She placed the baby pig down on a stuffed rabbit and prepared herself to leave the room (see Figure 14.3). It was mystifying how Niki had developed an internal

[2]In reviewing my notes, I found that I jumped ahead of Niki, luckily not far enough that it changed the course of her play. I went from her comment "Titty has no milk" (still protective of her mom, almost as if saying "The titty doesn't work, my mom does!") to a different statement, "The baby has no milk from Mommy." This comment definitely shifted the focus from the mother pig's teat to the baby. It also took the leap to talk about the "mommy" with no milk rather than staying with the teat. I remember discussing this with my supervisor and being aware that I needed to pay attention to my countertransferential responses and slight slips of the tongue that were meaningful and revealing.

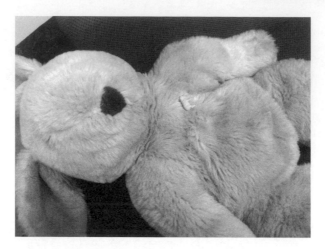

FIGURE 14.3. The bunny comforts the sad piglet.

clock; she seemed able to utilize the full 50-minute sessions with great precision.

The very next session she unfolded exactly the same play as she had the time before. One of the baby piglets unburied the mother, brought her out to the flat surface, and once again, the baby concluded that the mother had "no milk." This time when I repeated what Niki had said, I added, "I wonder how the baby pig feels that the mommy pig has no milk." Niki looked up at me, and I could see the distress in her eyes. She answered without hesitation, "The baby is sad and her tummy hurts." "Oh," I repeated, "the baby pig is sad and her tummy hurts." Niki went to sit on the couch next to the big stuffed rabbit where she had left the baby pig last time. To my surprise, since she had never touched or held this rabbit before this visit, Niki put it on her lap and began to smooth down the rabbit's fur, particularly at the head. She hugged it close to her before going to the door to leave. She reenacted this segment of the play about four more times, and each time she would hold and rock the rabbit a little bit longer and tighter. In addition, Niki started taking a little saucer and spoon, filling it halfway with sand, and spoon-feeding the rabbit "medicine food" before she put the rabbit back on the couch and said, "See you next time." Niki appeared to find reassurance in having a clear structure to follow. She had also begun to take charge of creating her own rituals in our therapy sessions.

During this period of time that Niki's play included uncovering the mother pig who lacked milk, Mrs. Tucker reported that Niki was exhibiting what she called "babyish behaviors." She noted that Niki was sometimes doing baby talk, was asking to be cuddled and rocked, and wanted to be close to her mother. Niki had also started fighting a little with Trisha and reverted back to earlier behavior of not wanting to play with her. Mother was curious about what was going on in therapy, and I simply replied that Niki seemed to be using play therapy very well and was currently involved in a series of play scenarios that seemed relevant and important to her. Mrs. Tucker never pressed for more information, perhaps sensing my reluctance to go into great detail.[3] I encouraged Mrs. Tucker to be especially responsive to Niki and, if she could, to find ways of spending a little more time nurturing her daughter after her therapy sessions.

It was abundantly evident by now that Niki was involved in posttraumatic play. This type of play allowed Niki to begin to acknowledge and address the difficult experiences of her young life in a once-removed fashion. The potential curative benefits of posttraumatic play were never clearer to me than they were watching Niki face the trauma of her mother's inability to nurture her. In essence, Niki set up in her play a recreation of her life experience: a mother who was not able to provide sufficient life sustenance for her child, a mother who could not see or respond to her child's pain. In addition, Niki was self-soothing and self-nurturing by holding and petting a large stuffed rabbit and by designating the rabbit as the sad baby piglet's caretaker. Not only was she taking care of herself by rocking and cuddling the rabbit, she also fed it in a very tender way before leaving each of her therapy sessions. Outside the therapy session she was reportedly more adept at getting her needs met by Mrs. Tucker (as well as her husband, to a lesser degree). So it was that Niki's fear, anxiety, and sadness began to be identified, experienced, and managed.

Resolution(s) Surface: An Alternative Food Source

Niki had yet one more surprise in store for me as I watched her play evolve with great curiosity. This one particular day she repeated the play sequence until the part when she states that the baby is sad that the

---

[3]These days I am much more willing to discuss the child's play themes in general terms, and I am more likely to inform parents of phases of treatment, especially the transition into posttraumatic play. I have found over the years that most parents are quite respectful of the play and willing to pay extra attention to children during challenging periods in their play work.

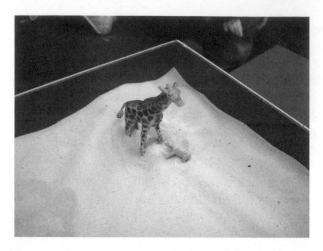

FIGURE 14.4. A new mommy surfaces in the opposite corner.

mother pig does not have milk. At this point, instead of going to sit on the couch with her stuffed rabbit, she went back to the shelf with the miniatures and pulled out a mother giraffe, which she placed parallel to the mother pig (see Figure 14.4). She took the baby piglet (who was sad) over to the mother giraffe, and she announced in the loudest voice I had ever heard from this child: "This giraffe mom has LOTS of milk!" (see Figure 14.5). I matched her enthusiasm as I repeated, "This mother

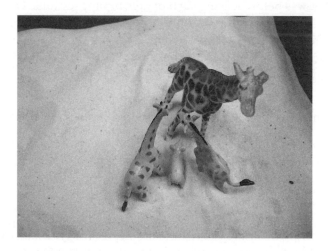

FIGURE 14.5. This mommy has milk for everybody!

giraffe has lots of milk!" Niki did not stop to hug the rabbit but did walk to the door as if ready to leave right then (a good 10 minutes before the end of the session). Somehow it felt right to leave just then, and so we did. This was one of the days that she waved goodbye and flashed a smile from the car. This was one of two full smiles I saw from Niki.

Possible Threat to the Food Supply

The next three sessions included Niki's mother giraffe, which was brought in at the conclusion of her usual story in the sandbox. But Niki also introduced her last miniature in the tray, a baby giraffe. At first, Niki herself seemed bewildered by the presence of the baby giraffe, and her affect was not so bright when she left these four miniatures in the sandbox. At the same time, she seemed compelled to repeat this sequence a few more times until, in the fifth session (of the baby giraffe sequences), Niki took the baby pig, walked it over to where the mother and baby giraffe were standing, and knocked over the baby giraffe (see Figure 14.6).

Niki seemed startled by what she had done and looked at me quickly. I said, "The baby pig bumped into the baby giraffe." Niki, with a twinkle in her eye, said, "She *knocked* her down." I was fascinated by the tussling between the baby pig and the baby giraffe and immediately reflected on all the times that Mrs. Tucker had wondered about how to improve the relationship between Niki and her new sister, Trisha. The next time Mrs. Tucker and I spoke, I asked her to tell me more about

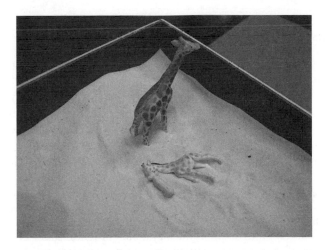

FIGURE 14.6. The babies battle for Mother and milk.

Niki's relationship with her sister—a subject about which Mrs. Tucker had a lot to say! She started out by saying that their sibling relationship had always been somewhat strained but that in the last month or so, it had improved dramatically. When I asked what she had observed, she told me that Niki was now seeking out Trisha, that she tolerated playing with her for longer and longer times, and most notably, that she did not whine or complain or get angry when she was attentive to Trisha. Mrs. Tucker mentioned how difficult it had been to ensure that Trisha was getting enough love and physical attention because Niki had always cried and seemed clingier whenever Trisha was around her mother. I asked Mrs. Tucker if she had any thoughts on what might have contributed to Niki's improved tolerance toward her sister, and she could not think of anything. As I hung up from our conversation, I felt quite intrigued with Niki's play that now included some play themes of apparent discord between the baby pig and the baby giraffe. It was as if playing out the conflict between the baby pig and the baby giraffe (projections of Niki and Trisha) and leaving it behind had allowed Niki to initiate less conflicted interactions with her sister at home.[4]

Resolution and Adaptation to the New Family

Niki did not persist in this overt conflict for much longer. After two more sessions, she announced, "This mommy has lots of milk for everybody!" Niki's declaration seemed earnest and definitive. This portion of her play was coming to an end.

Transitions and Closure

The end of this play occurred shortly after Niki's declaration of mother's abundance of milk. It appeared that she had resolved in her own mind that her sister Trisha was not a threat to her food supply and that Mother had enough milk for both children. It was thus interesting that Niki requested that her mother accompany her to her therapy sessions, a departure to our usual procedure. It had been 2 weeks since Niki had stopped playing in the sandbox for most of the session. The last two ses-

---

[4]I continue to be mystified about the circular loop of influence between children's real-life situation and the play scenarios they create in play therapy. Does the play therapy reflect real changes that are under way in a child's life? Or does the play reflect possibilities still to occur? Is the play a kind of rehearsal for behaviors that will soon emerge, or is the play a chronicling of what has occurred? Does the play, in fact, lay the groundwork so that change can occur?

sions she had played with the sand, as she had much earlier on, patting and sifting and making a smooth surface in which she placed her hand prints. From there, she played with some of the kitchen equipment as well as clay. She especially liked using the garlic press to make "spaghetti" for invited animal guests to eat. These appeared to be like tea parties where she would set out the full toy tea set and then she would serve spaghetti to her guests (no fluids).

In the third week of this play sequence she asked Mrs. Tucker to come with her to the therapy room, and Mrs. Tucker obliged after checking with me. Mrs. Tucker sat quietly as Niki showed her around the play therapy office, much as I had shown her and her mother during our first few sessions. Niki then asked mother to come over and touch the sand, and then she hid her own hands and asked her mother to find them. Mother made a playful game of it as she sought Niki's hands for quite a while, eventually finding them with great surprise on her face and in tone of voice. It was interesting to me that Mrs. Tucker turned to the stuffed rabbit on the couch on two occasions to ask the rabbit if he had seen Niki's hands. This produced a giggle in Niki, who said, "Mommy, he can't talk . . . rabbits don't talk!"

Then Niki told Mom to sit close to her because she wanted to tell her a story. Mrs. Tucker pulled up a chair and listened attentively as Niki told the tale of the mother pig. She narrated the following:

> "This is the mommy pig, and she has lots of babies. She came over here and she went inside the sand. Then her babies couldn't see her, and they said, 'Mommy, Mommy,' but she couldn't hear them . . . she had sand in her ears. And this baby fell on the floor [she picked up one of the pigs and threw him overboard], and see, the tree got on top of this baby, this baby drowned in the water. This pig found the mommy but the mommy has no milk."

She went and got the mother giraffe and yelled, "This mommy has lots and lots of milk, Mommy, this mommy is a good mommy!" She did not bring the baby giraffe into the tray, but she kept asserting that the mother giraffe had "lots of milk, lots for every baby." Mrs. Tucker understood how profound this play was and had a tear in her eye. "I'm so glad that this baby pig has lots of milk to drink." I thought it was so insightful of Mrs. Tucker to focus on the baby pig's needs at this moment. Niki then took her hand and said, "Now we have to give some milk to the rabbit." She went and got some sand in the saucer and brought the spoon over to Mrs. Tucker. Niki directed Mrs. Tucker to sit holding Niki on her lap, while Niki held the rabbit in her lap. This was the second full smile I saw Niki give, and she did so stretching her neck around to look at Mrs. Tucker, who of course responded with a wonderful smile of her own. This was a picture etched forever in my mind. It is one of those moments that motivates mental health professionals and makes our work worthwhile and superbly rewarding.

SUMMARY OF CLINICAL IMPRESSIONS AND FOLLOW-UP

Niki was a very young child who had endured malnutrition at the hands of a very unprepared and incapacitated young parent with her own history of abuse and neglect. She had recovered well physically from nonorganic failure to thrive; however, her psychological injuries were more long-lasting. Niki had been blessed to enter a foster home already prelicensed to adopt. The future adoptive parents, especially Mrs. Tucker, demonstrated relentless interest in this child, coming to the hospital to witness the child's recovery, something she was not required to do but that she felt was important in facilitating a smooth transition for Niki when she was placed in her foster home.

Niki had early signs of attachment problems and exhibited very clingy behaviors with the foster mother. In addition, she was quite hypervigilant, fearful, and void of emotional expression. Even her physical movements appeared hesitant and stilted, without fluidity of any kind. She avoided eye contact, was unable to cry to express discomfort, and literally needed to be held in her mother's arms round the clock for a few months. This child had never received proper nurturing or age-appropriate stimulation; she had spent most of her time alone, and when she was with her mother, she was treated as if she were an adult companion. One benefit of Tamara's talking with Niki as if she were much older was to stimulate her verbal language skills. When Mrs. Tucker began to work with her, Niki made great strides in language acquisition and expression. When Niki was upset, however, she had learned to wimper instead of cry, but her distress was apparent in her clingy and irritable behavior. As she began to gain strength and weight and become more mobile, Niki became more responsive to social contact. In particular, she tolerated touch from the nursing staff in the hospital and later from Mrs. Tucker, her husband, and her new older sister, Trisha.

Niki had the best possible home situation and the most stupendous fost-adopt parents I have ever met. She also had an extraordinary foster care and adoption worker from the Department of Social Services, and she began therapy with me when I had a very small caseload and dedicated all my time to thinking about and planning for Niki's treatment (with the benefit of a supervisor). Niki began therapy shortly after she was released from the hospital, where she had spent about 3 months. I had visited Niki in the hospital in order to decrease the stress of meeting yet another new person when she came for therapy. Niki knew me as the "puppet lady," because in those days I never went anywhere without big puppets or finger puppets.

As much as she had liked the puppets when she saw me in the hospital, when she came to my office, she was immediately fascinated with the sandbox. She spent quite a bit of time at first sifting and then patting down the sand to make a smooth surface. Eventually she began a story in the sandbox that seemed directly linked to her real life. She chose a mother pig from a shelf with miniatures representing various facets, roles, and relationships in life. She also chose baby piglets whose job it was to find the mother pig that Niki had buried in the sand. The babies appeared to face varied perils as they called out and searched for Mother, until eventually one little pig unburied the mother and helped to raise her to the smooth surface of the sand tray. Once out from under the sand, the mother lay on her side, displaying multiple nipples for feeding. One of the babies arrived at her mother's nipple, announcing that the mother had no milk. The baby piglet was both sad and suffering from a sore tummy. After repeating this sequence of play many times, Niki introduced a mother giraffe who had sufficient milk to feed the piglet and later a baby giraffe—the same one that later seemed to pose a threat and elicit aggression from the baby piglet. At the end, the conflict seemed to be resolved as the piglet felt reassured and declared that there would indeed be enough milk to go around.

This posttraumatic play brings the original distress to the forefront in a manner created and advanced by the child who has undergone the traumatic experience. Rather than the therapist introducing the specific way and the specific time that the child should address his or her past traumas, posttraumatic play often emerges spontaneously and serves the purpose of allowing the child the opportunity for gradual exposure and a measured tolerance of previously intolerable emotions. In fact, the pairing of a symbolic recreation with the safety of the therapy relationship and setting can have substantive and profound benefits. The child learns that the traumatic memory can be experienced and tolerated in the present without feeling the original pain.

In addition, because the child is in charge of the creation and retelling of the story, as well as the symbols that are selected and the projection that occurs, affect can be released and the power of the memory can be diminished. It is important to note that one of the greatest benefits of play is the quality of pretend, which mimics and yet suspends reality. When Niki chooses a pig to represent herself and then defines that pig as "sad" and having a "sore tummy," she has (safe) enough distance from the pain of the situation to find it tolerable. In other words, Niki gets to imagine that it is the pig who is sad and not herself and the pig who feels threatened and aggressive, not herself. In essence, this displacement affords Niki the opportunity to gradually own her painful emotions after first externalizing them in a manner that she can tolerate. Likewise, when the characters in her story release pain and find new resolutions to conflict, Niki is the beneficiary of such strides.

But more is happening here as Niki begins to experience her own sadness and fear and then takes steps to make herself feel better by holding and rocking the large stuffed rabbit. She even takes it one step further when she starts feeding the rabbit, ensuring that its basic needs are being met by her. In doing so, she takes both the "good caretaker" (nurturer) role as well as the role of the nourished, thus creating a symbolic dyad that she integrates as a real possibility. In fact, this possibility, this image of nurturing, is then created by Niki in vivo when her adoptive mother enters the room.

Niki chooses to tell her adoptive mother about her posttraumatic play and, by so doing, conveys a huge gesture of trust and closure to Mrs. Tucker. Niki exposes her fears and vulnerabilities to her new mother and confirms her ultimate confidence in her as well as the shift in loyalty that has taken place from Tamara to Grace.[5] As she does so, her bonding behaviors are not lost on her adoptive mother, who responds by celebrating Niki's joy in feeling loved and secure.

This case illustrates beautifully how well children can find unique ways of facing and processing their traumatic experiences. My job was to create a safe environment, provide some useful props, and witness her reality. I was cognizant of wanting to follow her pace and did not see my role as one of suggesting new themes or diverting her attention to something else. Finally, although I had very clear interpretations of

---

[5] Niki seemed to signal her understanding that her mother, Tamara, was simply limited in her ability to provide for her by asserting that it was the mother pig's teat that lacked milk. Conversely, when she declared the mother giraffe's abundance of her milk supply, she exclaimed, "This mommy has milk for everyone!" This very diminutive language subtlety may reflect a young child's amazing understanding of a highly complex issue (her mother's limited capacity to provide for her vs. mother's withholding of something that she possesses but chooses not to provide).

her play, I did not share those with her. To do so may have altered something in Niki's experience of her play work, and it felt very risky for me to interfere with this natural unfolding that took precisely the time and the direction it needed to take.

I have often been asked about the relative importance or desirability of bringing into conscious awareness specific aspects of Niki's story (or children's posttraumatic play, in general), and I will leave this issue for the reader to ponder. If, in fact, I had said to Niki something akin to "This is like what happened with you and your mommy," or if I had asked her if this story reminded her of something that had happened to her when she was a little baby, I often wonder what would have occurred. Would Niki have welcomed the question and made the immediate connection between her reality and her play. Or would she have objected that this pig was not her mother and that her mother was a good mommy, like Mrs. Tucker. In other words, would my making the connection have caused Niki to withdraw or to further understand what her play had meant. Given that I chose to avoid making those connections, I will never know the answer to that, but over the years I have pondered that question and come to the conclusion that these decisions are weighty ones to consider and could cause children to either embrace or reject their work. I prefer to err on the side of safety and trust that what is lurking in Niki's unconscious mind is what drives the play and thus what is already understood by her on some deep level. The other driving force at play is how Niki's behavior had changed and prospered during the course of therapy and most definitely in response to her new, stable, predictable, and nurturing environment.

Sixteen years later, I received an electronic communication from Mrs. Tucker, who had Googled my name and located me. She sent a JPG file of a lovely 20-year-old woman who had won a prize at a horseback riding show. She had a radiant smile in the picture and looked regal and self-assured as she posed with her horse. Mrs. Tucker informed me that Niki was a junior in college (she had skipped a grade), had an active social life, was academically successful, and had chosen to become a veterinarian. I couldn't help but smile remembering the play she had done as a very young child and how she had been loved and nurtured those animal miniatures back to health. Mrs. Tucker was still a foster parent, although now on an emergency basis only. She was older and felt that some of the children coming into care deserved parents who could keep up with them. Mrs. Tucker told me that she had remembered some of the advice that I had given her for years. Niki, however, no longer remembered me or the therapy of her very early years. Mrs. Tucker and

Niki had the opportunity to read this chapter and give permission for it to be published. Niki offered the following:

> "Dr. Gil, I can't say that I remember the play therapy that you describe in your chapter. But there is something strangely familiar about the story, as if it might have been a dream I once had. I think that if I had a child in a similar situation, I would want them to have play therapy because even now, so many years later, it feels like the most respectful thing to do for a young child. As you say, sometimes they really can lead the way. Thank you for honoring me with publication of this chapter and for remembering me after all these years. You might find it interesting to know that I have an extensive rabbit collection and my favorite book has always been *The Velveteen Rabbit* by Margery Williams [1999]. Take care, Niki."

REFERENCES

Gil, E. (1991). *The healing power of play: Working with abused children.* New York: Guilford Press.

James, B. (2008). *Handbook for treatment of attachment-trauma problems in children.* New York: Free Press.

Williams, M. (1999). *The velveteen rabbit: Or how toys become real.* New York: Harper Collins.

CHAPTER 15

Play and the Transformation of Feeling

Niki's Case

EVA-MARIA SIMMS

States parties recognize the right of the child to rest and leisure, to engage in play and recreational activities appropriate to the age of the child, and to participate freely in cultural life and the arts.
—ARTICLE 31, Convention on the Rights of the Child, United Nations

Traditionally, early childhood has been associated with play. From the philosopher Rousseau's claim that play is the child's work, through the poet Novalis's romantic view of the child's play world as the "golden age," to the educator Froebel's kindergarten movement and the psychologist Erik Erikson's term "play age" for early childhood, the connection between early childhood and play seemed well established and generally accepted by the end of the 20th century. In 1990 the United Nations ratified and legally protected child play in the international Convention on the Rights of the Child. It seems ironic that just as child play has achieved internationally protected status, it begins to vanish from American public life. Preschools and kindergartens are trading in their play corners for worksheets and desks, elementary and middle schools reduce leisure and playtime on the play grounds, parents are too afraid of traffic and abductions to let their children play in neighborhoods, and indoor play has been taken over by television and computer games. To find time and space for free play, unregulated and unstructured by adults, has become difficult for most children, especially in our educational institutions. Indeed, play has become antithetical to the goals of Western education.

In this chapter I illustrate the critical role of play in children's affective and cognitive development through a *phenomenological–structural* analysis of play as it unfolds over the course of a play therapy case. The case reveals many of the essential features of play and allows us to focus on the developmental trajectory from sensorimotor to symbolic play.

THE VITAL ROLE OF PLAY IN CHILDHOOD

Psychotherapists who work with children understand the transformative power of play. Rather than enjoyment and leisure, which are the hallmarks of ordinary play, pain and pathology are the driving forces of therapeutic play. This kind of play has an existential urgency: It provides a lifeline back into a world shared with others. Therapeutic play is play with an edge, stripped of all but its essential features.

The following passages by therapist Eliana Gil (as cited in James, 1994; see also Chapter 14, this volume) introduce us to her work with a 4-year-old child named Niki who suffered from failure to thrive as a result of profound parental neglect. We witness Niki's courageous struggle to work through her abandonment issues through play therapy, and in so doing, learn much about the vital role of play in children's lives.

In addition to malnutrition and untreated rashes and infections, Niki, at 4 years of age, could not walk, could barely talk, and was not toilet trained when she entered the foster care system:

> The foster mother reported that Niki was lethargic and passive. She did not cry, even when soiled or hungry. She preferred to stay in one spot, apparently uncomfortable with being out of her crib. She didn't seem interested in toys and usually clutched her blanket in her hands. Niki flinched when her foster mother came into the room in the morning. (Gil, as cited in James, 1994, p. 142)

Her therapist found her to be passive and unresponsive for many months, unattached to anyone and uninterested in the activities of other people:

Sitting next to her I would make sure she watched as I rolled a ball, cut a cardboard into shapes, played with water, built blocks, and built a variety of other things. She usually sat staring, with fingers of both hands in her mouth. (p. 142)

In the absence of caring adults, the horizon of a child's world is severely restricted. Neglected, uncared for children may not cry when hurt or upset because they do not expect a response from the world any more. They do not call out, in anticipation of a future gesture from their caregivers. Such children restrict their engagement with the world to familiar experiences: the minute shadings of a white crib, a distance that spans a few feet; the touch of others that confines itself to the feeling of a spoon on one's lips; or maybe the grasp of a hand under one's arms when placed on a potty chair. They perfectly adapt their senses to this restricted world. As a result, their sense of hearing, sight, touch, and taste become atrophied. After their release from isolation and neglect, they show autistic-like symptoms, and without intense therapeutic sensory work, their chances for succeeding in an ordinary family and school situation are not very good (Greenspan & Benderly, 1997).

Within this semiautistic world, play is replaced with repetitive, self-stimulating activities: rocking, head banging, flipping a light switch, or waving the fingers before the eyes. Unlike play, these activities are not modulated and varied, but are monotonously pursued without change in their structure. Normal play investigates the qualities of things as one encounters them, but autistic play limits the multiple possibilities inherent in a thing to action on just one exclusive feature. *Sensory defensiveness* implies that the horizon of possible modes of activity between self and world has been severely restricted. Play can arise only when children feel safe and cared for, when the halo of adult care lights up the world beyond the crib and makes it inviting instead of frightening.

Sensorimotor Play

Sensory experience and interaction with water, sand, blocks, scissors, and other things afford the young child the opportunity of being shaped by and shaping his or her particular environment. But to do so requires the courage to be challenged: water slips away, sand runs to nothing between one's fingers, scissors cut, and things resist. This type of play, which Piaget (1921/1951) termed *sensorimotor*, stimulates sensory and brain development. Rather than mere observation of the properties of objects, it entails direct experience, which in turn deepens the child's self-awareness. Children *discover* their fingers as they try to contain the sand or stack the blocks and their limitations when the sand is spilled or the block tower collapses. The most fundamental requirement of any type of play is the experience that I can change the structure of the world through my own engagement with it—and that I am changed in turn.

Niki's therapist models simple forms of play and tries to coax her out of the narrow circumference of her life in the crib by showing her that a playful engagement with things is safe. She opens up the possibilities inherent in the sand: it can be dug up or smoothed, hollowed or stacked, filtered or packed together. Experiencing the multiple possibilities inherent in objects is a precondition for play, and one quality that sets it apart from other human activities such as work or structured learning. When the sand responds to the touch of the hand, it makes suddenly visible the child's very own gesture. It becomes a possible location for self-expression and self-experience. It makes the child's intentionality visible: "Here *I want* to have a hollow in the sand. . . . and there. . . . do I want it to remain smooth?" Play becomes the location where *agency and selfhood are exercised without direct annunciation of the self* (Gadamer, 1996).

Initially, engaging in play is a big hurdle for Niki. For 4 months Niki keeps her fingers to herself as she learns how to participate in play by watching her therapist. The therapist is very aware that Niki needs the adult's constancy and the sameness of the small playroom. Niki first ventures into the world of play when she picks up two cups and pours sand from one into the other, a gesture that is followed by pouring water onto the sand. Filling and emptying, giving and receiving are two primary forms of human experience. The satisfaction of sensory sand play, its visceral pleasure, is enhanced by this primary experience of emptiness and fullness that Niki herself can now create. The sand flowing from the cup is more than an object to Niki. The outpouring and receiving of the cups is emotionally satisfying because it makes visible a principle of human existence, one that Niki as the unfilled infant has experienced in her previous life. Interaction with objects condenses the complexity of human emotions into a simple form, which then can be recreated and reproduced in drawing, play, language, and other symbolic expressions (Langeveld, 1968). Symbols arise in childhood—not in the mind but out of the *affective* encounter with the physical world.

Niki's initial inability to play, despite being in the "play age," highlights a number of structural elements of play. Play is a bodily, emotional, and mental engagement with the *possibilities* inherent in the physical world. These possibilities can only be taken up and explored when the child is *held* by a trusting and inviting relationship with adults (Erikson, 1950/1963). Adult neglect leads to autistic-type narrowing of the horizon of engagement, as the child fearfully avoids playing with the *possibilities of things*. Once the child takes up a playful relationship with the physical world, symbolism begins in the sensory–affective realm and only secondarily leads to cognitive understanding. The self is displayed and affirmed without directly announcing itself.

Symbolic Play

After playing with the sifting cups for quite a while, Niki achieves a significant breakthrough: She brings a mother pig with seven piglets into the sandbox. Out of the multiple forms that the sandbox offers, she chooses a particular one: Niki creates a world by turning the sandbox into a particular place and establishing a meaningful space for her piglets. In order to do this, she had to find the courage to break out of the narrow, repetitive, sensory experience of the sand and decide how to express herself. She tells us, in essence: "Out of all possibilities, the piglets and their mother are the first to inhabit my world, because their particular possibilities most closely mirror my need." Niki is awakening to the potentialities of her environment, and she steps into the clearing, allowing herself to be reflected back through her toys. The curtain upon the unfolding drama of mothers and babies has been opened, and the child cannot help but take up the narrative in her particular way.

> From this time forward her play took on different characteristics, becoming repetitive and exact. At every session for about three months, she buried the mother pig in the left hand corner of the sand tray. The piglets were placed in the opposite corner, and they took turns trying to find the mother pig. The child said nothing during this play, yet appeared to be absorbed in what she was doing, frequently showing a low-range affective variance. The piglets would go looking for the mother and would alternately fall in water and drown, climb and fall off a tree, fall off a bridge, and be unable to climb fences, mountains, or other obstacles. (Gil, as cited in James, 1994, pp. 142–143)

The endless journey of the piglets in search of their mother is deeply tragic. Niki has stepped into the world of symbolic play, and its affective power carries her along. Despite its almost unbearable sadness,

Niki perseveres with her script over and over. The young in search of Mother fall and drown and get stopped by mountains, trees, fences, and streams—it seems as if the whole world prevents them from getting what they need. The exact repetition of this painful game points to one of the key elements of play: Play is an emotional or *pathic* activity. Unlike cognitive or *gnostic* activities, which are articulate, process oriented, and focused on what we know about something, *pathic* activities are a feeling-toned communion with playthings. The pathic child experiences an immediate connection with his or her world (Buytendijk, 1976). Niki is not talking to her therapist to figure out how to live her life better (which would be a later, cognitive activity), but she is shaping the affective dimension of her life. Like a musician, she plays through the variations of her theme of "getting lost"; like a sculptor she goes over and over the layers to peel away the emotional form that lies under the surface. Her play differentiates the affective domain, and her toys help her find containers or gestures for the pain in her life. Unhurried play makes it possible for children to learn a silent symbolic language, prior to speech or even alongside the spoken word, which shapes and brings to visibility the affective threads that bind them, however tenuously, to things and people in their life.

"We play only with what is pathic in our presence" (Buytendijk, 1976, p. 129), what addresses our feeling life. The primary motivation for play lies in its power to let the child move in an externalized feeling world. Play evokes a world that is ineffable and profound. The feeling world the child displays through his or her toys goes beyond articulation in its complexity and depth. Play displays the affective life of the child, but, as in theater, there are some scripts that are more differentiated and satisfactory than others. It takes Niki 3 months to perfect her "searching for Mother" script. The first act, burying the mother, remains constant, but there are so many ways to get lost on the way to her!

> One day there was a major difference in Niki's repetitive scenario: None of the piglets drowned, fell down, or otherwise faced an overwhelming obstacle—they instead found and uncovered the mother pig! *Niki stopped abruptly, almost surprised by what she had done* and quickly moved away from the sand tray, indicating she was done for the day. (Gil, as cited in James, 1994, p. 143, emphasis added)

One quality of play, which, once again, Buytendijk articulated beautifully, is that we continue to play with something only *if it plays with us.* The unpredictable response of the ball, the many responses of the other players collapsed in a heap at the end of ring-around-the-rosies, the piglets exploring possible paths through the sand tray—all illustrate how playthings interact with the player and change the game. Niki is *surprised* when the piglets find and uncover their mother because the possibilities inherent in the sandbox go beyond the fixed game she has set up. At this juncture the sand tray becomes uncanny because the new constellation of playthings implies affective possibilities that are overwhelming. She arrests her symbolic play because she does not know if it is safe to step into the new world that is opened up: piglets *with* Mother. This is a fearful moment, an instant when the child gets a glimpse of the future: The piglets cannot go back now to getting lost. They must engage their mother. In her pathic world, the heroes find the Grail, but they get more than they bargained for. Finding the mother is not the end, but just the beginning, of another leg of the quest. It ushers in a new set of affective play gestures that symbolizes the relationship between mother and child.

> During the following session one piglet began the "search for the mother" ritual and found and uncovered her quickly. This time the child put the piglet next to the mother, looked up at me, and said, "titty no milk." She seemed genuinely sad, and her eyes watered up. I said "No milk for the baby," and the child responded tearfully, "Baby sad." She held a big stuffed rabbit in her lap for the rest of the session and rocked it and fed it with a plastic bottle. From time to time a single tear would fall on her cheek. (Gil, as cited in James, p. 143).

Niki's first verbal communicative act is the phrase: "titty no milk." It is the saddest and most hurtful insight of any abandoned child. Niki sums up what the mother's failure was: No milk signifies the absence of nourishment and intimacy, which in turn means the loss of the bond between mother and baby, which threatens her development and even her very survival. This is the tragic disappointment at the core of Niki's life experience. "Titty no milk"—it seems that her play with the piglets from the beginning has been working toward finding this emotional expression.

By playing in the sandbox she has elaborated the emotional ground in months of silent play, but finally words break through: "Baby sad." How skimpy these words seem compared to the full emotional impact of her play script! In response to these words she picks up the stuffed rabbit and comforts it by *rocking and feeding it*. Taking up the maternal gestures herself, Niki changes perspective and supplies to another what the pig failed to give the piglets, what her mother failed to give to her. We see here, once again, an affective form as it changes location from one thing to the next. She retreats from the pigs into the sphere of the stuffed rabbit because it is more intimate and immediate: The cloth rabbit can be hugged and touched; it is closer to all the senses than the toys in the sand tray. Holding and feeding are sensuous experiences and more primary than symbolic play. Niki's play narrative is eclipsed at this point because she needs more than symbolism. Her regression to holding the rabbit is a regression to a familiar experience: her blanket. But as she hugs the soft toy, she also feeds it and hence maintains the play space. She is not retreating into mute self-enclosure, as before. The sensuous and the symbolic come together and overlap without merging. Niki is comforted by the sensuousness of the rabbit's touch as she herself symbolically comforts another infant.

Niki plays not merely with material objects but with the affective dimension of the relationship between mother and infant as it reveals itself through the toys. In the world of play she can assume the maternal gestures herself while, at the same time, empathizing with the baby rabbit. The paradox of nurturing and abandonment is borne fully in Niki's Pietà-like cradling of the rabbit, while "from time to time a single tear would fall on her cheek."

Language has great difficulty unraveling the complexity of Niki's affective gestures. Her therapist, in a very unadorned way, allows for a very simple language to describe the events that are visible. Her sentences "The mother pig is buried. The baby pig fell from the tree" or "No milk for the baby" offer no other comfort but the communication that another human being is fully present and witnessing the drama unfold. Her language, which lifts into words the mute play of the child, is unobtrusive, allowing the child's own intentionality unfold. It simply restates an unadorned reality, and by so doing, respects the child's right to express her own suffering.

In the following therapy session Niki repeats the same process a number of times: The piglet finds the mother, there is no milk, the rabbit is stroked and fed.

> When the piglet found no milk the third time Niki did this play, Niki reached over and placed a mother giraffe in the opposite corner of the tray. She then picked up the baby giraffe, and the baby giraffe and the piglet seemed to nestle together next to the mother giraffe. "This mommy gots milk!" the child exclaimed. She again held the rabbit and stroked its

head, saying "There, there, . . . you awright." (Gil, as cited in James, 1994, p. 143)

After this session Niki's relationship with her therapist and foster mother became more engaged, and her play went beyond the piglets in the sand tray and included a whole variety of new forms. The narrative line of babies in search of mothers has come to its conclusion. The piglets, the baby rabbit, and Niki herself will be "awright."

Nikki's case powerfully highlights the potential of play to shift the feeling life of a child and to create a world that he or she understands and inhabits in a fuller way. Play is the creation of a symbolic world in all existential dimensions, and it allows for fluid experimentation with embodiment, coexistence, objects, spatiality, temporality. The *body* can be young or old, do or pretend to do what is not yet or never possible. *Others* can be real people who are imitated, or they might be purely pathic figures who are given an anthropomorphic form. *Things* transform from one into the other in metaphorical splendor, pushing the edge of what a particular thing is. *Space* allows for an imaginary world to be created and enacted, and yet there is a faithfulness to the most essential spatial forms (corner, nest, miniature, etc.). *Time* curls in on itself: It is nonlinear, past and future weave together, it is intuitive and unfettered by the need for timed production. Play follows the spell of the sensuous, is the lining, the curling over between natural and symbolic forms. It is essential for children at an age when they are not reflective, but learn by engagement.

EARLY CHILDHOOD AND THE STRUCTURES OF PLAY

Jean Piaget gave us a basic vocabulary for understanding childhood development that is still foundational to child psychology and education. I think one of his key insights about early childhood is that preschoolers are "egocentric"—that is, they do not distinguish between themselves and the world, and they are completely unreflective about themselves:

> Let us imagine a being, knowing nothing of the distinction between mind and body. Such a being would be aware of his desires and feelings but his notion of self would be undoubtedly much less clear than ours. Compared with us he would experience much less the sensation of the thinking self within him, the feeling of a being independent of the external world. The

knowledge that we are thinking of things severs us in fact from the actual things. But above all the psychological perceptions of such a being would be entirely different from our own. Dreams, for example, would appear to him as a disturbance breaking in from without. Words would be bound up with things and to speak would mean to act directly on these things. Inversely, external things would be less material and would be endowed with intentions and will. (Piaget, 1929/1951, p. 37)

For Piaget, the young mind confuses itself with the universe and is unconscious of its own self. When the child, around the age of 6, becomes more logical and reflective, the closeness to the world of things dissolves slowly and a more distant and self-aware human being emerges. Piaget thought that the child's entry into this new stage of cognitive development, which he termed the *concrete operational stage,* was fixed according to a biological timetable, and that no amount of hurrying could produce the loss of egocentrism and magical thinking without damaging the child. The experience of oneness with the world is a fact of early human development that needs to be respected.

Play, because of its affective, magical, prelogical relationship to things and people, is the perfect activity for a nondualistic, egocentric mind. Piaget's insight that the young child does not separate self from world and has very little understanding of an "inner" life has far-reaching implications for how we deal with Niki and other young children. For Niki, the world is not a panorama "out there"; rather, its openness and closedness, its invitation and repulsion are entwined with who she is. Her egocentrism, in Piaget's sense, means that in the beginning of her therapy she has no distance from her environment, and that the influence of the social world is immediate and profound. We understand the smallness of her world as a direct reflection of the smallness of her psychological life: No invitation from the world = no person there to be invited.

Niki's case and its analysis underscore seven characteristic features of play:

1. *Play requires a safe, predictable, and caring adult presence in the background,* without which, the child's horizon becomes constricted. Loving caregivers provide the sense of safety that emboldens the child to explore his or her environment and to risk being changed or shaped by it.

2. *Play follows the invitation of the sensuous world.* We find here a reversal of our common dualistic attitude that sees things as distant objects

out there, waiting to be manipulated by masterful adults. For the ego-centric child, things have their own intentionality: *Things play with the child*. Hence it is important to think about the qualities of play materials and what kind of play they invite. Is their structure and texture pleasing or exciting to the senses? Do they call for narrowly defined play scripts, or are they generous in what they allow the child to be?

3. *Play is an exercise in empathy.* Niki's exploration of the lost-piglet script reveals the close attention she pays to her playthings. She explores the possibilities inherent in the sand and the piglet figures, and out of their imaginary interaction new possibilities for action arise. Because young children do not have the preformed cultural explanations and concepts about the world that characterize adult thinking, their playful "magical" thinking is, in fact, a freer and unprejudiced investigation into the structure and symbolism of things. Play fosters an empathic relationship with things and people: The playing child allows him- or herself to be touched by them. The child probes their being, which is also a probing of his or her own being. The piglets are like Niki, and their victory draws a possible horizon for her own future victory. Play foster empathic observation, and it establishes an affective–ethical con-nection between the child and the physical and social worlds.

4. *Play explores and elaborates the affective dimension of the child's lived world.* For the young child, there is not a "physical world" out there, because his or her egocentrism does not see the world as other, but as extensions of him- or herself. When involved in her play, the child rear-ranges the visible world of things and also rearranges his or her feeling life.

The young child's egocentrism offers adults a wonderful opportu-nity: By the toys we offer, the stories we tell, the work we show them, the environments we create, we can influence our children's affective life immediately and profoundly. The young child absorbs what he or she sees without reflection, critique, or distance. Parents and teachers either issue the invitation to the child to step into a safe world and make something of it, or, in varying degrees, they foreclose the affective bond between the child and the world, as we saw in Niki's case.

5. *Symbols are discovered through an emotional and sensory contact with things and people before they become cognitive or linguistic.* Language is often insufficient to address the complexity of the affective domain, but play displays this complexity tangibly, over time and in all its paradoxical features. As Niki attaches her feelings to the piglet figures, her inter-action with them changes her feeling life in particular ways. The lost piglets become a *symbolic affective form* that is particularly suited to carry

out Niki's emotional project. It allows her to explore the subtleties and range of possible feelings as they are narrated through the pigs' adventures. The imaginative manipulation of toys restructures the child's experience of her own emotions. The landscape of feelings that ties her to people and things becomes elaborated and refined through her play. It seems to me that this is one of the most profound functions of play: It differentiates and represents the child's evolving emotional life.

6. *Play involves the creation of a meaningful, coherent world with ordered locations and scripts.* The play scripts Niki developed, like the play scripts of kindergarten children playing prince and dragon, or mother cat and kittens, are of an archetypal nature. Mother/father–baby, venturing forth into a dangerous world, getting lost in the woods, rescuing people, fighting against evil—these are all typical plots for young children's play. By elaborating and individualizing these scripts, the child traverses an emotional human landscape and in the process articulates his or her feeling and thinking life.

7. *Play is the locus of the child's developing capacity for intentionality; the self is revealed and affirmed in the play-world without directly announcing itself.* Play thus honors the child's egocentrism by allowing awareness without self-awareness, self without self-reflection. We saw Niki display and affirm herself by developing and inhabiting a world of her own creation. She chose the pig and piglets, she made the trees, ditches, and walls. Play makes her emotional intentions visible. It allows for a symbolic space where the prereflective child can show herself *without directly announcing it.* The pleasure of play is driven by the satisfaction that the world I have created in my play reflects myself. Its failings in apathy and boredom, or in the extreme form of autistic repetition, are also a failing of the self. Play, to paraphrase Rousseau, is truly the child's work, because in play the child changes the world and him- or herself. Play requires that adults give children the freedom to build their own imaginary worlds free from adult expectation and instruction, but never too far removed from a protective adult presence.

FROM PLAY TO LITERACY

The structural analysis of Niki's play has revealed that play has an important function in educating the child's feeling life. Play in a preschool or kindergarten is not a waste of time in the antechambers of literacy, but an activity that is not only appropriate but essential for the egocentric, nondualistic child. It teaches the child attention, observation, and empathy; it awakens symbolic capacity and provides images for a varied emotional life; and it strengthens the child's sense of agency, intentionality, and selfhood.

The neglect or even disdain for play in American education has deep roots. Decades ago Piaget was asked by American educators how to speed up the developmental process in preoperational, young children. This has become known as the "American Question." Piaget's reply was: "But why would you want to do that?" I share Piaget's puzzlement, together with Spock, Brazelton, Elkind, and Greenspan.

Yet Piaget himself, despite his careful attention and understanding of early childhood thought, often disparages young children's mental activity. From the beginning of his research work, Piaget found children to exhibit forms of thinking that threatened adult logic. He evaluated the young child's egocentrism mostly in negative terms when compared to adult cognition: It is an "absence of consciousness of the self" and a "failure to differentiate between the self and the world" (Piaget, 1929/1951, p. 35). The child's adherence to observation of the physical world without distinguishing it from the self leads to a form of realism, which, for Piaget, is an "anthropocentric illusion" and leads to "all those illusions which teem in the history of science" (p. 34). Even though Piaget showed much sensitivity to the texture of child thought, in the final analysis he dismissed it as merely a step to a higher adult logic. As Johnson so aptly summarizes: "For Piaget, the young child is a primitive *scientist*, with an immature set of hypotheses about the nature of reality" (Johnson, 1995, p. 47). Piaget's dismissive attitude has clouded the minds of educators, who, against Piaget's own advice, try to hurry our children through this "preoperational" stage, which is merely a waiting room where one wastes time on the way to the good stuff.

Play is the first casualty in hurrying up our children because, on the surface, it seems to be unproductive and a waste of time. Would time not be better spent in adult structured, educational activities so that we can give our children a head start in the three R's?

Let us explore this premise by considering the precursors to literacy. Literacy is much more than the acquisition of a mechanical skill; indeed, it restructures the psychological life of young children. As Ong (1982) and Eisenstein (1979) have pointed out in their social and historical studies, the acquisition of writing technology transforms consciousness, not only in the cultural acquisition of print, but also in the lives of our young children. The cultural shift from orality to literacy is mirrored in each child's experience when he or she learns to read (Egan, 1998). A competent reader has to develop the following: a capacity for physical, emotional, and mental self-restraint; a tolerance for delayed gratification; a sophisticated ability to think conceptually and sequentially; a preoccupation with both historical continuity and the future; and a high valuation of reason and hierarchical order (Postman, 1994). On a practical level, children who learn to read have to sit still and restrict physical and mental attention to a small space, memorize arbitrary symbols, stay focused on a purely mental activity, think and see sequentially, give up their social interactions, pay attention to their teacher, and enter a purely symbolic world that is not mediated by human voice or presence. In order to be a competent reader, the child has to restructure the way he or she lives in the world. With the shift from audible interactions to visual text comes subtler changes in the way reality is experienced. Walter Ong (1982, p. 73) beautifully evokes the difference between a world shaped through the activities of either the ear or the eye, a shift that also applies to oral child culture:

> In a primarily oral culture where the word has its existence only in sound, with no reference whatsoever to any visually perceptible text, and no awareness of even the possibility of such a text, the phenomenology of sound enters deeply into human being's feel for existence, as processed by the spoken word. For the way in which the world is experienced is always momentous in psychic life. The centering action of sound (the field of sound is not spread out before me but is all around me) affects man's sense of the cosmos. For oral cultures, the cosmos is an ongoing event with man at its center. Man is the *umbilicus mundi*, the navel of the world (Eliade, 1958, pp. 231–235, etc.). Only after print and the extensive experience with maps that print implemented would human beings, when they thought about the cosmos or the universe or "world," think primarily of something laid out before their eyes, as in a modern printed atlas, a vast surface or assemblage of surfaces (vision presents surfaces) ready to be "explored."

The process of learning to read decenters the child from the "*umbilicus mundi*," the participatory, egocentric oneness with the world. Reading and the educational rituals that accompany it send children on their way to becoming the rational, distanced, analytical observers that Piaget had in mind as the endpoint of development, the stage he labeled *formal operations.*

Reading is an essential aspect of Western human development because it produces a particular self that functions relatively well in our technologically sophisticated societies and knows how to handle the vast array of symbolic material that characterizes a literate culture. But it is also clear that the qualities required of a good reader are in stark opposition to the egocentric nature of young children's thinking and experiencing. Our children need time in the "oral" world to develop the mental and emotional capacities that will turn them into creative, self-reflective, socially responsible adults who have the motivation and will to realize their projects (Simms, 2008). By pushing literacy into the kindergartens and preschools and by eliminating time and space for play, we prevent our children from developing emotional sophistication, an intelligence that relies on its own observation, an ethical bond with the people and things around them, and a faith in their own will and ability to create worlds—maybe with better scripts than the ones we provide them with today.

ACKNOWLEDGMENT

This chapter is reprinted from "Play and the Transformation of Feeling: Niki's Case," in S. Olfman, Ed. *All work and no play. How educational reforms are harming our preschoolers* (pp. 177–191). Westport, CT: Greenwood Publishing. Copyright 2003 by Eva-Maria Simms. Reprinted with permission.

REFERENCES

Buytendijk, F. J. J. (1976). *Wesen und Sinn des Spiels* [*The nature and meaning of play*]. New York: Arno Press.

Egan, K. (1998). *The educated mind: How cognitive tools shape our understanding.* Chicago: University of Chicago Press.

Eisenstein, E. (1979). *The printing press as an agent of change: Communications and cultural transformations in early-modern Europe.* New York: Cambridge University Press.

Eliade, M. (1958). *Patterns in comparative religion.* New York: Sheed & Ward.

Erikson, E. H. (1963). *Childhood and Society.* New York: Norton. (Original work published 1950)

Gadamer, H.-G. (1996). *Truth and Method* (2nd ed.) (J. Weinsheimer & D. G. Marshall, Trans.) New York: Continuum.

Greenspan, S. I., & Benderly, B. L. (1997). *The growth of the mind: And the endangered origins of intelligence.* New York: Addison-Wesley.

James, B. (1994). *Handbook for treatment of attachment-trauma problems in children.* New York: Lexington Books.

Johnson, A. (1995). Constructing the child in psychology: The child as primitive in Hall and Piaget. *Journal of Phenomenological Psychology, 26*(2), 35–57.

Langeveld, M. J. (1968). *Studien zur Anthropologie des Kindes* [*Studies in the philosophical anthropology of the child*]. Tuebingen, Germany: Max Niemeyer Verlag.

Ong, W. J. (1982). *Orality and literacy. The technologizing of the word*. New York: Routledge.

Piaget, J. (1951). *The child's conception of the world* (J. Tomlinson & A. Tomlinson, Trans.). Savage, MD: Littlefield Adams. (Original work published 1929)

Postman, N. (1994). *The disappearance of childhood*. New York: Vintage Books.

Simms, E.-M. (2008). The child in the world: Embodiment, time, and language in early childhood. Detroit: Wayne State University Press.

Index

Page numbers followed by an *f* or *n* indicate figures or notes.